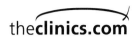

SURGICAL CLINICS
OF NORTH AMERICA

Critical Care
for the General Surgeon

GUEST EDITORS
Juan Carlos Puyana, MD
Matthew R. Rosengart, MD, MPH

CONSULTING EDITOR
Ronald F. Martin, MD

December 2006 • Volume 86 • Number 6

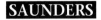

An Imprint of Elsevier, Inc.
PHILADELPHIA   LONDON   TORONTO   MONTREAL   SYDNEY   TOKYO

W.B. SAUNDERS COMPANY
A Division of Elsevier Inc.

1600 John F. Kennedy Blvd., Suite 1800, Philadelphia, PA 19103-2899

http://www.theclinics.com

SURGICAL CLINICS OF NORTH AMERICA
December 2006
Editor: Catherine Bewick

Volume 86, Number 6
ISSN 0039–6109
ISBN 1-4160-3916-3

Surgical Clinics of North America (ISSN 0039–6109) is published bimonthly by Elsevier Inc., 360 Park Avenue South, New York, NY 10010-1710. Months of publication are February, April, June, August, October, and December. Business and Editorial Offices: 1600 John F. Kennedy Blvd., Suite 1800, Philadelphia, PA 19103-2899. Customer Service Office: 6277 Sea Harbor Drive, Orlando, FL 32887-4800. Periodicals postage paid at New York, NY and additional mailing offices. Subscription prices are $220.00 per year for US individuals, $347.00 per year for US institutions, $110.00 per year for US students and residents, $270.00 per year for Canadian individuals, $424.00 per year for Canadian institutions, $286.00 for international individuals, $424.00 per year for international institutions and $143.00 per year for Canadian and foreign students/residents. To receive student/resident rate, orders must be accompanied by name of affiliated institution, date of term, and the *signature* of program/residency coordinator on institution letterhead. Orders will be billed at individual rate until proof of status is received. Foreign air speed delivery is included in all *Clinics* subscription prices. All prices are subject to change without notice. POSTMASTER: Send address changes to *Surgical Clinics*, Elsevier Periodicals Customer Service, 6277 Sea Harbor Drive, Orlando, FL 32887-4800. **Customer Service: 1-800-654-2452 (US). From outside of the US, call 1-407-345-1000.**

The *Surgical Clinics of North America* is also published in Spanish by McGraw-Hill Interamericana Editores S.A., P.O. Box 5-237 06500 Mexico D.F. Mexico; and in Portuguese by Interlivros Edicoes Ltda., Rua Comandante Coelho 1085, CEP 21250, Rio de Janeiro, Brazil; and in Greek by Paschalidis Medical Publications, Athens Greece.

The *Surgical Clinics of North America* is covered in *Index Medicus, EMBASE/Excerpta Medica, Current Contents/Clinical Medicine, Current Contents/Life Sciences, Science Citation Index,* and *ISI/BIOMED.*

Printed in the United States of America.

CONSULTING EDITOR

RONALD F. MARTIN, MD, Staff Surgeon, Department of Surgery, Marshfield Clinic, Marshfield, Wisconsin; Lieutenant Colonel, United States Army Reserve, Medical Corps

GUEST EDITORS

JUAN CARLOS PUYANA, MD, FACS, FRCSC, FACCP, Associate Professor of Surgery and Critical Care; and Director of Research, Innovative Medical & Information Technology Center, University of Pittsburgh Medical Center, Pittsburgh, Pennsylvania

MATTHEW R. ROSENGART, MD, MPH, Assistant Professor, Department of Surgery, University of Pittsburgh Medical Center, Pittsburgh, Pennsylvania

CONTRIBUTORS

VISHAL BANSAL, MD, Fellow, Surgical Critical Care, Department of Surgery, University of California at San Diego, San Diego, California

TIMOTHY G. BUCHMAN, MD, PhD, Harry Edison Professor, Department of Surgery, Washington University School of Medicine, St. Louis, Missouri

DAVID CABA, MD, MS, Postdoctoral Associate, Department of Surgery, University of Pittsburgh, Pittsburgh, Pennsylvania

DAVID CRIPPEN, MD, FCCM, Associate Professor and Medical Director, Neurovascular Critical Care, Department of Critical Care Medicine, University of Pittsburgh Medical Center, Pittsburgh, Pennsylvania

MICHAEL DONAHOE, MD, Associate Professor of Medicine, Division of Pulmonary, Allergy, and Critical Care Medicine, University of Pittsburgh School of Medicine, Pittsburgh, Pennsylvania

ALBERTO GARCIA, MD, Chief, Trauma Division, Hospital Universitario del Valle; Chief, Emergencies Unit, Clinica Valle el Lili; and Professor, Department of Surgery, Universidad del Valle, Cali, Colombia

MAXIM D. HAMMER, MD, Assistant Professor of Neurology, The Stroke Institute, University of Pittsburgh Medical Center, Pittsburgh, Pennsylvania

GINA HOWELL, BA, Medical Student, University of Pittsburgh, Pittsburgh, Pennsylvania

DAVID T. HUANG, MD, MPH, The CRISMA Laboratory (Clinical Research, Investigation, and Systems Modeling of Acute Illness), Departments of Critical Care Medicine and Emergency Medicine, University of Pittsburgh, Pittsburgh, Pennsylvania

JASON R. LEONG, DO, Senior Critical Care Medicine Fellow, Department of Critical Care Medicine, University of Pittsburgh, Pittsburgh, Pennsylvania

JASON A. LONDON, MD, MPH, Assistant Professor, Division of Trauma and Emergency Surgery, Department of Surgery, University of California, Davis Medical Center, Sacramento, California

AVERY B. NATHENS, MD, PhD, MPH, Associate Professor, Department of Surgery, University of Washington; Director of Surgical Critical Care, Harborview Medical Center, Seattle, Washington

JUAN B. OCHOA, MD, FACS, Associate Professor, Departments of Surgery and Critical Care, University of Pittsburgh, Pittsburgh, Pennsylvania

CARLOS A. ORDOÑEZ, MD, Assistant Professor, General Surgery; Assistant Professor, Trauma and Critical Care, Universidad del Valle; and Director of Trauma/Surgical Intensive Care Unit, Fundación Clínica Valle del Lili, Cali, Colombia

PATRICIA A. PENKOSKE, MD, Instructor, Department of Anesthesia, Washington University School of Medicine, St. Louis, Missouri

MICHAEL R. PINKSY, MD, CM, Dr hc, Professor of Critical Care Medicine, Bioengineering, and Anesthesiology, Department of Critical Care Medicine, University of Pittsburgh School of Medicine, Pittsburgh, Pennsylvania

PATRICIO M. POLANCO, MD, Postdoctoral Fellow, Division of Trauma, Department of Surgery, University of Pittsburgh School of Medicine, Pittsburgh, Pennsylvania

JUAN CARLOS PUYANA, MD, FACS, FRCSC, FACCP, Associate Professor of Surgery and Critical Care; and Director of Research, Innovative Medical & Information Technology Center, University of Pittsburgh Medical Center, Pittsburgh, Pennsylvania

MATTHEW R. ROSENGART, MD, MPH, Assistant Professor, Department of Surgery, University of Pittsburgh Medical Center, Pittsburgh, Pennsylvania

VAISHALI DIXIT SCHUCHERT, MD, Assistant Professor, Departments of Critical Care and Surgery, University of Pittsburgh, Pittsburgh, Pennsylvania

MATTHEW J. SENA, MD, Assistant Professor, Division of Trauma and Emergency Surgery, Department of Surgery, University of California, Davis Medical Center, Sacramento, California

KRISTEN C. SIHLER, MD, MS, Assistant Professor of Surgery, Section of General Surgery, University of Michigan Health System, Ann Arbor, Michigan

SAMUEL A. TISHERMAN, MD, FACS, FCCM, Associate Professor, Department of Surgery, and Department of Critical Care Medicine, University of Pittsburgh, Pittsburgh, Pennsylvania

CONTENTS

> Critical care medicine was born from the selective pressures of human disease, and with the perseverance and foresight of a select few pioneers, has become an independent field of medicine. This introduction travels back in time to evaluate those visionaries and their landmark contributions. Advancements in caring for the critically ill and organ failure occurred during the wars of the twentieth century. Landmark advances in the management of respiratory paralysis occurred in the polio epidemic of the 1940s. It was during this era that the world's first ICU was developed. Contemporary critical care differs considerably from that which marked its birth. Much of the technology we currently employ is assumed: invasive hemodynamic monitoring, mechanical ventilation, antisepsis, and antibiotics.

> Severe secondary peritonitis carries significant mortality, despite advancements in critical care support and antibiotic therapies. Surgical management requires a multidisciplinary approach to guide the timing and the number of interventions necessary to eradicate the septic foci and create optimal healing with the fewest complications. Research is needed regarding the best surgical strategy for very severe cases. The use of deferred primary anastomosis seems

safe in patients presenting with hemodynamic instability and hypoperfusion. These patients have a high risk of anastomotic failure and fistula formation. Allowing for aggressive resuscitation and judicious assessment of the progression of local inflammation are safe strategies to achieve the highest success and minimize serious and protracted complications in patients who survive the initial septic insult.

The Relationship between the Surgeon and the Intensivist in the Surgical Intensive Care Unit

Patricia A. Penkoske and Timothy G. Buchman

When a patient enters the intensive care unit, the admitting surgeon also enters a new environment. In some hospitals, the surgical intensive care unit (SICU) is "closed"—critical care providers manage care; in others the unit is "open," and the admitting surgeon is in charge. A third system is the "mixed" model of ICU administration; a collaborative approach. This article addresses concerns and conflicts that frequently arise between admitting surgeons and intensivists. It is written from the perspective of two surgeon-intensivists who have been in both roles. Recent behavioral and social research on ICU conflicts and their resolution is reviewed, and new strategies for conflict resolution are also presented.

Critical Care Issues in the Early Management of Severe Trauma

Alberto Garcia

Violent trauma and road traffic injuries kill more than 2.5 million people in the world every year, for a combined mortality of 48 deaths per 100,000 population per year. Most trauma deaths occur at the scene or in the first hour after trauma, with a proportion from 34% to 50% occurring in hospitals. Preventability of trauma deaths has been reported as high as 76% and as low as 1% in mature trauma systems. Critical care errors may occur in a half of hospital trauma deaths, in most of the cases contributing to the death. The most common critical care errors are related to airway and respiratory management, fluid resuscitation, neurotrauma diagnosis and support, and delayed diagnosis of critical lesions. A systematic approach to the trauma patient in the critical care unit would avoid errors and preventable deaths.

Basic Ventilator Management: Lung Protective Strategies

Michael Donahoe

Acute respiratory failure is manifested clinically as a patient with variable degrees of respiratory distress, but characteristically an abnormal arterial blood partial pressure of oxygen or carbon dioxide. The application of mechanical ventilation in this setting can be life saving. An emerging body of clinical and basic research, however, has highlighted the potential adverse effects of positive pressure ventilation. Clinicians involved with the care of critically ill patients must recognize and seek to prevent these complications using lung-protective ventilation strategies. This article discusses the basic concepts of mechanical ventilation, reviews the categories of ventilator-associated lung injury, and discusses current strategies for the recognition and prevention of these adverse effects in the application of mechanical ventilation.

Ventilator-associated pneumonia (VAP) is a significant nosocomial infection affecting up to one third of patients requiring mechanical ventilation, and is associated with significant attributable morbidity and mortality. Clinicians should have a heightened clinical suspicion for VAP with diagnostic goals focusing on accuracy; gathering of lower respiratory tract culture; and appropriate and timely initial antibiotic therapy. Early and adequate antibiotic therapy is important to optimize the management of patients with VAP. The incidence and etiologic patterns of the major pathogens causing VAP must be taken into account when making empiric antibiotic therapy choices. Subsequent de-escalation and prescription of an appropriate duration of therapy guided by clinical response and culture results may lead to decreased morbidity and future antibiotic resistance.

The hemodynamic monitoring of a surgical patient acquires a major relevance in high-risk patients and those suffering from surgical diseases associated with hemodynamic instability, such as hemorrhagic or septic shock. This article reviews the fundamental physiologic principals needed to understand hemodynamic monitoring at the bedside. Monitoring defines stability, instability, and response to therapy. The major hemodynamic parameters measured and derived from invasive hemodynamic monitoring, such as arterial, central venous, and pulmonary catheterization, are discussed, as are its clinical indications, benefits, and complications. The current clinical data relevant to hemodynamic monitoring are reviewed and discussed.

Sepsis and septic shock are not uncommon conditions in the surgical intensive care unit. Sepsis is a generalized activation of the immune system in the presence of clinically suspected or culture-proven infection. Severe sepsis is sepsis with organ system dysfunction. Septic shock is sepsis with hypotension (systolic blood pressure <90 mm Hg) without other causes. Although the incidence of sepsis is increasing, the case fatality rate is falling. This improvement in outcome is in part due to bold initiatives like the Surviving Sepsis Campaign from the Institute for Health care Improvement. In this article the authors present the epidemiology of severe sepsis and evidence-based guidelines for its treatment, with a focus on the surgical patient.

Dr. Stanley Dudrick invented total parenteral nutrition in 1968, providing a desperately needed therapy to those patients who could not eat. It has since saved thousands of patients worldwide. Nutrition interventions (NI) in surgical/trauma and critically ill patients have evolved dramatically during the last 20 years from a supportive therapy to a clear therapeutic role. Like any other form of therapy, NI will benefit patients when adequately indicated and prescribed. NI, however, may cause significant side effects and harm when poorly ordered. This article reviews the indications for the prescription of the different forms of NI available to the clinician caring for the surgical patient.

Hyperbilirubinemia, or jaundice, is common in the ICU, with incidence up to 40% among critically ill patients. Unfortunately, it is poorly understood in the critically ill, and too often presents a diagnostic dilemma to the ICU physician. Causes of jaundice in the ICU are multiple; the etiology in any given patient multifactorial. Acute jaundice can be a harbinger or marker of sepsis, multisystem organ failure (MSOF), or a reflection of transient hypotension (shock liver), right-sided heart failure, the metabolic breakdown of red blood cells, or pharmacologic toxicity. The persistence of jaundice is associated with a significant increase in patient morbidity and mortality. Acute ICU jaundice is best divided into obstructive and nonobstructive. This stratification directs subsequent management and therapeutic decisions

Cardiovascular failure in critically ill patients carries a high mortality. Identification and treatment of the underlying etiology simultaneously with prompt therapy are indicated to avoid the consequences of prolonged shock. Physicians should assess patients using all available clinical, radiologic, and laboratory data to avoid the pitfalls associated with use of single measures of regional or global perfusion. Continued evidence of inadequate perfusion despite fluid resuscitation warrants consideration of placement of a pulmonary artery catheter or pharmacologic support of the cardiovascular system. Finally, the dynamic nature of physiology in critically ill patients requires constant patient reassessment and flexibility in treatment to tailor therapy individually as the pathologic state evolves.

FORTHCOMING ISSUES

RECENT ISSUES

The Clinics are now available online!

www.theclinics.com

SURGICAL
CLINICS OF
NORTH AMERICA

Surg Clin N Am 86 (2006) xiii–xv

Foreword

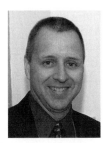

Ronald F. Martin, MD
Consulting Editor

There are many reasons to love the discipline of surgery. It is a discipline of intellectual challenges, physical labors, and fairly rapid results from many endeavors, and an opportunity to live in a world that many will only catch a glimpse of. I, like many others, enjoy nearly all of the above, though perhaps the shine that many of these events have historically held for me has altered its luster as time has passed. But what really fascinates me most about surgery is the irony. Irony, in my opinion, drives our discipline. For example, we as surgeons frequently do not really *need* to know exactly what is wrong with a given patient as long as we know, more or less, exactly what needs to be done for the patient. As a matter of fact, most of what we do in the operating room, under different circumstances, would be considered assault. Yet, in our privileged roles, we are requested to inflict some small measure of mayhem to hopefully provide a greater long-term good.

The ICU is an environment full of irony. One of the common events that lead a patient to the ICU, the *code*, has to be one of the most ironic propositions we encounter. Strangely, the sicker one becomes, and the nearer unto death, the decisions and practices that a physician has to employ become simpler and more straightforward. The list of approved Advanced Cardiac Life Support or Advanced Trauma Life Support guidelines can be reduced in algorithmic form to a few laminated cards that a house officer can easily fit in her pocket or use as bookmark. This event that is so often dramatized on television and in movies, where life itself hangs in the balance, is usually handled by the judicious employ of a few consensus guidelines by a small group of caregivers who frequently have never met the

doi:10.1016/j.suc.2006.10.005
surgical.theclinics.com

patient. At some level "code" guidelines are so fundamental that it does not matter how the patient came to find himself in the position of needing to be resuscitated. Now the irony: assuming the "code" results in an alive patient, we find ourselves moving from a position of minimal choices to one of very complicated choices usually involving very highly trained super-specialists.

When I began training, my first lesson in critical care was "Air goes in and out, blood goes round and round, and oxygen is good." The person who taught me that was one of the most brilliant physicians I have ever worked with and certainly the best intensivist I ever met. Needless to say, his understanding of the matter far exceeded mine, so I think he made it simple for me to start with. Yet, in many ways, the points that he made about keeping people alive depending on a sophisticated understanding of the simple basic principles have not changed all that much.

The current intensive care environment allows us sophistication previously unavailable. In some cases, we do not even "need" to be physically present. The virtual ICU is a reality (please again note the irony). Most parameters of organ performance can be measured intermittently or continuously, and the data stream can be monitored remotely, as can streaming video of the actual patient. Trends can be analyzed by software programs and recommendations generated by decision tree analysis. Even in the cases in which we are present, there seems to be a trend toward data collection and analysis replacing examination and observation in the management of the critically ill patient.

As one of the authors in this issue writes, "Critical care sometimes creates amalgams of life-in-death: a state of being unable to participate in human life, unable to die." In another example of irony, we have the capacity to create a third answer to a traditionally binary question: are we alive? The creation of this meta-state of animation has lead to some very thorny financial and political problems. The small-scale problem of Terry Schiavo (not really critical care but emblematic) played out in the large-scale arena of congressional politics showed the public disparity of views on how personal decisions could and should be made. Meanwhile, the large-scale problem of medical funding for an "all comers" health care system remains largely unresolved.

The percentage of health care dollars spent in the last several months of human life in the United States is staggering. Given that the supply of funds for the entire health care system is likely to decrease, we are again forced to consider the concept of value. Exactly how much is it worth to extend life by how much? And is some life extension, based on quality of life, worth some greater amount than others? These are serious societal questions that need serious answering. Many of us think that we physicians should be best suited to provide the answers or at least lead the framework, but we have not. The serious debate over utility versus futility has never gained traction. Is it because our interests are conflicted, the needs of our individual patients versus the needs of the group? Is it because the question is too hard to answer? Are we so death averse (again, the ultimate irony) that we cannot bring ourselves to address the questions? Are there perverse financial incentives to not want the question resolved? I wish I knew, but I do not.

The big question of what we should do may not be resolvable in the immediate future or ever. The solutions may be forced upon us without option, as death used to be. What I would suggest is that to decide what one *should* do, one must first have a realistic understanding of what one *can* do. Drs. Puyana and Rosengart have assembled a truly excellent collection of articles that should give the reader greater insight into what we *can* do. It is up to the rest of us to engage in becoming educated and educating others so that we may all decide what we *should* do. I leave you with one last example of irony, a collection of subspecialty articles written for general surgeons. But after all, we generalists will invariably deal with those who are critically ill, or be involved with someone becoming critically ill as a result of our efforts. Enjoy.

Ronald F. Martin, MD
Department of Surgery
Marshfield Clinic
1000 North Oak Avenue
Marshfield, WI 54449, USA

E-mail address: martin.ronald@marshfieldclinic.org

SURGICAL
CLINICS OF
NORTH AMERICA

ELSEVIER
SAUNDERS

Surg Clin N Am 86 (2006) xvii–xviii

Preface

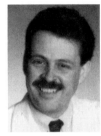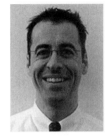

Juan Carlos Puyana, MD   Matthew R. Rosengart, MD, MPH
Guest Editors

Management of the critically ill patient has evolved at an exceedingly fast pace over the last two decades. New insights into the processes of inflammation and infection, in combination with advances in pharmacology, ventilator management, and monitoring techniques, have rapidly changed the landscape of how we provide intensive care. The number of specialists now referred to as "intensivists" continues to increase, and current critical care programs are evolving into independent departments. Furthermore, new standards of care for providing critical care are being revisited as a result of initiatives such as the Leapfrog group and the recommendations resulting from the Institute of Medicine report on medical errors and safety. These events have generated a new approach to quality control and improved safety along the spectrum of medical care, starting in our ICUs. However, the number of surgeons applying to programs for subspecialty surgical critical care training is decreasing. Although it is difficult to predict the influence of these changes on the practice of the general surgeon, it is likely that surgeons will need to invest more time so as to remain knowledgeable in the field and that there will be a greater dependence on non-surgeon intensivists for provision of care. For these reasons we feel that the current issue of critical care for the general surgeon is timely. We wanted to cover several aspects of common pathologic entities that require intensive care within the purview of a general surgical practice. Space constraints limit the current critical care therapies discussed; however, we hope that the topics selected

doi:10.1016/j.suc.2006.10.001   *surgical.theclinics.com*

for this issue will be of interest to our readers and, more importantly, that they will provide useful and practical information.

Juan Carlos Puyana, MD
Matthew R. Rosengart, MD, MPH
University of Pittsburgh Medical Center
200 Lothrop Street
Pittsburgh, PA 15213-2356, USA

E-mail addresses: Puyanajc@upmc.edu (J.C. Puyana);
rosengartmr@upmc.edu (M.R. Rosengart)

ELSEVIER
SAUNDERS

Surg Clin N Am 86 (2006) 1305–1321

SURGICAL
CLINICS OF
NORTH AMERICA

Critical Care Medicine: Landmarks and Legends

Matthew R. Rosengart, MD, MPH

*Department of Surgery, University of Pittsburgh Medical Center Presbyterian,
Pittsburgh, PA15213, USA*

Critical care medicine was born from the selective pressures, or evolution if you will, of human disease, and in combination with the perseverance and foresight of a select few pioneers, has become the independent field of medicine as we regard it today. Its true origin, not surprisingly, is difficult to establish. Florence Nightingale described the benefits of creating an individual facility for the care of postoperative patients; however, it was the establishment of a three-bed unit for postoperative neurosurgical patients by Dr. W.E. Dandy at the Johns Hopkins Hospital that heralded the development of intensive care in the United States.

Ironically, though not uncommonly, subsequent advancements in caring for the critically ill occurred during the wars of the twentieth century. Insight into the pathophysiology of organ failure gleaned from treating the severely injured provided a large impetus to the development of intensive care. Identifying shock and instituting appropriate intravascular fluid resuscitation (eg, saline, colloid) was well-established at the conclusion of World War I, and the techniques of blood transfusion became operant during World War II [1]. Surgical improvisation led to technical advances and the immediate survival of previously lethal injuries, yet necessitated prolonged supportive therapy for ultimate recovery. Shock wards were established to resuscitate and care for soldiers injured in battle or undergoing surgery, and postoperative patients were admitted to recovery rooms to facilitate nursing care. The subsequent reduction in morbidity and mortality resulted in the spread of recovery rooms to nearly every hospital by 1960 [1,2].

A discussion of the development of intensive care would be incomplete without mentioning the polio epidemic of the late 1940s, from which landmark advances in the management of respiratory paralysis occurred. It is

This work supported by NIH grant K12HD049109-01.
E-mail address: rosengartmr@upmc.edu

also during this era that many report that the world's first intensive care unit, as defined as "a ward where physicians and nurses observe and treat 'desperately ill' patients 24 hours a day," was developed by Dr. Bjorn Ibsen in Copenhagen in 1953 [3]. The first patient admitted to that unit at 6 PM on December 21st, 1953 was a 43-year-old-man who had unsuccessfully attempted to hang himself.

> "He was agitated, confused and cyanotic with laboured respiration. Temperature 38.6°C and pulse 136. An x-ray showed bilateral infiltrates and oedema of the lungs. It was felt that fatal cardiopulmonary failure was imminent. Oxygen via facemask and when oxygen saturation decreased..., with positive pressure ventilation from a bag and mask, was started. Furthermore, the patient was given one unit of blood (500 mL), isotonic glucose (1000 mL), and an antibiotic (Aureomycin) [3]."

He ultimately succumbed to multiple organ dysfunction. By the late 1950s, ICUs had been established in a quarter of large community hospitals, and by the late 1960s, this proportion had expanded to a majority. In 1986 the American Board of Medical Specialties approved a certification of special competence in critical care for the four primary boards: anesthesiology, internal medicine, pediatrics, and surgery. In the years that ensued, critical care significantly reduced the allocation of resources (length of stay, cost), and by 1997 more than 5000 ICUs were operational across the United States [2].

Contemporary critical care differs considerably from that which marked its "birth." Much of the technology we currently employ is assumed: invasive hemodynamic monitoring, mechanical ventilation, antisepsis, and antibiotics. In this introduction the author travels back in time to evaluate those visionaries and their landmark contributions, which have enabled the development of intensive care as both unit to care for the critically ill and philosophy for managing them.

Mechanical ventilation

The majority of patients requiring intensive care need ventilatory support [4,5]. Little thought is entertained when considering the efforts that culminated in enabling this technology, which has not only saved millions, but has also enabled striking advances in the field of surgery.

Recording of the use of mouth-to-mouth resuscitation can be traced back to the initial recordings of history. *The Old Testament* describes the successful resuscitation of a dead child by the Prophet Elisha. In the sixteenth century, the Swiss alchemist and physician Paracelsus first provided artificial ventilation to both animals and dead humans using fireplace bellows [6,7]. The Belgian professor of anatomy Andreas Vesalius explored this concept in 1543, as detailed in his classic work *De Humanii Corporis Fabrica*, in which he details the ability to ventilate dogs and pigs after thoracostomy/thoracotomy using a fireplace bellows [6–8].

For the centuries that followed, advancements in positive-pressure ventilation (PPV) were hindered by the inability to maintain secure tracheal canulation through which ventilation could be achieved. In the nineteenth century, O'Dwyer reported orotracheal intubation with metal tubes for use in cases of diphtheria; these canulae had expanded upper ends that wedged the tube into the glottis. Similarly, Matas described his intermittent positive-pressure ventilator (IPPV), which employed a metal laryngeal canula that was guided by extrinsic palpation into the trachea [7,9–12]. Continued efforts to develop the instrumentation for and perfect the techniques of laryngoscopy and to develop entotracheal tubes were conducted, yet the difficulties encountered were discouraging, and emphasis shifted to the development of subatmospheric (negative pressure) devices.

In 1864 Alfred F. Jones of Lexington, Kentucky built a body-enclosing tank ventilator, which many consider the first "iron lung" [6]. In 1904, Sauerbach endorsed the differential pressure method that used subatmospheric pressure applied to the entire patient, emphasizing that it obviated the issues of pneumthorax inherent to thoracic surgery and the hazards of PPV [6,13,14]; however, the chamber was large, necessitating the accommodation of both surgeon and patient, and subsequent investigations revealed that ventilation was inadequate and that supplemental oxygen was needed [7]. Though it gained widespread acceptance in Europe, it was never popular in the United States, yet it still marked a significant contribution, the concepts of which would prove invaluable during the 1947 to 1948 polio epidemic of Europe and North America.

In 1918 Dr. Steuart first constructed an airtight wooden box specifically for the treatment of polio, sealed at the shoulders and waist with clay and powered by a motor-driven bellows [13]. In 1929, Dr. Cecil Drinker, a Harvard University professor of physiology, combined efforts with his brother Philip and developed the negative-pressure tank ventilator, which became known as the "iron lung" (Fig. 1) [15,16]. This monumental discovery was a serendipitous idea generated while observing a colleague measure the breathing of an anesthetized cat enclosed in a metal box sealed at the neck. Drinker recreated the experimental model. He paralyzed the cat, yet this time pumped air in and out of the box; he was able to sustain the cat for hours. Drinker approached consolidated Gas and Electric company, which at the time was supporting research development to improve methods for managing patients of electric shock and gas poisoning; the company gave him $500 to pursue his ideas.

It would be during the late 1940s, as polio ravaged both Europe and North America, that the Drinker tank ventilator would be first used to provide ventilatory support to a child at Boston City Hospital who had been stricken with respiratory paralysis caused by polio.

"On his way through the wards, Phillip saw children dying of suffocation induced by polio; he could not forget the small blue faces, the terrible

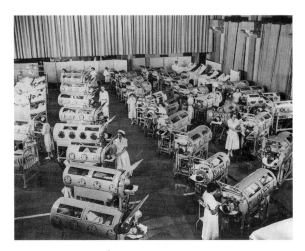

Fig. 1. Iron lungs in auditorium. (*Reprinted from* Rancho Los Amigo National Rehabilitation Center, Downey, CA; and the Polio Survivors Association, Downey, CA; with permission.)

gasping for air … yet when the machine was perfected, the first patient happened to be a little girl from Children's hospital … . Phil had the machine moved into the ward near the child's bed so she could see it and get used to the loud whine of the motor. Early next morning, the hospital called Phil. By the time he reached the hospital the child was in the machine unconscious. The staff had been afraid to turn on the power. Phil started the pump and in less than a minute saw the child regain consciousness. She asked for ice cream. Phil said he stood there and cried." –Catherine Drinker Bowen [13]

The tanks became widely accepted and employed as a life-saving measure. During this mass deployment, several serious disadvantages became apparent. Aside from being bulky and costly, the pressure gradient was reversed between the right atrium and peripheral veins, patient access was restricted, and atelectasis was common. The most serious problems involved the hazards of an unprotected airway.

Further evolution of these mechanical devices continued to occur. During the Copenhagen polio epidemic of 1952, tracheostomy and continuous manual ventilation by IPPV replaced the cuirass or body respirator. Lassen [17] and Ibsen [18], who were responsible for coordination of this massive effort, emphasized basic principles of airway management: protection, humidification, avoidance of elevated oxygen tension, and meticulous physiotherapy. Concomitant with adoption of these principles, polio mortality fell from 80% to 25% [6,19]. The successful application of positive-pressure ventilation led to the design of a large number of volume-cycled and time-cycled ventilators in Scandinavia, Germany, and the United Kingdom and established IPPV as a standard ventilation practice.

The introduction of the Salk and Sabin vaccines brought eradication of polio; however, controlled airway management and positive-pressure mechanical ventilation had become established standards of practice. Further advancements would occur in the operating theater. Development and use of modern anesthesia ventilators began with Giertz, a Swedish surgeon and a former assistant of Saurerbruch. He collaborated with an otolaryngologist who had developing a series of endotracheal and endobronchial tubes and conceived the idea for an air-driven ventilator, the spiropulsator [6]. This machine incorporated the motor of a vacuum cleaner motor and the flasher mechanism used in nautical light buoys. Dr. Ernst Morch, unable to obtain a spiropulsator in Denmark, developed his own machine, which embodied a piston and cylinder mechanism [6]. This machine became the first clinically proven ventilator and was routinely used in thoracic surgery.

The eventual impetus for American adoption of controlled ventilation came from cardiothoracic surgery laboratories demonstrating the superiority of PPV in providing efficient oxygenation and carbon dioxide elimination. One of the first widely available American ventilators was the Jefferson ventilator developed at Jefferson Medical College in Philadelphia. As surgeons and anesthetists recognized and accepted the benefits of controlled automatic ventilators other machines were developed (Morch, Bennett, Bird "Mark 4") and became available [6].

Antisepsis

By the mid-nineteenth century, surgery had traversed the theoretical and had become a reality. The discovery of anesthetics (chloroform, nitrous oxide) eliminated the trepidation of pain, and the incidence of surgery was accelerating at an exponential pace. Now death consequent to wound sepsis remained the primary fear, and its incidence paralleled that of surgery itself.

Joseph Lister (1827–1912) was born in Essex, England to a wealthy Quaker family (Fig. 2) [20,21]. His father and mother possessed keen interests in science, and in experimentation and education, respectively, and his father was granted membership in the Royal Society of Fellows. At age 17 Lister entered University of College in London, progressed into medical school in 1848, and upon graduating with honors in 1852, was appointed to a surgical internship at the Edinburgh Royal infirmary under the tutelage of Dr. James Syme. Here he questioned the contemporary perspectives of the etiology of wound suppuration, which were that wound sepsis was due to elements in gases of the air, the "contagions and miasmas." Expounding upon his observations that wound sepsis typically afflicted those patients who had open wounds, he reasoned that the elements responsible for suppuration gained access through breaks in the skin [20,21].

In 1860 he accepted the position of Professor of Surgery at Glasgow. The following year a new surgical facility was constructed with the hopes of reducing the incidence of operative sepsis and its high associated mortality.

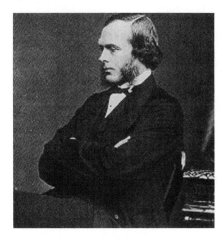

Fig. 2. Photo of Joseph Lister (1827 to 1912).

Lister was placed in charge of this project, efforts which proved to be in vain when Lister reported that between 45% and 50% of his amputation cases died from sepsis between 1861 and 1865 [20,21].

During this period, toward the end of the Civil War, Louis Pasteur was demonstrating that fermentation resulted from small microbes, rather than gases of the air as was currently believed. A colleague relayed these observations to Lister, who incorporated them into his current hypotheses to ultimately develop the "germ theory." Lister reasoned that fermentation mirrored the processes of wound suppuration, and speculated that these same microbes were the etiology of wound sepsis. He also incorporated this theory with the results of an engineer named Crooks who had eliminated the malodor of sewage (ie, fermentation) in Glasgow by adding carbolic acid. In the next year, Lister would reduce the incidence of wound sepsis by applying dressings soaked in carbolic acid and wrapped in tin foil. In 1867 he would present to the British Medical Association that his wards at the Glasgow Royal Infirmary had remained clear of sepsis for 9 months, and in 1870 Lister's antiseptic techniques would save the lives of many soldiers during the Franco-Prussian war [20,21].

These impressive results would still be insufficient to sway the current doctrines regarding air contamination as the cause of wound suppuration. In 1877 Robert Koch made the instrumental discovery that the microbes that Pasteur demonstrated in the air did exist. Koch observed that infected sheep's blood grew tiny organisms shaped like rods (*Bacillus* anthrax), which could inoculate and infect other sheep. A young German surgeon, Dr. von Bergmann, and his assistant, Dr. Schimmelbusch, demonstrated that these microbes were present on the patient's skin, the surgeon's hand, and even the surgical instruments, and that heating the instruments would sterilize them (Fig. 3).

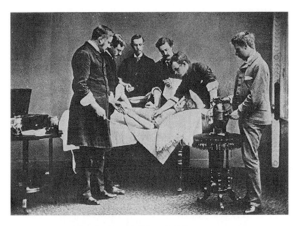

Fig. 3. Joseph Lister's laboratory.

In 1877, as Chair of Clinical Surgery at King's College, Lister introduced antisepsis to surgery, and simultaneously eliminated the smell of wound sepsis and those who denounced his theories. That same year, under aseptic technique, Lister performed an open patella repair, an intervention that previously had often resulted in death [20]. News of the operation was widely publicized and its success was instrumental in forcing surgical opinion throughout the world to accept that his methods greatly added to the safety of operative surgery. In the years that ensued, Lister continued to pioneer the field of antisepsis, finding that sterilizing catgut sutures in carbolic acid and cutting them short to the knot would prevent infection. He also learned that their duration could be prolonged by treatment with chromic.

Despite these landmark advancements, his greatest attribute, many note, was a keen awareness of his own limitations and a strong sense of humility and modesty. Lister himself would criticize his prior research and recommendations for wound care, and subsequently embrace newer methods, including steam and chemical sterilization of instruments and the importance of hand washing. As many of his carbolic compounds were extremely caustic to both wound and surgeons' hands, Lister himself would serve as "human subject," bandaging his hands to find the right balance of antiseptic solution that would not irritate the skin [20,21]. In 1897 Lister was made Baron Lister of Lyme Regis, and in 1891 the Institute of Preventative Medicine was established.. His wife died in 1892, and Lister retired from general practice the following year, dying in February of 1912 in Walmer, Kent.

Antibiotics

Sir Alexander Fleming (1881–1955) was born on a farm at Lochfield in Ayrshire (Fig. 4). He was locally educated and after 2 years at the Kilmarnock Academy, moved to London. During employment in a shipping office,

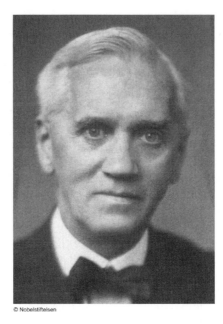

© Nobelstiftelsen

Fig. 4. Sir Alexander Fleming. (Courtesy of © The Nobel Foundation, Stockholm, Sweden: 1945; with permission.)

Fleming inherited some money from an uncle, which, under the recommendations of his physician brother Tom, he invested in medical education at St. Mary's Hospital in London. He qualified with distinction in 1906, and had the opportunity of becoming a surgeon. By chance, the captain of the rifle club, wishing to capitalize upon Fleming's talent in marksmanship, encouraged his appointment to the research department at St. Mary's, where he became assistant bacteriologist to Sir Almroth Wright, a pioneer in vaccine therapy and immunology. He gained an MB and then a BSc with Gold Medal in 1908 [22–24].

Fleming served throughout World War I as a captain in the Army Medical Corps. It was perhaps these wartime experiences, during which he witnessed the death of many soldiers from septicemia, that served as sufficient impetus to dedicate his studies to identifying antibacteriological compounds. At the time, the antiseptics employed were more deleterious to the host immunological system than the targeted pathogen, an effect Fleming demonstrated through a series of elegant experiments. Despite this, most army physicians continued to administer antiseptics [22,23].

As Fleming continued his investigations, Dr. Cecil Paine, a former student, first demonstrated the value of penicillin. Paine would successfully treat a pneumococcal infection that involved the lacerated eye of a local miner, obviating the typical need of enucleation. Several other cases were equally notable. Though he never published his results, he did discuss his penicillin work with a newly arrived professor pathology, Dr. Howard Florey, who would later prove pivotal in enabling the mass production of penicillin (Fig. 5).

By 1928, Fleming was studying the properties of staphylococci, and though regarded as a brilliant researcher, he was also considered careless. Upon returning from vacationing, Fleming discarded many culture dishes contaminated with fungus in disinfectant. In demonstrating his research endeavors to a visitor, he retrieved some of the unsubmerged dishes, whereupon he noted a penumbra of bacterial inhibition surrounding a mold that had accidentally contaminated the plate [22,23]. Unbeknownst to him, a spore of *Penicillium notatum* had drifted in from a neighboring mycology lab. Fleming isolated an extract from the mold, correctly identified it as from the penicillium family, and named the agent penicillin. He published his discovery in 1929 in the *British Journal of Experimental Pathology* to little acclaim. Fleming subsequently encountered difficulties in culturing *Penicillium*, and even greater hardship in refining it. His impression was that this would not be an important contribution to the management of infections; however, his perspective would suddenly change with the dramatic cure of Keith Rogers by the administration of penicillin.

In 1939 a team of scientists at Sir William Dunn School of Pathology in Oxford led by the Australian-born physiologist Dr. Howard Florey pursued

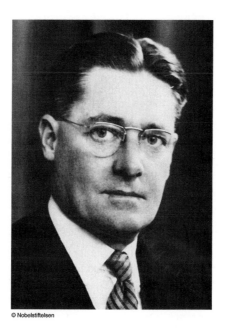

© Nobelstiftelsen

Fig. 5. Sir Howard W. Florey. (Courtesy of © The Nobel Foundation, Stockholm, Sweden: 1945; with permission.)

the task of isolating and purifying penicillin. The team had previously done work with Fleming's lysozyme, and Florey had read Fleming's paper that described the antibacterial effects of penicillin. Ernst Chain, a talented chemist, worked out the processes necessary to isolate and concentrate the compound (Fig. 6). He also correctly theorized the structure. After the team had developed a method of purifying penicillin to an effective first stable form in 1940, several clinical trials ensued, and their amazing success inspired the team to develop methods for mass production and mass distribution in 1945. By D-day of World War II there was enough penicillin for every soldier who needed it; by the conclusion of the war it had saved millions of lives. Soon, too, pneumonia, syphilis, gonorrhea, and scarlet fever would suddenly become treatable [22,23,25,26].

The serendipity of September 1928 heralds the initiation of modern antibiotics. Concomitant with these early discoveries, Fleming remarked upon many other observations that have become tenets of modern medicine and infectious disease. Fleming discovered that bacterial resistance emerged in the presence of either insufficient concentrations of drug or insufficient durations of administration, and cautioned against the use of penicillin in the absence of an appropriate diagnosis. Fleming was knighted in 1944, and in 1945 Fleming, Florey, and Chain jointly received the Nobel Prize in Medicine. Florey received great honor from his peerage for his

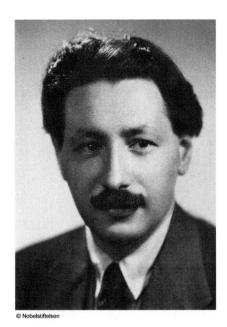

© Nobelstiftelsen

Fig. 6. Ernst B. Chain. (Courtesy of © The Nobel Foundation, Stockholm, Sweden: 1945; with permission.)

monumental work in making penicillin available to the public and saving millions of lives in WWII, becoming a Baron.

Fleming died in 1955 and was buried as a national hero in the crypt of St. Paul's Cathedral in London [24]. Interestingly, Fleming was a long member of the Chelsea Arts Club, a private club for artists of all genres, founded in 1891 at the suggestion of the painter James McNeil Whistler. Fleming was admitted to the club after he made "germ paintings," in which he drew with a culture loop using spores of highly pigmented bacteria. The bacteria were invisible while he painted, but when cultured made bright colors:

Serratia marcescens—red
Chromobacterium violaceum—purple
Micrococcus luteus—yellow
Micrococcus varians—white
Micrococcus roseus—pink
Bacillus spp—purple

Hemodynamic monitoring

Though it is to H.J.C. Swan (1922–2005) and Willian Ganz (1919–present) that we attribute the honor of developing the pulmonary artery catheter (PAC) by associating the instrument with their names, it is in fact R.D. Bradley who first described in 1964 the use of a miniature flow-directed PAC and its use in critically ill patients [27,28]. In collaboration with M.A. Branthwaite, he described the assessment of cardiac output by thermal dilution, using a thermistor mounted on the tip of the catheter; however, it was adapting a balloon to the tip, as first demonstrated by M. Lategola, that enabled Swan and Ganz to develop the flow-directed PAC to measure pulmonary artery occlusion pressure (Paop) as we understand it today [29].

The paths leading to the union of Swan and Ganz deserve interest equaling that surrounding the history of their research contributions. H.J.C. Swan was born in 1922 in Ireland; both of his parents were physicians [30]. During his undergraduate studies at St. Vincent's college in Dublin, he developed meningitis and lapsed into a coma. His mother, through the administration of sulfa drugs, cured him. Upon graduating in 1939, he pursued education at the University of London, St. Thomas's hospital, receiving an MB in 1945. After a 3-year tour of service in the Royal Air Force, he pursued a research fellowship at the University of London, where he was awarded a PhD in physiology in 1951. He was elected a Fellow of the Royal College of Physicians of London and began to study the vascular response to symphomimetic agents, investigations that would culminate in many publications and significant notoriety in the field of cardiology. In 1951, he emigrated to America to work at the Mayo Clinic under the tutelage of Dr. Earl Wood. His research endeavors would continue to be fruitful, and in collaboration with Dr. Wood he would play an integral role in the development of indicator dilution techniques, using indocyanine green for the measurement of cardiac output and detection of intracardiac shunts. In 1956 he was naturalized as a US citizen, and a decade later he relocated to Los Angeles to assume the directorship of the Division of Cardiology at the Cedar-Sinai Medical Center at University of California. It was here that he hired William Ganz [31].

William Ganz was born in Czechoslovakia in 1919 [30]. His medical studies commenced at Charles University in Prague in 1937, but were postponed during World War II because of military commitments [31]. He received his medical degree in 1947, graduating with the highest honor. Thereafter, he trained in medicine under the tutelage of Dr. Weber at the City Hospital in Prague, and subsequently became Director of Coronary Research at the Cardiovascular Research Institute in Prague, a position he retained until 1966. During this period, he developed a method for the measurement of regional blood flow, including coronary sinus blood flow, as well as cardiac output measurement using thermodilution techniques. In 1960, he was awarded the CSc (Candidate of Sciences, equivalent to PhD) title by the Czechoslovakian Academy of Sciences. Dissatisfied with life in a communist system, Dr. Ganz emigrated to the United States in 1966 with his wife Magda and two sons Tomas and Peter. He settled in Los Angeles, where he joined Dr. Swan in the Department of Cardiology of the Cedars of Lebanon Hospital. In 1968 they began to work together on the development of a flow-directed catheter [31].

Dr. Swan's conception of the flow-directed PAC occurred in a brief moment of enlightenment during an outing with his children in Santa Monica [31]. In the days preceding this event, he had used, to little success, a Bradley thermodilution catheter in managing an elderly patient. Dr. Swan noted that amongst the sedentary sailboats in the harbor, a large spinnaker was moving through the water at a reasonable speed. He contemplated that a sail or parachute anchored to the end of a highly flexible catheter might facilitate the safe passage of the device into the pulmonary artery. This original proposal triggered the concept to attach an inflatable balloon to the tip of a highly flexible catheter. Through the support of Edwards Laboratory, the company that had developed the Starr-Edwards heart valve and the Fogarty embolectomy catheter, he manufactured the first flow-directed pulmonary artery catheter [30–32]. Dr. Ganz piloted their invention in an anesthetized dog. Upon balloon inflation the catheter floated through the right heart into the pulmonary artery, "wedging" itself into a small arterial branch. The transduced waveform represented the pressure in the distal pulmonary artery. Their landmark discovery detailing the human use of this catheter was published in the *New England Journal of Medicine* in 1970 [31,32]. In the decades that ensued, the catheter gained universal acceptance and widespread use in the management of all critically ill patients. Though its use has come under scrutiny, there is little doubt as to the ramifications that this discovery has had in facilitating hemodynamic monitoring in a variety of clinical settings.

Vasopressors and inotropes

"... neither by reasoning, nor by actual demonstration of the facts, can you convince some people that an opinion which they have accepted on authority is wrong." –William Horatio Bates

Care of the critically ill patient would be close to impossible without the use of vasopressor support. In May 1886, Williams Bates reported the discovery of a substance produced by the adrenal gland in the New York Medical Journal, unaware of the degree to which he would facilitate the care of critically ill patients in the century to follow.

William Horatio Bates (1860–1931) was born in 1860 in Newark, New Jersey [33]. He obtained his undergraduate degree from Cornell University in 1881, and his medical degree from the College of Physicians and Surgeons in 1885. New York City proved to be his home, as he established clinical practices at the Manhattan Eye and Ear hospital, Bellevue hospital, the New York Eye infirmary, the Northern dispensary, and the Northeastern dispensary. He served as an instructor in ophthalmology at the New York Post-Graduate Medical School from 1886 to 1891. Bate's research interests mirrored his clinical emphasis, the eye, and in 1896 he resigned from clinical practice to focus upon his scientific investigations. In the laboratory, Bates proved that the normal fixation of the eye is central, but never stationary, and the techniques he developed to treat poor eyesight were based upon his theory of accommodation and training the patient in the dual art of relaxing and focusing the eyes. He also developed a method for imaging the curvature of the globe. His research would culminate in the publication of *Perfect Eyesight Without Glasses* in 1919, which contradicted contemporary ophthalmologic doctrine and thus necessitated publication at his own expense [33].

In 1894, while seeking to determine the therapeutic effect on the eye of the active principles of the ductless glands, Bates discovered the stringent and hemostatic properties of the aqueous extract of the suprarenal capsule, later commercialized as adrenalin. In 1896 he announced this discovery in a paper read before the New York Academy of Medicine, though he never isolated the specific compound or provided a name.

It was not until 1895 that a Polish physiologist isolated and identified the compound. Napoleon Cybulski (1854–1919) was born into a wealthy family in 1854 and received a silver medal from the Minsk Secondary School in 1875. He subsequently enrolled at the Military Medical Academy in St. Petersburg, where he graduated *eximia cum laude* in 1880. He excelled in the scientific community, primarily because of his research efforts in cardiovascular physiology, and in 1885 was appointed chair of the Department of Physiology at the Faculty of Medicine of Jagiellonian University, a distinguished honor he held until 1919. One of his greatest achievements was the construction of a device for precise measurements of blood movement in the vessels—the photohemotachometer—which provided a better insight into the physiology and pathophysiology of the circulatory system. In the field of endocrinology, Cybulski, together with Wladyslaw Szymonowicz, discovered that extracts of the adrenal glands contained substances that elevate blood pressure in 1895. They too did not provide a name. In 1897, in the United States, John Abel prepared crude adrenal extracts and gave them the name epinephrine. Interestingly, however, none of the extracts "behaved" like the parent compound. In 1901 it was again identified and described by the Japanese scientist Jokischi Takamine, who named it adrenaline and patented the compound. Park, Davis and Company market the isolated compound under the name Adrenalin®; and it is from these two original sources that we derive the two names: adrenalin and epinephrine.

Cardiopulmonary resuscitation

"When given a choice—take both!" –Peter J. Safar

Peter J. Safar (1924–2003) was and is the "Father of cardiopulmonary resuscitation (CPR)"(Fig. 7). He was born in Vienna, Austria in 1924, to physician parents; his father practiced surgery and his mother pediatrics. Perhaps it is not surprising that he pursued a career in medicine and received his MD from the University of Vienna in 1948. In 1950, he relocated to New

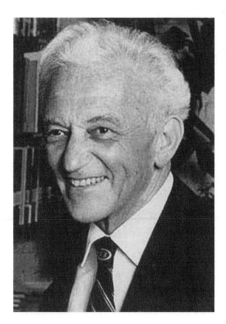

Fig. 7. Peter J. Safar. (Courtesy of the Safar Center for Resuscitation Research, University of Pittsburgh, Pittsburgh, PA; with permission.)

Haven, Connecticut to continue his studies at Yale. "While at Yale," he remarked, "I realized surgery would not advance without better life support ... . And you learn life support in anesthesiology" [34]. Subsequently, he completed a residency in anesthesiology at the University of Pennsylvania, graduating in 1952.

Upon completing his training, Safar traveled to Peru with his wife, Eva, to direct the anesthesiology department at the National Cancer Institute in Lima [34]. Shortly thereafter, he returned to the United States to establish and direct the department of Anesthesiology at Baltimore City Hospital in Maryland. There his research focused upon translating methods of resuscitation from the medical arena to the environment of the general public (ie, mass disasters, cardiac arrest), and in doing so fathered "life-supporting first aid" or as it is known today, CPR. Safar emphasized establishing control of the patient's airway and breathing by tilting back the head, opening the mouth, and using mouth-to-mouth breathing, documenting these maneuvers as steps "A" (airway) and "B" (breathing)" in resuscitation. When he combined this with closed-chest cardiac massage, "C" (circulation), he established the "ABCs" of basic life support, and in doing so, had created CPR. He worked hard to popularize the procedure around the world, and collaborated with a Norwegian company to create "ResusciAnne," the first CPR training mannequin.

In 1961 Safar moved to the University of Pittsburgh to establish yet another anesthesiology department; one that has become the largest in the nation. While at Pittsburgh, Safar identified the need to establish a facility that could provide continuous life support for critically ill medical and postoperative patients who required ongoing multisystem physiologic support, in addition to those who remained comatose after CPR. Subsequently, he developed the United States' first critical care medicine program and paramedic ambulance service. In 1966, Safar's research was forced to shift focus to identifying a method for cardiopulmonary cerebral resuscitation; his 11-year old daughter, Elizabeth, died from an anoxic neurological insult caused by an asthma attack. His efforts generated novel new therapies and investigations that employ hypothermia to preserve neurological function and extend the critical time for life-saving medical and surgical interventions.

Safar's passions culminated in contributions to medicine that solidify him as one of the fathers of critical care medicine. He, along with several other pioneers, cofounded the Society of Critical Care Medicine in 1972, which has grown to a membership of 13,000 representing 80 countries. Before his death in 2003, he had been recognized by the German Academy of Natural Sciences Leopoldina, the Austrian Academy of Sciences, the Russian Academy of Medical Sciences, had received the American Heart Association CPR Pioneer Award, and had been nominated for the Nobel Prize in medicine three times. Many remark of his tireless advocacy of human rights, or for what he termed "peace medicine." "Humanism is more than Greek and Latin," Safar said. "It should mean all that focuses on the goodness of

Homo sapiens, ranging from the sanctity of human life, to an appreciation of the humanities" [34].

References

[1] Society IC. Evolution of intensive care in the UK. Available at: www.ics.ac.uk/downloads/ history.pdf. Accessed July 16, 2006.

[2] Society of Critical Care Medicine. History of critical care. Available at: http://www.sccm.org/ SCCM/Patient-Family+Resources/History+of+Critical+Care/. Accessed July 16, 2006.

[3] Berthelsen PG, Cronqvist M. The first intensive care unit in the world: Copenhagen 1953. Acta Anaesthesiol Scand 2003;47(10):1190–5.

[4] Dasta JF, McLaughlin TP, Moody SH, et al. Daily cost of an intensive care unit day: the contribution of mechanical ventilation. Crit Care Med 2005;33(6):1266–71.

[5] Carson SS, Cox CE, Holmes GM, et al. The changing epidemiology of mechanical ventilation: a population-based study. J Intensive Care Med 2006;21(3):173–82.

[6] Somerson SJ, Sicilia MR. Historical perspectives on the development and use of mechanical ventilation. AANA J 1992;60(1):83–94.

[7] Grenvik A, Eross B, Powner D. Historical survey of mechanical ventilation. Int Anesthesiol Clin 1980;18(2):1–10.

[8] Vesalius A. De Humani Corporis Fabrica. Basileae, Switzerland; 1543. p. 659.

[9] O'Dwyer J. Fifty cases of croup in private practice treated by intubation of the larynx, with a description of the method an do fthe dangers incident thereto. Med Rec 1887;32:557–61.

[10] O'Dwyer J. Intubation of the larynx. New York Medical Journal 1885;42:145–7.

[11] Matas R. History and methods of intralaryngeal insufflation for the relief of acute surgical pneumothorax. Trans South Sug gynecol Assoc 1899. p. 52–84.

[12] Matas R. Intralaryngeal insufflationfor the relief of acute surgical pneumothorax. Its history and methods with a description of the latest devices for this purpose. JAMA 1900;34:1468–73.

[13] Dunphy LM. "The steel cocoon." Tales of the nurses and patients of the iron lung, 1929– 1955. Nurs Hist Rev 2001;9:3–33.

[14] Sauerbruch F. Pathologie des offenen Pneumothorax und de Grundlagen meines Verfahrens zur seiner Ausehaltung. Mitteilungen fur Grenzgebiete der Medizin und chir urgie 1904;8: 399–411 [in German].

[15] Drinker P, Shaw L. An apparatus for the prolonged administration of artificial respiration. J Clin Invest 1929;7:229–47.

[16] Drinker P, McKhann C. The use of a new apparatus for prolonged administration of artificial respiration. JAMA 1929;92:1658–60.

[17] Lassen HC. A preliminary report on the 1952 epidemic of poliomyelitis in Copenhagen with special reference to the treatment of acute respiratory insufficiency. Lancet 1953;1(1):37–41.

[18] Ibsen B. Treatment of respiratory complications in poliomyelitis; the anesthetist's viewpoint. Dan Med Bull 1954;1(1):9–12.

[19] Snider GL. Historical perspective on mechanical ventilation: from simple life support system to ethical dilemma. Am Rev Respir Dis 1989;140:S2–7.

[20] Parker S. Joseph Lister (1827–1912). Available at: www.surgical-tutor.org.uk/default-home.htm?surgeons/lister.htm ~ right. Accessed July 31, 2006.

[21] Francoeur JR. Joseph Lister: surgeon scientist (1827–1912). J Invest Surg 2000;13(3):129–32.

[22] The Nobel Foundation. Sir Alexander Fleming. Available at: http://nobelprize.org/ nobel_prizes/medicine/laureates/1945/fleming-bio.html. Accessed July 31, 2006.

[23] The Nobel Foundation. Nobel Lectures, Physiology or Medicine 1942–1962. 1964.

[24] Brown K. Penicillin man: Alexander Fleming and the antibiotic revolution. Stroud, Gloucestershire (UK): Sutton Publishers; 2004.

[25] The Nobel Foundation. Ernst B. Chain. Available at: http://nobelprize.org/nobel_prizes/ medicine/laureates/1945/chain-bio.html. Accessed July 31, 2006.

[26] The Nobel Foundation. Sir Howard W. Florey. Available at: http://nobelprize.org/nobel_prizes/medicine/laureates/1945/florey-bio.html. Accessed July 31, 2006.

[27] Bradley RD. Diagnostic right-heart catheterisation with miniature catheters in severely ill patients. Lancet 1964;67:941–2.

[28] Achan V. Another European view: the origin of pulmonary artery catheterization. Crit Care Med 1999;27(12):2850–1.

[29] Lategola M, Rahn H. A self-guiding catheter for cardiac and pulmonary arterial catheterization and occlusion. Proc Soc Exp Biol Med 1953;84(3):667–8.

[30] Swan HJ, Ganz W. Hemodynamic monitoring: a personal and historical perspective. Can Med Assoc J 1979;121(7):868–71.

[31] Palmieri TL. The inventors of the Swan-Ganz catheter. H.J.C. Swan and William Ganz. Curr Surg 2003;60(3):351–2.

[32] Swan HJ, et al. Catheterization of the heart in man with use of a flow-directed balloon-tipped catheter. N Engl J Med 1970;283(9):447–51.

[33] The National cyclopaedia of American biography, vol. 24. White JT, editor. New York: p. 383–4.

[34] Mitka M, Peter J. Safar, MD: "father of CPR," innovator, teacher, humanist. JAMA 2003; 289(19):2485–6.

ELSEVIER
SAUNDERS

SURGICAL
CLINICS OF
NORTH AMERICA

Surg Clin N Am 86 (2006) 1323–1349

Management of Peritonitis in the Critically Ill Patient

Carlos A. Ordoñez, MD[a], Juan Carlos Puyana, MD[b],*

[a]Universidad del Valle, Fundación Clínica Valle del Lili, Autopista Simón Bolívar,
Carrera 98 No. 18-49, Cali, Colombia
[b]Division of Trauma and General Surgery, University of Pittsburgh Medical Center
Presbyterian, Suite F-1265, 200 Lothrop Street, Pittsburgh, PA 15213, USA

The terms peritonitis, intra-abdominal infection, and abdominal sepsis are not synonymous, yet sometimes they are used indistinctly to define similar clinical states. Peritonitis is defined as an inflammatory process of the peritoneum caused by any irritant/agent such as bacteria, fungi, virus, talc, drugs, granulomas, and foreign bodies. Intra-abdominal infection is defined as the local manifestations that occur as a consequence of peritonitis. Intra-abdominal sepsis entails a systemic manifestation of a severe peritoneal inflammation.

The clinical spectrum of peritonitis may also be classified according to the pathogenesis as primary, secondary, or tertiary peritonitis. Alternatively, a more localized phenomenon in peritonitis is the formation of abscesses, a condition characterized by the isolation and walling off of the infectious process from the rest of abdominal cavity [1–3].

The mortality of an intra-peritoneal infection in the early 1900s was close to 90%. This condition was managed nonoperatively until Kishner introduced the basic principles of surgery in intra-abdominal infections: (1) elimination of the septic foci, (2) removal of necrotic tissue, and (3) drainage of purulent material. By the 1930s, mortality had been reduced to 50%. With the introduction of antibiotics, the mortality continued to decrease slowly. The use of cephalosporins by the early 1970s was associated with a reduction of mortality to less than 30% to 40%. Subsequent advances in the understanding of physiology, the monitoring and support of the cardiopulmonary

Funded in part by Fogarty International Center NIH Grant No. 1 D43 TW007560-01.
* Corresponding author.
E-mail address: puyanajc@upmc.edu (J.C. Puyana).

systems, the rational use of new drugs, and ICU care aided in stabilizing mortality at around 30% [1,4].

There is no controversy regarding the standard treatment that includes control of the source and intra-abdominal lavage (washing); however, in patients who have advanced peritonitis, the source of the infection may not be completely eradicated with a single operation. Thus controversy arises, specifically regarding issues such as time and frequency of repetitive laparotomies, and management of the open wound/abdomen. Furthermore, the aggressive resuscitation required in these patients causes gut and abdominal wall edema that may be associated with increased intra-abdominal pressure, worsened by a premature closing of the abdominal wall. To date, it is clear that the reduction of mortality below 20% has been the result of a better understanding of the role of damage control, prevention of intra-abdominal compartment syndrome, and improved antibiotic alternatives with broad-spectrum newer medications [5–15].

Anatomy and physiology of the peritoneum

The peritoneum is a single layer of mesothelial cells resting on a basal membrane, and a bed of conjunctive tissue formed by adipose cells, macrophages, fibroblasts, lymphocytes, and some elastic fibers of collagen. The abdominal cavity is covered by the parietal peritoneum and it turns into the visceral peritoneum to cover the abdominal viscera. The total surface of the peritoneum is approximately 1.7 m^2. In normal conditions it is sterile, and it contains 50 mL of yellow fluid, which contains a few macrophages; mesothelial cells generally and lymphocytes. Most of the peritoneal membrane behaves like a passive barrier, semipermeable to the bidirectional diffusion of water and most solutes. The total surface of interchange of the peritoneal cavity is approximately 1 m^2. Unlike liquids and most solutes, larger particles are eliminated through the larger orifices that exist between the specialized mesothelial cells that cover the lymphatic conduits on the diaphragmatic surface of the peritoneal cavity. These intracellular orifices correspond to fenestrations of the basal membrane, and together serve as conduits of the peritoneal cavity to the underlying lymphatic drainage system of the diaphragm, called "lakes" or "lagoons." The reabsorption of particles or bacteria is only possible in the subdiaphragmatic peritoneal surface through numerous stomas or intracellular lagoons, to which a network of lymphatic vessels flows into the diaphragmatic lacunas. These lacunas have a diameter of 8 to 12 microns, subject to variations depending on the diaphragmatic movements and the changes of thoraco-abdominal pressure. Smaller particles, such as bacteria that by general are approximately 2 microns in diameter, are readily absorbed through diaphragmatic lacunes into the thoracic duct. Intra-peritoneal fluid and exudates circulate constantly in the cavity toward the decanting zones via gravity, and toward the subphrenic spaces by the suction caused by diaphragmatic contraction.

This works like a suction pump. It accelerates the flow during inspiration, and diminishes or restrains it during expiration, and it is probably the most important mechanism in charge of the "defensive" cleansing of the peritoneum [1,4].

After peritoneal inoculation of bacteria in dogs, the micro-organisms can be identified within 6 minutes in the thoracic duct and within 12 minutes in the bloodstream. This is the first mechanism of peritoneal defense, and after the insaturation of a peritoneal infection, bacteremia can occur. If the host is healthy or bacteremia is not massive, it will be controlled without any other systemic repercussion. If, on the contrary, the host is jeopardized or bacteremia is very great, a systemic inflammatory response with commitment of the patient (sepsis) can be produced [16,17].

Simultaneously to the first physical contact between the bacteria and the peritoneum, there is an associated injury to the mesothelial cells, with subsequent activation of inflammatory mediators, which will activate both cellular and humoral immunological responses.

The initial response of the peritoneum against the bacterial contamination is characterized by hyperemia and increased exudates of fluid with phagocytes into the peritoneal cavity. In this initial stage these are predominately macrophages. Neutrophils arrive within 2 to 4 hours, and become the predominant cells of the peritoneal cavity by the first 48 to 72 hours. These cells release great amount of cytokines such as interleukin (IL)-1, IL-6, and tumor necrosis factor (TNF), leukotriens, platelet activating factor, C3A and C5A, that promotes even more local inflammation. The combined effect of these mediators contributes to observed inflammatory response during peritonitis. As there is destruction of the bacteria, the lipo-polysacharids of gram-negative *Enterobacteria* constitute a powerful stimulus for further generation of inflammatory cytokines [18,19].

As a consequence of this inflammation there is production of fibrinogen in the septic foci, with fast formation of fibrin, creating a mesh of fibrin that temporarily reduces and blocks the reabsorption of fluid from peritoneal cavity and "traps" bacteria. This phenomenon may generate the formation of an abscess. In addition, the omentum migrates toward the inflamed area and aids in delivering mediators and cells to facilitate the abscess formation. The most common location is the subphrenic areas.

This response can be controlled and the peritonitis can be resolved, or it may continue to produce a residual or persistent peritonitis or may form an abscess. Therefore, there are three defense mechanisms in the peritoneum against the bacteria that have contaminated it, but these three mechanisms also have paradoxical effects in the organism. The first one, the early mechanical elimination of the bacteria through the diaphragmatic gaps, may in fact produce bacteremia, that if massive, will generate septic shock and eventually death. The second, the liberation of large exudates, rich in phagocytic cells and opsoninas, may also produce a severe displacement of fluids and proteins toward this "third space," which would cause a state of hipovolemia and shock with loss of albumen toward the peritoneal cavity.

The systemic response of to a severe bacterial peritonitis will then include the liberation of catecholamines, and an increase of the secretion of hormones adrenocorticoids, as well as the secretion of aldosterone and antidiuretic hormone. The hemodynamic alterations that are observed in patients who have peritonitis have several causes. The hypovolemia decrease the extracellular volume by the massive shift of fluids toward the peritoneal cavity, producing a decrease in cardiac index, increase of the resistance vascular peripheral, and oxygen consumption increase in the periphery. IL-2 and IL-8 favor cell recruitment; this stimulus of the cell abduction is so profound that pancytopenia can be observed some 4 to 6 hours after the initial stimulus. It has been difficult, however, to show the direct correlation between the magnitude of the septic answer and the concentration of circulating cytokines [20–23].

Classification of intra-abdominal infection

Primary peritonitis

Primary peritonitis is an inflammation of the peritoneum by an extraperitoneal source, frequently occurring from hematogens dissemination. It occurs in children and adults, and can endanger life, particularly in patients who have cirrhosis or in children who have nephrosis. Primary or spontaneous peritonitis relates to the deterioration of the immune defenses of the guest. It is generally produced by a single micro-organism, and the main pathogens in adults are the coliforms. In fact, 70% of these infections they are caused by *Escherichia coli*, 10% to 20% by gram-positive cocci, and 10% by anaerobes. The management includes antibiotics and fluid resuscitation. Occasionally the patient may have to undergo surgery, usually as a diagnostic laparotomy characterized by finding purulent material with gram-positive cultures without obvious perforation or abscesses in solid organs [1,24].

Secondary peritonitis

This is an infection that results from an inflammation or mechanical break of the integrity of the intestinal or the urogenital tract or solid organs, thus exposing the peritoneal cavity to the resident flora of the gastrointestinal (GI) tract.

Secondary peritonitis is classified as acute peritonitis by perforation, postoperative peritonitis, or post-traumatic peritonitis.

Acute peritonitis by perforation

This is the most common type of acute intra-abdominal. Almost 80% of cases result from necrosis of the digestive conduit [1–4]. The perforation of the small intestine caused by the inflammation and necrosis of the intestine, such as in typhoid fever and mesenteric ischemia secondary to the intestinal obstruction, occurs initially as a paralytic ileus, with subsequent progression to necrosis and perforation. Peritonitis caused by appendicitis in most cases presents as a localized peritonitis that if left long enough, may become a generalized peritonitis. Close to 22% of peritonitis is secondary to inflammation of the colon (diverticulitis and colitis); less common causes are perforations of the colon by cancer, incarcerated hernia, or intussusceptions. Necrotizing pancreatitis may be associated with subsequent peritonitis if there is contamination or infection of the necrotic pancreas and or exudates.

Postoperative peritonitis

The incidence of postoperative peritonitis occurs in 1% to 20% of patients undergoing laparotomy, and its occurrence is related to the primary reason for laparotomy and other risk factors that are discussed below. The most common cause of postoperative peritonitis is anastomotic failure/leak. In the majority of the cases there is a delay in diagnosis. As a general rule, symptoms are evident between the fifth and the seventh postoperative days, contributing to a very high mortality. The infected intestinal content and the proteolytic enzymes leak into the peritoneal cavity, inflaming it and producing the local and systemic response described above just as the diagnosis is performed. Morbidity and mortality also depend on the anatomical location and the magnitude of the leak. Thus, for example, it is more difficult to repair a duodenum that is fixed and leaks toward the retro-peritoneum than a leak in the distal small bowel or colon that can be easily externalized. In some instances of postoperative peritonitis, the anastomosis may be intact; however, the patient may remain sick because of residual peritonitis from diverse causes. Among them is the inadequate drainage of the initial septic focus, in which the surgeon failed to drain completely, or more commonly, the peritoneum does not have the sufficient defense capacity to control the problem [1,2,25].

Post-traumatic peritonitis

Peritonitis in trauma patients may occur because of missed injures, such as mesenteric tear with loss of blood supply and subsequent ischemia and intestinal perforation. This type of intra-abdominal infection is usually serious because of the delay in diagnosis, especially in patients who have multiple injuries and associated traumatic brain injury. Patients who suffer a penetrating trauma by sharp weapon or by firearm, with an acute abdomen, are operated on immediately and the injury is controlled. Generally, the intra-abdominal infection secondary to contamination seen in penetrating traumatism is a function of the time lapsed between the injury and the surgery. Only a third of the patients who have penetrating trauma of the colon have contamination of the cavity peritoneal that requires treatment with antibiotics [26–28].

Tertiary peritonitis

Tertiary peritonitis is defined as a persistent or recurrent intra-abdominal infection, after an apparently adequate treatment of a primary or secondary peritonitis. The standard treatment of secondary peritonitis consists of draining the septic focus to remove the necrotic material and to prevent the reaccumulation of pus with an adequate management of antibiotics from 5 to 7 days. If, having completed adequate surgical and antibiotic treatment, the infection persists or recurs after 48 hours, then it can be considered as a tertiary peritonitis. Furthermore, the term tertiary or recurrent peritonitis may also be used when there is persistent infection after a third reintervention for secondary peritonitis that has been managed with staged or planned relaparotomies. The microbiology of this infection is characterized by low virulence germs or sterile peritonitis. The flora changes with time, and the local mechanisms of defense of the abdominal cavity are overwhelmed. Ongoing organ dysfunction should indicate inadequate drainage or unidentified focus. This presentation is classically seen in immune-compromised patients. The patient is septic, showing a hyperdynamic cardiovascular state, fever, and failure to thrive. The operative findings are characterized by lack of formation of abscess and rather diffuse exudates without fibrin-purulent membranes, and the appearance is of a liquid more or less clear. Cultures of this fluid reveal coagulase negative *Staphylococcus*, enterococcus, *Pseudomonas*, yeast, and *Enterobacter* among others. The septic foci are rarely amenable to percutaneous drainage, and they are in difficult locations within the abdomen. An inexperienced surgeon may describe a sero-sanguineous fluid, and may conclude that the abdominal cavity is clean and even think that that the laparotomy was unnecessary; however, these patients usually experience a severe systemic response immediately after the procedure, with tachycardia, hypotension, and bacteremia. It is therefore necessary to aggressively manage the immediate postoperative resuscitation in the ICU with fluids combined with inotropic and vasopressor support. Progressive multiple organ dysfunction with death may follow if this cycle is not controlled [29–33].

The management of tertiary peritonitis should be done in the ICU, and should be performed by a multidisciplinary team. The patient will require metabolic and nutritional support, as well as hemodynamic and respiratory care; early physical therapy is ideal. An opportune and timely decision to adjust antibiotics according to the most recent culture report of blood and of the abdominal cavity should be made in conjunction with the surgeon and the intensivist. From the surgical viewpoint, the decision for on-demand relaparotomy should be made in advance, and decisions for reoperation should not be delayed. If the decision has been made for management with an open abdomen with planned laparotomy using a mesh, then it should be decided when to suspend the repeated lavages of the abdominal cavity, because these can cause more damage than benefit after the fifth or sixth procedure. Antimicrobial therapy should not exceed 14 days, except in patients who have fungal infections [34–38].

Diagnosis

The diagnosis of peritonitis is a clinical diagnosis, based mostly on history and physical examination. The main symptom in all cases is abdominal pain. The pain can be sharp or insidious; often the pain is constant and intense, and is aggravated with movement. The majority of patients lie still, with their knees bent and the head raised; these maneuvers diminish the tension of the abdominal wall and alleviate the pain. Anorexia, nausea, and vomiting are frequent symptoms. Nevertheless, depending on the etiology of the peritonitis and of their time of evolution, the symptoms can vary. The majority of patients are seen in poor general conditions, showing a sharp and severe illness. The temperature is usually above 38° centigrade, but patients who have septic shock may have hypothermia. Tachycardia and the decrease in the amplitude of the pulse are indicatives of hypovolemia, and they are common in the majority of patients. Patients present with a high cardiac output and decreased systemic vascular resistance. They may have increase pulse pressure. Pain to palpation is the most characteristic sign of peritonitis, to both deep and superficial touch. Initially there is voluntary guarding; subsequently the muscular wall undergoes an involuntary and severe spasm. Bowel sounds may or may not be present, and they may resemble an early ileus. Localized peritonitis generates pain localized toward the inciting organ. Percussion of the abdomen may aid in accurately localizing the place of maximum peritoneal irritation. Rectal examination, although indispensable in the physical examination, rarely orients toward the origin of the peritonitis. In the first hours of peritoneal irritation the pain may be intense, but to the extent that time elapses, the pain becomes more insidious and more difficult to assess. A high index of suspicion may be the difference in making an early rather than a late diagnosis with dire consequences. The patient may have an elevated white cell count greater than 11,000 cells per mL with left shift. Leucopenia suggests generalized sepsis and is associated with a poor prognosis. Blood chemistry may be normal, but in serious cases it may indicate severe dehydration, such as increased blood ureal nitrogen (BUN) and hypernatremia. Metabolic acidosis helps in the confirmation of the diagnosis. A urinalysis is indispensable to rule out urinary tract infection, pyelonephritis, and nephrolithiasis. Plain film of the abdomen is not ordered routinely. When obtained, however, it could reveal paralytic ileus with bowel distension or air fluid levels. An upright chest radiograph is useful if perforated viscera is suspected. Free air in the abdomen may occur in 80% of cases of duodenal ulcer perforation, but it is observed with less frequency when there is colon, small bowel, or intraperitoneal rectum perforation [1,39–42].

When the diagnosis is made clinically, an abdominal CT only delays the surgical intervention. Nevertheless, an abdominal CT can be useful in for suspected recurrent or undrained infection in the postoperative period. Velmahos and colleagues [43] recommend obtaining an abdominal CT in critically ill post-trauma patients who have sepsis of unknown origin. The CT usually aids in guiding therapy in two of every three cases. Abdominal ultrasound (US) may also aid in working up patients who have postoperative septic complications. Depending on the operator, fluid collection may be identified; however, this finding by itself may be nonspecific. The greatest advantage of US is that it can be done at the bedside. Bowel loops may be identified by their peristalsis, and bedside percutaneous drainage may be done in some cases, thus facilitating the procurement of samples for cultures. Go and coworkers [44] performed a comparative study to validate the use of US versus CT in patients who had postoperative intra-abdominal sepsis. They showed that CT is the procedure of choice in these patients, and that US may used in selected cases.

Diagnostic peritoneal lavage

Diagnostic peritoneal lavage (DPL) is a trustworthy and safe method for the diagnosis of generalized peritonitis, specifically in patients who do not have conclusive signs on physical examination, who have poor medical history, or who have sedation or post brain injury, advanced age, or spinal cord injury. Patients on steroids or immune-compromised patients may or may not give conclusive results in the DPL. A positive DPL (greater than 500 leukocytes/mL) suggests peritonitis.

Laparoscopy has been used, and there have been recent reports about its efficacy. It is useful in selected cases that have similar characteristics as those described for DPL. The limiting step is the ability of creating an adequate optical cavity in patients who have abdominal distension, anasarca, or previous surgery/scars. Finally, the gold standard diagnostic intervention continues to be exploratory laparotomy. The risks of an added surgery versus the benefits of obtaining a diagnosis are critical to aid in making an individual decision. In summary, the clinical assessment takes precedence over diagnostic tests that may delay a life-saving intervention. One must avoid unnecessary delays that will ultimately compromise the patient's physiology and will impact the ability to successfully resuscitate the patient after surgery.

Treatment

The management of severe peritonitis is complex and requires a multidisciplinary approach. The surgeons and intensivists must work together with practitioners in nutritional support, personal respiratory therapy, infectious disease, and radiology. The use of standard protocols for resuscitation and hemodynamic/ventilatory support to facilitate overall management should have a positive impact on outcome. The authors have developed a strict surgical management protocol with aggressive interventional approach to eradicate septic foci in the abdomen (AAST).

When the decision for re-exploration is made because of patient deterioration or failure to thrive associated with early organ dysfunction, an aggressive preoperative resuscitation is implemented, including management with mechanical ventilation with low tidal volumes (6–8 mL/kg), placement of a pulmonary artery catheter (PAC), and judicious fluid resuscitation. Elderly patients require more aggressive cardiac monitoring, and may need perioperative support to maintain an adequate cardiac output. These patients may also require monitoring of intra-abdominal pressure to prevent and identify abdominal compartment syndrome. Once the patient is adequately resuscitated, he is taken to the operating room.

Goals of resuscitation

As a general guideline, the authors use the following parameters to guide resuscitation: (1) central venous pressure (CVP) and pulmonary occlusion pressure (POP) between 8 and 12 mmHg, (2) mean arterial pressure (MAP) greater than 65 mmHg, (3) urine output greater than 0.5 mL/Kg/h, and (4) a mixed venous O_2 saturation greater than 70%.

The authors attempt to correct the patient's compromised hemodynamic and respiratory status, and in most cases achieve these parameters within 6 hours of ICU care. Effective circulatory volume and inotropic/vasopressor support are often needed. We use dobutamine, and we aim for a hemoglobin above 7 gr/dL. Transfusions of packed red cells are given when there is active bleeding or if the mixed oxygen saturation is less than 70% and the hemoglobin is less than 7. We use crystalloids, and a patient may easily require three to six liters in the first hours, depending on the state of the patient and the illness. Blood glucose is also closely monitored, aiming to maintain values around 220 mg/dL. All patients receive prophylactic medications, including ranitidina or omeprazol for stress ulcer prevention and subcutaneous heparin for prevention of thromboembolic disease if there is no evidence of coagulopathy. Enteral nutrition is preferred to intravenous as soon as possible. The use of low-dose steroids for 7 days is indicated if the state of shock persists despite adequate resuscitation, or if there is poor response to vasopressors or adrenal insufficiency [45–57].

Antibiotic therapy should be initiated as soon as possible. The initial therapy is administered on an empirical basis. The selection of antimicrobial agents should be based on the suspicion of the responsible micro-organisms and the capacity of the antibiotics to reach adequate levels in the peritoneal cavity. Generally upper GI tract perforations are associated with gram-positive bacteria, which are sensitive to cephalosporin and penicillins. Perforations of the distal small bowel and colon generally present with polimicrobial aerobic and anaerobic bacteria.

Secondary peritonitis is characterized by positive cultures with combinations of the following flora: *E Coli, Streptococcus, Enterobacter* spp, *Klebsiella* spp, enterococci, *Pseudomona aeruginosa, Proteus* spp, *Staphylococci aurous*, and epidermides. The are *Bacteroides fragilis, Clostridium* spp and *Peptostreptococci*. Antifungal therapy should be used if their presence is documented in the peritoneal cavity [58–60].

In cases of moderate or community-acquired peritonitis, monotherapy may be sufficient. In these cases the authors suggest the use of ampicillin/sulbactam or ertapenem. Combined therapy is best guided by the local ICU/hospital antibiogram. The first line of therapy may differ from one institution to the next, and may include anti-anaerobic medications such as metronidazol or clindamicina, combined with aminoglycsides in selected cases (gentamycin or amikacyn), ciprofloxacyn and third- or fourth-generation cephalosporins (ceftriaxona or cefotaxime).

In severe cases and patients who have high risk of nosocomial infections, the authors use initial monotherapy with piperacillin—tazobactam, or carbapenem type (imipenem or meropenem). The alternative is the use of fourth-generation cephalosporin and metronidazole.

Careful attention to dosing must be given and corrective measurements implemented daily according to drug levels, because many of these patients have unsteady volume of distribution caused by marked fluid shifts [61–65]. The duration of therapy should be established and guided by the surgical findings. The absence of fever, elevated white count, or left shift may aid in discontinuing antibiotic therapy because the incidence of recurrence is low when these parameters have been met. If leukocytes and rectal temperature are normal for 48 hours, they can be suspended by postoperative day 4, depending on the pathology that produced the peritonitis [66,67]. The incidence of recurrent intra-abdominal sepsis has been reported as high as 33% to 50% in patients who remain febrile and have persistent leukocytosis. The 1996 European consensus recommends short as possible duration of antibiotic use, depending on the condition that caused the peritonitis, without exceeding 5 days [68].

Surgical management

The goals of surgical treatment are eliminating the cause of the contamination, reducing the bacterial inoculum, and preventing persistent or recurrent sepsis. The surgical approach is best made via a midline incision to ensure adequate and complete exploration of the abdominal cavity. Diligent hemostasis and thorough exploration are of primary importance. Suctioning of all fluid cavities is done and quantified. Samples are taken for Gram's stain fungal studies and culture. In general terms, control is achieved by excluding or resecting the perforated viscera. If a colonic perforation is found, the proximal segment is externalized with a col and a mucous fistula is made on the distal segment. In cases that have small bowel perforation, resection is followed by primary anastomosis whenever possible. Not infrequently, the small bowel may require entry both of the proximal and distal segment, especially if the peritoneal contamination is severe and the viability of the bowel is doubtful. The other fundamental objective in the surgical treatment of peritonitis consists in reducing the size of the bacterial load to prevent sepsis and recurrent reaccumulation of purulent material. A thorough lavage of the abdominal cavity removing all detritus and particles should be done. Special attention should be given to areas where abscess may form such as the pelvis, the gutters, and the subphrenic spaces. These areas should be carefully exposed and debrided, avoiding bleeding by excessive peeling of the fibrin [1–4]. Warm saline solution is used until a clear return is obtained. The authors do not recommend using iodine or other chemical agents to lavage the peritoneal cavity, because they may compromise the local inflammatory response. Excess fluid must be suctioned as well.

In closing the abdominal cavity, ideally the fascia should be reapproximated with nonabsorbable material. The skin should be left open and covered with wet gauze dressings for a period from 48 to 72 hours. The incidence of wound infection is close to 42% in these cases; however, if the wound is clean after 3 to 4 days, a secondary closure of the skin maybe attempted, depending of the underlying cause of peritonitis [8,23,69–71].

Some patients may not improve despite adequate initial operative management. These patients may require several laparotomies to achieve the goals listed above. Therefore the surgeon should decide during the first or "index" laparotomy whether or not the patient may benefit from a reoperation, which could be done either as needed or through a planned/scheduled reintervention [72–76]. Postoperative peritonitis has a very high mortality, ranging from 30% to 50%. High mortality may be caused in part by delayed diagnoses and delayed reintervention of complications with associated organ dysfunction. The mortality and morbidity associated with aggressive reoperation strategy in complicated patients who have peritonitis has been reported in the literature. Because the decision to reoperate may not always be done soon enough, several authors suggest the use of open abdomen or strict daily re-exploration to avoid delays in management. During the 1980s this was a procedure recommend often. More recent reviews indicate that laparotomy on demand may be as beneficial and may have lower morbidity; however, there is no definitive evidence indicating which strategy is better [77–85].

Re-laparotomy "on demand"

The authors refer to relaparotomy on demand (ROD) when the decision for further intervention is not planned in a fixed or scheduled manner, but is rather based on the clinical progress of the patient during the immediate postoperative course. These patients manifest clinical evidence of an intra-abdominal complication characterized by generalized peritonitis or abscess.

These complications can manifest at any time, as early as during the first week postoperative. The most common scenario is a patient who has ongoing septic picture, caused by a persistent peritonitis with reaccumulation of pus. Some suggest that these patients may have ongoing immunosupression and are more susceptible to endotoxemia or true "translocation." Most commonly these patients develop new pathogens and manifest a variety of symptoms suggesting ongoing infection. The surgeon must be very attentive and have a high index of suspicion. The clinical presentation may include persisting pain, prolonged ileus, abdominal distension, or intolerance to enteral nutrition. Patients may have persistent fever and leucocytosis, as mentioned earlier. The surgeon should make the diagnosis within the first 48 hours after any of these nonspecific findings occur and avoid waiting until the fifth or seventh postoperative day, even though some authors suggest that anastomotic failure or leaks may take that long to manifest themselves. Koperna and Schulz [86] showed that patients reoperated after 48 hours had mortality significantly higher than those operated earlier (76.5% versus 28%; $P = .001$); however, the timing of the relaparotomy did not have any repercussion on survival in those patients who had an acute physiology and chronic health (APACHE) II score greater than 26. This finding suggested that under these circumstances of severely impaired physiology the early operation had little effect.

Unfortunately, the symptoms described above may be a manifestation of systemic inflammatory response (SIRS). Furthermore, patients may manifest respiratory distress syndrome and renal dysfunction as well. The most challenging dilemma for the surgeon is to decide whether or not these findings are the result of an untreated abdominal source. Therefore the decision to reoperate is extremely difficult. The clinical criteria are subjective. The authors frequently obtain feedback from all those involved in the daily care of the patient, including the intensivist, infectious disease consultant, and the radiologists. Early postoperative changes in the CT may be difficult to interpret. After a laparotomy there is distortion of the planes, and there may be fluid collections that can be blood, serum, saline solution, intestinal liquid or pus that can complicate the diagnosis even further. Yet the radiologist is key to guide the surgeon to perform a limited exploration, or to avoid the surgery if a transcutaneous approach is safe and effective. Occasionally the surgeon is obliged to carry out a complete exploration [6]. The advantage of deciding to do a laparotomy on demand at the time of the index laparotomy is that the patient is not submitted to unnecessary surgery or anesthesia. The most serious disadvantage is when a needed reintervention is done late, when the patient's underlying physiology is compromised and has progressed to deterioration and multiple organ dysfunction. Lamme and colleagues [87] compared these two strategies in a retrospective study of 278 patients. The ROD had a mortality of 21.8% (n = 197) compared with 36% in the planned relaparotomy (PR) group ($P = 0.016$). The average numbers of surgeries in the ROD group was 0.9/patient compared with

1.3 in the PR group. Fifty-four percent of the patients assigned to ROD did not need a relaparotomy.

A meta-analysis of all reports on ROD and PR for secondary peritonitis showed that there is not a significant difference in mortality when these two modalities are compared [88]. Hutchins and coworkers [89] found that the combined positive predictive value of the clinical assessment made in concert with the input from the laboratory and radiological data as well as the assessment made by the intensivist and the surgeons is close to 83%. In this study the hospital mortality was 43% and the average time for execution of the relaparotomy was 5 days. Not surprisingly, outcome was highly associated to age and organ dysfunction [89].

Planned re-laparotomy

The decision to re-explore the abdomen is made during the initial surgery. The patient is programmed to undergo a repeat laparotomy every 24 hours until the septic focus is fully controlled. Daily debridement and lavage is performed removing all necrotic tissue via a "laparostomy" or open abdomen. To have easy access to the abdomen, a protective nonadhesive mesh is use to cover the bowel. The indications for PR at the authors' institutions are to cover the bowel. The indications for PR at universidad del valle, Fundación Clínica valle del Lili and the University of Pittsburgh are

Failure in obtaining an adequate control of the source during the laparotomy index
Inadequate or poor drainage
Diffuse fecal peritonitis
Hemodynamic instability
Reassessment of the anastomosis (tenuous)
Intra-abdominal hypertension

The authors use a mesh for staged abdominal repair [7]. We achieve adequate control after two to three reinterventions planned every 24 hours. The advantages of PR in our opinion are the ability to clean and treat the whole abdominal cavity as a giant abscess. By placing a mesh with Velcro (Velcro, Manchester, New Hampshire) we do not add unnecessary straining on the skin or the fascia that otherwise would be necessary in some cases of ROD. The very approach of PR should avoid the occurrence of abdominal compartment syndrome and intra-abdominal hypertension. The technique itself requires that the surgeon be extremely gentle; ideally the same surgeon who performed the index laparotomy should do the subsequent procedures. He or she decides whether to break all the interloop adhesions and possible collections, and should know how accessible some of the areas in the peritoneum may be. The amelioration of the inflammatory response, the presence of clean granulation tissue, and the reduction of the systemic response should all aid in deciding when to discontinue the PR and when to proceed with removing the mesh and closing the abdomen. In the authors' experience, we accomplish this stage with two to three laparotomies. At this point, we remove the Velcro or zipper that we use occasionally, and in most patients the wound is then covered with a Bogota bag, allowing for formation of granulation tissue underneath. In most of our cases, the authors carry on the subsequent laparostomies in the ICU under general anesthesia using intravenous agents [6,8]. Alternatively, the PR strategy can be modified by using a vacuum pack system as another technique that may facilitate reduction of the size of the wound, and in some cases facilitate closure of the fascia. Additional advantages of the vacuum pack include managing the possible intra-abdominal hypertension and better control of drainage and fluid production from the wound. Several reports have been published regarding the use of the vacuum pack system [90–92]. In the authors' institutions we prefer the method described by Barker and coworkers [93]. In the initial step during the index laparotomy when a decision for PR is made, a large sheet of polyethylene is used that is displayed laterally all the way into the colic gutters bilaterally, thus preventing the bowel from adhering to the abdominal cavity. Then several small cuts are made on the plastic sheet and the plastic sheet is covered with three or four abdominal surgical towels. On top of the surgical towels, two Jackson-Pratt drains are placed and these are then covered with two more abdominal surgical towels. In some patients the authors close the skin partially with 1-0 vicryl and a large adhesive dressing is used to cover the abdominal wall. We place a negative pressure close to 100 to 150 mm Hg.

The disadvantages of PR include higher requirements of anesthesia and surgery; increased manipulation of the viscera that may result in fistula formation, evisceration, increased loss of fluid, electrolyte, and proteins; and potential contamination with exogenous flora. This is a more labor-intensive approach and requires great dedication from the multidisciplinary team. Several studies suggest the use of APACHE II to assess the level of physiologic compromise on a daily bases. There have been reports indicating that PR reduces significantly the mortality in patients who have APACHE II scores ranging between 10 to 25. Patients who have initial APACHE II scores greater than 26 have a high mortality regardless of the strategy used, and patients who have APACHE II scores less than 10 have a good prognosis regardless of the approach used, PR or ROD [7,94–96].

Our multidisciplinary team in Cali, Colombia has been working with a protocolized approach to these patients over the last 10 years, and we have accumulated experience of 267 patients who had severe peritonitis managed with the PR approach. The demographic and clinical characteristics of our population are summarized in Tables 1, 2 and 3. The number of laparotomies used in the PR strategy has diminished in our hands, because we have realized over time that most times an adequate lavage and debridement is completed by the third procedure (see Table 2).

Table 1
Demographic and clinical characteristics of patients with peritonitis 1995–2004

Total number	267
Age (years)	52.2 ± 20
Male gender, %	62.5
APACHE II, %	
0–10	24
11–25	70.4
26–35	5.6
Median APACHE II, %	14
Source of infection, %	
Colon	33.3
Small bowel	22.5
Liver biliary tract	8.6
Stomach—duodenum	10.5
Pancreas	13.9
Others	11.3
Number of re-laparotomies	
Mean ± SD	4 ± 3
Median	3
Length of hospital stay, days	
Mean ± SD	25.7 ± 18
Median	20
Length of ICU stay, days	
Mean ± SD	15.8 ± 13
Median	12
Fistula, %	15.3
Septic shock, %	54.3
ARDS, %	30
Days on ventilator	
Mean ± SD	9.5 ± 11
Median	6
Mortality, % (95% CI)	19.9 (15.1–24.7)

Abbreviations: ARDS, acute respiratory distress syndrome; CI, confidence interval.

The source of infection in this group of patients was colon pathology in 33% of the cases: 22.5% from the small bowel, 22% from hepatobiliary and pancreas sources, 10.5% from stomach and duodenum, and 5% originated from appendicitis. Cultures obtained during the index laparotomy yielded negative results in 25% of the cases, most likely because of previous use of antibiotics. *E coli* was found in the 23% of the patients, enterococci in the 11.6%, *Pseudomona* in 7.7%, *Klebsiella* in 6%, *Staphylococcus* in 5.1%, and other bacteria in 21%. The authors used combination metronidazol-cefotaxime in 43% of the cases, imipenem in 11.3%, carbapenem alone in 20.6%, and combination carbapenem with fluconazol or vancomiyn in 8.6%. The overall mortality was 19.9%, (95% confidence interval [CI],15.1–24.7) and multiple regression analyses revealed age older than 50 years, APACHE II greater than 25, and septic as independent predictors of death (see Table 3).

Table 2
Comparison between patients from 1995–1999 with patients operated on from 2000–2004

	1995–1999	2000–2004	P
Number	102	165	–
Age	53.9 ± 18	51 ± 20	0.24
Male gender, %	61.8	63	0.83
APACHE II			
0–10	23.5	24.2	0.89
11–25	65.7	71.6	0.3
26–35	7.8	4.2	0.2
Median, APACHE II, %	14	14	–
Source of infection, %			
Colon	39.2	33.3	0.93
Small bowel	16.7	26.1	0.07
Liver biliary tract	7.8	9.1	0.68
Stomach—duodenum	12.7	9.1	0.85
Pancreas	16.7	12.1	0.29
Others	12.8	10.3	0.79
Number of relaparotomies			
Mean ± SD	4.9 ± 3.8	3.4 ± 2.3	0.00007
Median			
Length of hospital stay, days			
Mean ± SD	27.2 ± 19	24.8 ± 18	0.3
Median	22	20	
Length of ICU stay, days			
Mean ± SD	18 ± 14	14.4 ± 11.6	0.08
Median	14	11	
Fistula, %	16.5	14.2	0.19
Septic shock, %	52.9	55	0.72
ARDS, %	49	18.2	<0.0001
Days on ventilator			
Mean ± SD	12 ± 12	8 ± 9	0.04
Median	9.5	5	
Mortality, % (95% CI)	28.4 (19.6–37.1)	14.5 (9.1–19.1)	0.0005

Abbreviation: CI, confidence interval.

In the authors' hands, PR is a safe and viable technique. We experienced a reduction in mortality from 28.4% seen during the period 1995 to 1999 to a mortality of 14.5% (95% CI, 9.1–19.1) from the year 2000 until now. We were able to diminish the number of relaparotomies to 3.4 ± 2.3. It is likely,

Table 3
Predictors of death multivariate analysis

Variable	OR	95% CI	P
Age > 50 years	1.02	1.001–1.04	0.037
APACHE II > 25	1.06	0.99–1.13	<0.05
Period before year 2000	1.98	0.78–3.41	0.3
Septic shock	17.7	6.2–50.7	0.0001

Abbreviations: CI, confidence interval; OR, odds ratio.

however, that the reason for this lower mortality is not merely the result of diminishing the number of laparotomies, but rather the combined effect of a protocolized management that included aggressive resuscitation and improved metabolic, ventilatory, and hemodynamic support [45,53,54,97].

Intraoperative management and surgical approach to bowel anastomosis: the role of deferred early anastomosis

Control of the source of infection and prevention of further contamination can be achieved quickly by performing an ostomy. This procedure is strongly indicated, especially in the face of massive contamination, hemodynamic instability, and hypoperfusion. The bowel can be exteriorized at any level, most commonly as a colostomy or an ileostomy, and in some cases as a distal or even proximal jejunostomy. Yet these ostomies could became a source of significant morbidity in those patients who survive the acute phase of peritonitis. Complications range from electrolyte and fluid imbalance to skin and wound complications such as hernias and stenosis, as well as serious psychological problems. Furthermore, there is a significant morbidity associated with the surgical approach to re-establish bowel continuity [98,99]. Primary anastomoses of the small bowel are done routinely in patients who have peritonitis caused by small bowel pathology. In patients who have peritonitis secondary to perforated diverticulitis, the decision to perform a primary anastomosis should be based on an individual basis, according to the patient's stability and the surgeon's judgment [100–103]. More recently, primary colonic anastomosis has been advocated in the setting of acute trauma of the colon [104–111]. In trauma, the risk of intra-abdominal infection is independent of the surgical procedure, as shown by Demetríades and colleagues [112], who recommend primary anastomosis in most cases. These data, however, cannot be extrapolated to cases of advanced peritonitis.

De Graaf and coworkers [113] described the use of primary anastomosis as a feasible technique in the management of severe secondary peritonitis in critically ill patients; its use, however, has been limited because of the high risk of failure and leak, which in these patients may result in worsening sepsis, multiple organ dysfunction syndrome (MODS), and death. The determinants that dictate whether or not a patient should undergo primary repair or undergo exteriorization of the bowel are

Hemodynamic stability
Extent of inflammation of the peritoneal cavity
Viability of the bowel

The bowel should not be anastomosed in the face of severe contamination or diffuse peritonitis; in the setting of a failed anastomosis (postoperative peritonitis); in cases who have severe edema of the bowel, severe malnutrition, chronic use of steroids, mesenteric ischemia; and during the initial phases of damage control surgery.

The concept of performing a deferred primary anastomosis (DPA) in septic patients who have peritonitis stems from the authors' experience with the concept of staged laparotomy and damage control in trauma patients. Despite the use of damage control in trauma patients, the mortality-associated damage control has been reported above 40% in some series [114–120].

The authors implemented a protocol of damage control in septic patients who had peritonitis and followed our patients in a prospective observational and descriptive study at the Fundación Valle de Lilí in Cali, Colombia, from November 2000 to May 2004 [121]. Our protocol was designed with the objective of performing definitive management of the bowel whenever possible. Specific criteria were defined and patients were submitted to DPA, thus minimizing the numbers of ostomies. The inclusion criteria were

- Severe peritonitis with hemodynamic instability and sepsis
- Septic shock
- Aged 18 years and older

Patients were excluded if they died in the first 24 hours, or if the bowel anastomosis and definitive closure of the abdomen was accomplished during the first-index laparotomy.

All patients were operated within 6 hours of arrival to the emergency room. They underwent aggressive resuscitation, and were submitted to bowel resection and ligature. The abdominal cavity was lavaged and the pus drained. They were placed in the authors' planned laparotomy schedule, explained above, and managed in the ICU as described earlier. When the peritonitis was controlled, a DPA was performed using either a GIA 80 automatic suture device or a hand-sewn anastomosis with vicryl 3-0 continuous suture in a single plan (Figs. 1–4) [122–125].

The demographic data of 26 patients submitted to DPA are depicted in Table 4. Fifteen patients underwent small bowel resection in the initial surgery (57.7%), and 11 (42.3%) had a colon resection. The abdominal wall

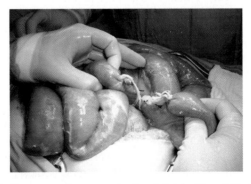

Fig. 1. Temporary closure proximal and distal with umbilical tape.

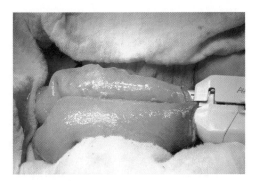

Fig. 2. Side-to-side anastomis with GIA 80 4.8.

was closed with a Velcro mesh as described earlier. The average number of relaparotomies until peritonitis was controlled was four. The relaparotomies were performed every 24 hours. The authors performed 14 anastomoses in the small bowel, five colo-colonic anastomoses, and four ileo-colonic anastomoses. Three patients could not undergo bowel anastomosis because of severe protracted inflammation. Eighteen anastomoses were done with stapler; 5 were hand- sewn. All patients underwent one-more-look relaparotomy to ascertain the integrity of the anastomosis before closing the abdomen. Twenty patients had septic shock, and 4 patients developed acute respiratory distress syndrome (ARDS). The most frequent micro-organisms were *E coli*, followed by *Candida albicans* and *Pseudomona aeruginosa*. Only 3 patients developed fistulas. The first patient had a colonic leak colon that closed in the first 5 days without surgery. Two fistulas of the small bowel were difficult to manage and required prolonged support with total parenteral nutrition (TPN). One patient closed spontaneously in 3 months and the third one was taken to the surgery for resection of the fistula 4 months

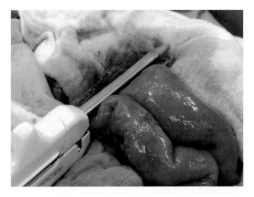

Fig. 3. GIA 80 4.8 stapled anastomosis to close bowel ends.

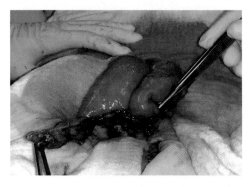

Fig. 4. Anastomosis completed.

later. Twenty patients received TPN while their bowel was ligated, and enteral nutrition was given to 24 patients about 30 hours after the anastomosis was accomplished. We closed the fascia in 14 patients, 11 underwent skin closure only, and one died before closing.

The mortality was 11.6% (3 patients). Twenty three patients left the hospital alive. The causes of death were line sepsis in one patient, a cardiac event in the second, and the third patient died of multiple organ dysfunction and gut failure with untreatable fistulas (Table 5).

The results of this study indicate that damage control and DPA in severe peritonitis is a viable technique. The numbers of ostomies was reduced, and this was accomplished with a low mortality.

Closure of the abdominal wall

The technique to close the abdomen is decided on during the last relaparotomy when the Velcro mesh is removed. Ideally by this time there is

Table 4
Characteristics of patients who underwent deferred primary anastomosis

Number	26
Age, mean, years	54.5
Male, %	61.5
Type of peritonitis, %	
Secondary	30.7
Post-traumatic	6.7
Postsurgery	61.6
Median, APACHE II, %	14.5
ICU, LOS, mean, days	17.9
LOS hospital, mean, days	27

Abbreviation: LOS, length of stay.

Table 5
Overall outcome in 26 patients with deferred primary anastomosis

Outcome	n	%
Primary success	20	77
Fistula	3	11.5
Stoma	3	11.5
Mortality at 28 days	3	11.5

formation of granulation tissue, and in most patients the bowel is adhered to the abdominal wall.

The authors contemplate the following options:

- Remove the Velcro mesh, bring the fascia together with no tension, and leave the skin open.
- Place a plastic bag (Bogota bag) on the abdominal cavity and suture it to the abdominal wall (skin or fascia); wait a few more days for granulation tissue to form.
- Close the skin only because the fascia is adhered and cannot be closed. An incisional hernia repair is done 6 months later.
- When the granulation has been completed and is not possible to close the fascia or the skin, then a split-thickness skin graft is placed over the laparostomy with subsequent correction of the incisional hernia.
- In some cases is possible to "shrink" the defect by bringing the Velcro closer and closer until the last relaparotomy, at which point the foci can be sutured. The authors achieved closing of the fascia in the 50% of the cases of 267 patients managed with Velcro [8,126].
- Using a vacuum pack system in 33 of our patients, the authors were also able to close the fascia in 50% of them and skin in the other 50%. Clearly the vacuum pack has the added advantages of maintaining sterility of the cavity, facilitating prompt access to the abdomen, preventing loss of domain, preserving the quality of the fascia, facilitating wound care by sucking the drainage around the wound, and diminishing the chance of intra-abdominal hypertension and the syndrome of abdominal compartment (Sistema vacuum pack en peritonitis severa. Carlos A. Ordóñez, MD, personal communication, 2006).

The authors do not advise closing by doing an extensive dissection of the fascia, nor do we use a mesh at this time to prevent colonization. [8,126]. When the patient is totally recovered, in approximately 6 to 8 months, a repair of the incisional hernia is performed.

Summary

Severe secondary peritonitis is an entity that continues to carry a significant mortality, despite advancements in critical care support and antibiotic therapies. Surgical management is pivotal and requires a multidisciplinary approach to guide the timing and the number of interventions that may be necessary to eradicate the septic foci and create the optimal conditions for healing with the fewest possible complications. Further research is needed to determine the best surgical strategy for very severe cases. The use of DPA seems to be a safe option in patients presenting with hemodynamic instability and hypoperfusion. These patients have a high-risk anastomotic failure and fistula formation. Allowing for aggressive resuscitation and judicious assessment of the progression of the local inflammation are safe strategies to achieve the highest success and minimize serious and protracted complications in patients who survive the initial septic insult.

References

[1] Wittmann DH, Walker AP, Condon RE. Peritonitis, intra-abdominal infection, and intra-abdominal abscess. In: Schwartz SI, Shires GT, Spencer FC, editors. Principles of surgery. 6th edition. New York: McGraw-Hill; 1994. p. 1449–84.

[2] Wittmann DH, Shein M, Condon RE, et al. Management of secondary peritonitis. Ann Surg 1996;224(1):10–8.

[3] Schein M, Saadia R. Peritonitis: contamination and infection, principles of treatment. In: Schein M, Rogers P, editors. Schein's common sense emergency abdominal surgery. 2nd edition. New York: Springer; 2005. p. 95–101.

[4] Wittmann DH. Intra abdominal infections: pathophysiology and treatment. New York: Marcel Dekker Publisher; 1991. p. 8–75.

[5] Rotstein OR, Nathens AB. Peritonitis and intra-abdominal abscesses. In: Wilmore D, et al, editors. ACS surgery. principles and practice. New York: WedMD Inc; 2002. p. 1239–62.

[6] Schein M, Saadia R, Rosin D. Re-laparotomy and laparostomy for infection. In: Schein M, Rogers P, editors. Schein's common sense emergency abdominal surgery. 2nd edition. New York: Springer; 2005. p. 395–410.

[7] Wittmann DH. Newer methods of operative therapy for peritonitis: open abdomen, planned relaparotomy or staged abdominal repair (STAR). In: Tellado JM, Christou NV, editors. Intra-abdominal infections. Madrid (Spain): Harcourt; 2000. p. 153–92.

[8] Ordóñez CA, Franco JE. Peritonis y sepsis intra-abdominal. In: Ordóñez CA, Ferrada R, Buitrago R, editors. Cuidado intensivo y trauma. Bogotá (Colombia): Editorial Distribuna; 2003. p. 667–84 [in Spanish].

[9] Marshall J, Innes M. Intensive care unit management of intra-abdominal infection. Crit Care Med 2003;31(8):2228–37.

[10] Schein M. Surgical management of intra-abdominal infection: is there any evidence? Langenbecks Arch Surg 2002;387(1):1–7.

[11] Holzheimer RG, Gathof B. Re-operation for complicated secondary peritonitis—how to identify patients at risk for persistent sepsis. Eur J Med Res 2003;8(3):125–34.

[12] Malangoni M. Contributions to the management of intra-abdominal infections. Am J Surg 2005;190(2):255–9.

[13] Malbrain M, Deerenb D, De Potterc T, et al. Intra-abdominal hypertension in the critically ill: it is time to pay attention. Curr Opin Crit Care 2005;11(2):156–71.

[14] Sugrue M. Abdominal compartment syndrome. Curr Opin Crit Care 2005;11(4):333–8.

[15] Malbrain M, Chiumello D, Pelosi P, et al. Incidence and prognosis of intra-abdominal hypertension in a mixed population of critically ill patients: a multiple-center epidemiological study. Crit Care Med 2005;33(2):315–22.

[16] Holzheirmer RE, Shein M, Wittmann DH. Inflammatory response in peritoneal exudates and plasma of patients undergoing planned relaparotomy for severe secondary peritonitis. Arch Surg 1995;130(12):1314–9 [discussion: 1319–20].

[17] Schein M, Wittmann DH, Holzeimer R, et al. Hypothesis: compartmentalization of cytokines in intra abdominal infection. Surgery 1996;119(6):694–700.

[18] Tang GL, Kuo CD, Yen T, et al. Perioperative plasma concentrations of tumor necrosis factor alpha and interleukin-6 infected patients. Crit Care Med 1996;24(3):423–8.

[19] Riche F, Cholley B, Panis Y, et al. Inflammatory cytokine response in patients with septic shock secondary to generalized peritonitis. Crit Care Med 2000;28(2):433–7.

[20] Baue AE. Multiple organ dysfunction syndrome. Arch Surg 1997;132(7):703–7.

[21] Merrell RC. The abdomen as source of sepsis in critically ill patients. Crit Care Clin 1995; 11(2):255–72.

[22] León A, Torres M, Montenegro G. Infección intra-abdominal. In: Gómez A, Alvarez C, León A, editors. Enfermedades infecciosas en UCI. Una aproximación basada en la evidencia. Bogotá (Colombia): Editorial Distribuna; 2004. p. 293–353 [in Spanish].

[23] Patiño JF, Quintero G, Baptiste S. Infección quirúrgica. In: Patiño JF, editor. Lecciones en cirugía. Bogotá (Colombia): Editorial Médica Panamericana; 2000. p. 105–17 [in Spanish].

[24] Laroche M, Harding G. Primary and secondary peritonitis: an update. Eur J Clin Microbiol Infect Dis 1998;17(8):542–50.

[25] Johnson CC, Baldessarre J, Levison ME, et al. Peritonitis: update on pathophysiology, clinical manifestations, and management. Clin Infect Dis 1997;24(6):1035–45 [quiz: 1046–7].

[26] Rogers PN, Wright IH. Postoperative intra-abdominal sepsis. Br J Surg 1987;74(11):973–5.

[27] Bartlett JG. Intra abdominal sepsis. Med Clin North Am 1995;79(3):599–617.

[28] Martin RF, Rossi RL. The acute abdomen an overview and algorithms. Surg Clin North Am 1997;77(6):1227–43.

[29] Wittmann DH. Tertiary peritonitis. In: Tellado JM, Christou NV, editors. Intra-abdominal infections. Madrid (Spain): Harcourt; 2000. p. 143–52.

[30] Cercenado E, Garcia-Garrote F. Therapeutic challenges of tertiary peritonitis. In: Tellado JM, Christou NV, editors. Intra-abdominal infections. Madrid (Spain): Harcourt; 2000. p. 179–92.

[31] Nathens AB, Rotstein OD, Marshall JC, et al. Tertiary peritonitis: clinical features of a complex nosocomial infectoin. World J Surg 1998;22(2):158–63.

[32] Meakins JL. Surgical infection in art. Arch Surg 1996;131(12):1289–95.

[33] McClean KL, Sheehan GJ, Harding GK, et al. Intra abdominal infection: a review. Clin Infect Dis 1994;19(1):100–16.

[34] Reemst PT, Van Goor H, Goris RJ, et al. SIRS, MODS, and tertiary peritonitis. Eur J Surg Suppl 1996;(576):47–8 [discussion: 49].

[35] Borráez OA. Peritonitis terciaria. In: Quintero G, Nieto JA, Lerma C, editors. Infección en cirugía. Bogotá (Colombia): Editorial Médica Panamerican; 2001. p. 238–44 [in Spanish].

[36] Schein M, Marshall J. LIRS, SIRS, Sepsis, MODS and tertiary peritonitis. In: Schein M, Rogers P, editors. Scheińs common sense emergency abdominal surgery. 2nd edition. New York: Springer; 2005. p. 415–23.

[37] Malangoni MA. Evaluation and management of tertiary peritonitis. Am Surg 2000;66(2): 157–61.

[38] Rosengart M, Nathens A. Tertiary peritonitis. Current treatment options in infectious diseases 2002;4:403–09.

[39] Nieto JA. Sepsis abdominal. In: Quintero G, Nieto JA, Lerma C, editors. Infección en cirugía. Bogotá (Colombia): Editorial Médica Panamericana; 2001. p. 213–29 [in Spanish].

[40] Uribe R. Sepsis abdominal. Tópicos en Medicina Intensiva 2003;2(3):195–203 [in Spanish].

[41] Cohen J, Brun-Buisson C, Torres A, et al. Diagnosis of infection in sepsis: an evidence-based review. Crit Care Med 2004;32(Suppl 11):S466–94.

[42] Cheadle W, Spain D. The continuing challenge of intra-abdominal infection. Am J Surg 2003;186(5):15S–22S.

[43] Velmahos G, Kamel E, Berne T, et al. Abdominal computed tomography for the diagnosis of intra-abdominal sepsis in critically injured patients. Arch Surg 1999;134(8):831–6 [discussion: 836–8].

[44] Go H, Baarslaga H, Vermeulenb H, et al. A comparative study to validate the use of ultrasonography and computed tomography in patients with post-operative intra-abdominal sepsis. Eur J Radiol 2005;54(3):383–7.

[45] Annane D, Sebille V, Bellissant E. Corticosteroids for patients with septic shock. JAMA 2003;289(1):43–4.

[46] Dellinger P, Carlet J, Masur H, et al. Surviving sepsis campaign guidelines for management of severe sepsis and septic shock. Crit Care Med 2004;32(3):858–73.

[47] Paugam-Burtz C, Dupont H, Marmuse J. Daily organ-system failure for diagnosis of persistent intra-abdominal sepsis after postoperative peritonitis. Intensive Care Med 2002; 28(5):594–8.

[48] Marshall J, Maier R, Jimenez M, et al. Source control in the management of severe sepsis and septic shock: an evidence-based review. Crit Care Med 2004;32(11):S513–26.

[49] Levy M, Fink M, Marshall J, et al. 2001 SCCM/ESICM/ACCP/ATS/SIS International Sepsis Definitions Conference. Crit Care Med 2003;31(4):1250–6.

[50] Mulier S, Penninckx F, Verwaest C, et al. Factors affecting mortality in generalized postoperative peritonitis: multivariate analysis in 96 patients. World J Surg 2003;27(4):379–84.

[51] Marshall J, Innes M. Intensive care unit management of intra-abdominal infection. Crit Care Med 2003;31(8):2228–37.

[52] van Goor H. Interventional management of abdominal sepsis: when and how. Arch Surg 2002;387:191–200.

[53] Rivers E, Nguyen B, Havstad S, et al. Early goal-directed therapy in the treatment of severe sepsis and septic shock. N Engl J Med 2001;345(19):1368–77.

[54] Van den Berghe G. Intensive insulin therapy in critically ill patients. N Engl J Med 2001; 345(19):1359–67.

[55] Paugam-Burtz C, Dupont H, Marmuse JP, et al. Daily organ-system failure diagnosis of persistent abdominal sepsis after postoperative peritonitis. Intensive Care Med 2002; 28(5):594–8.

[56] Anaya DA, Nathens AB. Risk factors for severe sepsis in secondary peritonitis. Surg Infect (Larchmt) 2003;4(4):355–62.

[57] Blot S, De Waele J. Critical issues in the clinical management of complicated intra-abdominal infections. Drugs 2005;65(12):1611–20.

[58] Burnett RJ, Haverstock DC, Bellinger PE, et al. Definition of the role of enterococcus in intra abdominal infection: analysis of a prospective randomized trial. Surgery 1995; 118(4):716–21 [discussion: 721–3].

[59] Mainous MR, Lipsett PA, ÓBrien M, et al. Enterococcol bacteremia in the surgical intensive care unit. Arch Surg 1997;132(1):76–81.

[60] Sawyer RG, Rosenlof LK, Adams RB, et al. Peritonitis into the 1990's: changing pathogens and changing strategies in the critically ill. Am Surg 1992;58(2):82–7.

[61] Solomkin JS, Reinhard HH, Dellinger EP, et al. Results of a randomized trial comparing sequential intravenous/oral treatment with ciprofloxacin plus metronidazole to imipenem/cilastatin for intra abdominal infections. Ann Surg 1996;223(3):303–15.

[62] Nathens AB, Rotstein OD. Antimicrobial therapy for intra abdominal infection. Am J Surg 1996;172(6A):1S–6S.

[63] Chang DC, Wilson SE. Meta-analysis of the clinical outcome of carbapenem monotherapy in the adjunctive treatment of intra-abdominal infections. Am J Surg 1997;174(3):284–90.

[64] Solomkin JS. Antibiotic resistance in postoperative infections. Crit Care Med 2001; 29(Suppl 4):N97–9.

[65] Solomkin J, Yellin A, Rotstein O, et al. The Protocol 017 Study Group. Ertapenem versus piperacillin/tazobactam in the treatment of complicated intra-abdominal infections: results of a double-blind, randomized comparative Phase III trial. Ann Surg 2003;237(2):235–45.

[66] Álvarez-Lerma F, Palomar M, Grau S. Management of antimicrobial use in the intensive care unit. Drugs 2001;61(6):763–75.

[67] Visser MR, Bosscha K, Olsman J, et al. Predictors of recurrence of fulminant bacterial peritonitis after discontinuation of antibiotics in open management of the abdomen. Eur J Surg 1998;164(11):825–9.

[68] Consensus: recommended duration of antibiotic administration. Eur J Surg Suppl 1996;(576):1–75.

[69] Nathens AB, Rotstein OD. Therapeutic options in peritonitis. Surg Clin North Am 1994; 74(3):677–92.

[70] Christou NV, Barie PS, Dellinger EP, et al. Surgical Infection Society Intra Abdominal Infection Study: prospective evaluation of management techniques and outcome. Arch Surg 1993;128(2):193–8 [discussion: 198–9].

[71] Marshall JC, Christou NV, Meakins JL. The gastro intestinal tract: the "undrained abscess" of multiple organ failure. Ann Surg 1993;218(2):111–9.

[72] Wittmann DH, Aprahamian C, Bergstein JM, et al. Etappenlavage, advanced diffuse peritonitis managed by planned multiple laparotomies utilizing zippers slide fastener, and Velcro for temporary abdominal closure. World J Surg 1990;14(2):218–26.

[73] Hau T, Ohmann C, Wolmershauser A, et al. Planned relaparotomy vs relaparotomy on demand in the treatment of intra abdominal infections. Arch Surg 1995;130(11):1 [discussion: 1193–6, 1196–7].

[74] Adkins AL, Robbins J, Villalba M, et al. Open abdomen management of intra-abdominal sepsis. Am Surg 2004;70(2):137–40 [discussion: 140].

[75] Ordóñez CA, Ferrada R, Flórez G, et al. Abdomen abierto en sepsis intra-abdominal. Malla de nylon con cierre. Panamerican Journal of Trauma 1989;1(1):16–21 [in Spanish].

[76] Borráez OA. Abdomen abierto. In: Quintero G, Nieto JA, Lerma C, editors. Infección en cirugía. Bogotá (Colombia): Editorial Médica Panamericana; 2001. p. 230–7 [in Spanish].

[77] Ordóñez CA, García A, Flórez G, et al. Uso de la malla en abdomen abierto, en sepsis intra-abdominal. Revista Columbiana de Cirugía 1995;10(2):101–8 [in Spanish].

[78] Bosscha K, Hulstaert PF, Visser MR, et al. Open management of the abdomen and planned reoperations in severe bacterial peritonitis. Eur J Surg 2000;166(1):44–9.

[79] Schein M. Planned reoperations and open management in critical intra-abdominal infections: prospective experience in 52 cases. World J Surg 1991;15(4):537–45.

[80] Aprahamian C, Wittmann DH, Bergstein JM, et al. Temporary abdominal closure (TAC) for planned relaparotomy (etappenlavage) in trauma. J Trauma 1990;30(6):719–23.

[81] Rakic M, Popovic D, Rakic M, et al. Comparison of on-demand vs planned relaparotomy for treatment of severe intra-abdominal infections. Croat Med J 2005;46(6):956–63.

[82] Agalar F, Eroglu E, Bulbul M, et al. Staged abdominal repair for treatment of moderate to severe secondary peritonitis. World J Surg 2005;29(2):240–4.

[83] Özgüç H, Yilmazlar T, Gürlüler E, et al. Staged abdominal repair in the treatment of intra-abdominal infection: analysis of 102 patients. J Gastrointest Surg 2003;7(5):646–51.

[84] Biswajit M. Staged abdominal repair (STAR) operation: how I did it. Indian J Surg 2004; 66(3):182–4.

[85] Lamme B, Mahler C, van Hill J, et al. Relaparotomie bei sekundärer. Peritonitis Programmier te Relaparotomie oder Relaparotomie on demand? Chirurg 2005;76(9):856–67 [in German].

[86] Koperna T, Schulz F. Relaparotomy in peritonitis: prognosis and treatment of patients with persisting intra-abdominal infection. World J Surg 2000;24(1):32–7.

[87] Lamme B, Boermeester M, Belt E, et al. Mortality and morbidity of planned relaparotomy versus relaparotomy on demand for secondary peritonitis. Br J Surg 2004;91(8):1046–54.

[88] Lamme B, Boermeester MA, Reitsma JB, et al. Meta-analysis of relaparotomy for secondary peritonitis. Br J Surg 2002;89(12):1516–24.

[89] Hutchins R, Gunning P, Nuala Lucas N, et al. Relaparotomy for suspected intraperitoneal sepsis after abdominal surgery. World J Surg 2004;28(2):137–41.

[90] Mille P, Meredith W, Johnson J, et al. Prospective evaluation of vacuum-assisted fascial closure after open abdomen planned ventral hernia rate is substantially reduced. Ann Surg 2004;239(5):608–14 [discussion: 614–6].

[91] Suliburk J, Ware D, Balogh Z, et al. Vacuum-assisted wound closure achieves early fascial closure of open abdomens after severe trauma. J Trauma 2003;55(6):1155–60.

[92] Garner G, Ware D, Cocanour C, et al. Vacuum-assisted wound closure achieves early fascial closure of open abdomens after severe trauma. Am J Surg 2001;182(6):630–8.

[93] Barker D, Kaufman H, Smith L, et al. Vacuum pack technique of temporary abdominal closure: a 7-year experience with 112 patients. J Trauma 2000;48(2):201–6 [discussion: 206–7].

[94] Bohnen JM, Mustard RA, Oxholm SE, et al. APACHE II score and abdominal sepsis: a prospective study. Arch Surg 1988;123(2):225–9.

[95] Knaus WA, Draper EA, Wagner DP, et al. APACHE II: a severity of disease classification system. Crit Care Med 1985;13(10):818–29.

[96] Koperna T, Schulz F. Prognosis and treatment of peritonitis. Arch Surg 1996;131(2):180–6.

[97] Hotchkiss R, Karl I. Medical progress: the pathophysiology and treatment of sepsis. N Engl J Med 2003;348(2):138–50.

[98] Carlsson E, Berglund B, Nordgren S. Living with an ostomy and short bowel syndrome: practical aspects and impact on daily life. J Wound Ostomy Continence Nurs 2001;28(2): 96–105.

[99] Edwards DP, Leppington-Clarke A, Sexton R, et al. Stoma-related complications are more frequent after transverse colostomy than loop ileostomy: a prospective randomized clinical trial. Br J Surg 2001;88(3):360–3.

[100] Schilling MK, Maurer CA, Kollmar O, et al. Primary vs. secondary anastomosis after sigmoid colon resection for perforated diverticulitis (Hinchey Stage III and IV): a prospective outcome and cost analysis. Dis Colon Rectum 2001;44(5):699–703 [discussion: 703–5].

[101] Gooszen AW, Gooszen HG, Veerman W, et al. Operative treatment of acute complications of diverticular disease: primary or secondary anastomosis after sigmoid resection. Eur J Surg 2001;167(1):35–9.

[102] Zorcolo L, Covotta L, Carlomagno N, et al. Safety of primary anastomosis in emergency colo-rectal surgery. Colorectal Dis 2003;5(3):262–9.

[103] Biondo S, Jaurrieta E, Marti Rague J, et al. Role of resection and primary anastomosis of the left colon in the presence of peritonitis. Br J Surg 2000;87(11):1580–4.

[104] Curran TJ, Brozota AP. Complications of primary repair of colon injury: literature review of 2964 cases. Am J Surg 1999;177(1):42–7.

[105] Gonzalez RP, Falimirski ME, Holevar MR. Further evaluation of colostomy in penetrating colon injury. Am Surg 2000;66(4):342–6 [discussion: 346–7].

[106] Bulger EM, McMahon K, Jurkovich GJ. The morbidity of penetrating colon injury. Injury 2003;34(1):41–6.

[107] Singer MA, Nelson RL. Primary repair of penetrating colon injuries: a systematic review. Dis Colon Rectum 2002;45(12):1579–87.

[108] Gonzalez RP, Merlotti GJ, Holevar MR. Colostomy in penetrating colon injury: is it necessary? J Trauma 1996;41(2):271–5.

[109] Sasaki LS, Allaben RD, Golwala R, et al. Primary repair of colon injuries: a prospective randomized study. J Trauma 1995;39(5):895–901.

[110] Murray JA, Demetriades D, Colson M, et al. Colonic resection in trauma: colostomy versus anastomosis. J Trauma 1999;46(2):250–4.

[111] Maxwell RA, Fabian TC. Current management of colon trauma. World J Surg 2003;27(6): 632–9.

[112] Demetriades D, Murray JA, Chan L, et al. Penetrating colon injuries requiring resection: diversion or primary anastomosis? An AAST prospective multicenter study. J Trauma 2001;50(5):765–75.

[113] De Graaf JS, van Goor H, Bleichrodt RP. Primary small bowel anastomosis in generalized peritonitis. Eur J Surg 1996;162(1):55–8.

[114] Rotondo M, Schwab CW, McGonigal M, et al. "Damage control": An approach for improved survival in exsanguinations penetrating abdominal injury. J Trauma 1993;35(3): 375–82 [discussion: 382–3].

[115] Rotondo MF, Zomies DH. The damage control sequence and underlying logic. Surg Clin North Am 1997;77(4):761–77.

[116] Schreiber M. Damage control surgery. Crit Care Clin 2004;20(1):101–18.

[117] Sugrue M, D'Amours SK, Joshipura M. Damage control surgery and the abdomen. Injury 2004;35(7):642–8.

[118] Shapiro M, Jenkins D, Schwab W, et al. Damage control: collective review. J Trauma 2000; 49(5):969–78.

[119] McPartland K, Hyman N. Damage control: what is its role in colorectal surgery? Dis Colon Rectum 2003;46(7):981–6.

[120] Johnson J, Gracias V, Schwab W, et al. Evolution in damage control for exsanguinating penetrating abdominal injury. J Trauma 2001;51(2):261–9 [discussion: 269–71].

[121] Ordóñez CA, Pineda JA, Arias R, et-al. Curso clínico de la peritonitis severa en pacientes críticamente enfermos tratados con sutura primaria diferida. Revista Colombiana de Cirugía, in press [in Spanish].

[122] Takeyama H, Sato M, Akamo Y, et al. Keyhole procedure: a new technique for intestinal anastomosis with a large opening and less tissue trauma, using both circular and linear staplers. Surgery 2003;133(3):345–8.

[123] Moriura S, Kobayashi I, Ishiguro S, et al. Continuous mattress suture for all hand-sewn anastomoses of the gastrointestinal tract. Am J Surg 2002;184(5):446–8.

[124] Burch J, Franciose R, Moore EE, et al. Single-layer continuous versus two-layer interrupted intestinal anastomosis: a prospective randomized trial. Ann Surg 2000;231(6):832–7.

[125] Demetriades D, Murray J, MD, Chan L, et-al. Handsewn versus stapled anastomosis in penetrating colon injuries requiring resection: a multicenter study. J Trauma 2002;52(1): 117–21.

[126] Ordóñez CA, Arias R, Granados M, et al. Mortalidad y morbilidad de la peritonitis secundaria con re-laparotomía planeada. Rev Colomb Cir 2006;21:124–32 [in Spanish].

ELSEVIER
SAUNDERS

SURGICAL
CLINICS OF
NORTH AMERICA

Surg Clin N Am 86 (2006) 1351–1357

The Relationship between the Surgeon and the Intensivist in the Surgical Intensive Care Unit

Patricia A. Penkoske, MD[a],[*],
Timothy G. Buchman, MD, PhD[b]

[a]Department of Anesthesia, Washington University School of Medicine,
660 South Euclid Street, St. Louis, MO 63108, USA
[b]Department of Surgery, Washington University School of Medicine,
660 South Euclid Street, St. Louis, MO 63110, USA

When a patient enters the intensive care unit, either postoperatively or after an acute event, the admitting surgeon also enters a new environment. In some hospitals, the surgical intensive care unit (SICU) is "closed," where critical care providers manage their care, and in others the unit is "open," and the admitting surgeon is the one in charge. A third system is the "mixed" model of ICU administration, where there is a collaborative "co-attending" approach. This article is written from the perspective of two surgeon-intensivists who have been in both roles. It addresses areas of concern and conflict that frequently arise between admitting surgeons and intensivists. In doing this, areas of research that may help to explain why differences in the approach to a patient exist are discussed. ICU conflicts and their resolution have been the subject of recent behavioral and social research that are reviewed. New strategies for conflict resolution are also presented.

Illustrative case history

Mr. X, a 75-year-old male, has chronic obstructive pulmonary disease, stable chronic renal insufficiency, congestive heart failure with an ejection fraction of 30%, and Type II diabetes mellitus. He has had an uneventful laparoscopic right colectomy by Surgeon Y, and has been admitted to the

* Corresponding author.
E-mail address: pattypenkoske@yahoo.com (P.A. Penkoske).

SICU for postoperative management of fluids. He meets discharge criteria and is transferred to the surgical ward the next day. Three days later, he becomes acutely ill with an anastomotic leak, returns to the operating room for washout and colostomy, and is readmitted to the SICU. Although his sepsis initially responds to aggressive critical care, he develops multiple organ dysfunction syndrome. Two weeks after the emergency surgery, he remains dependent on mechanical ventilator support, and his renal failure has progressed to the point where renal replacement therapy (dialysis) seems imminent. His wife presents the patient's advance directives, including a living will in which he states that extraordinary supports should not be used to prolong his life if there is no meaningful chance of returning to good health.

This case is but one instance of an increasingly common pattern of initial success, significant deterioration, and ICU readmission for support of multiple dysfunctional systems. During the initial success period, conversations and decisions revolve around processes of care—transfusion targets, which antibiotic to administer, timing of extubation, and so on. The reason for this technical focus is that both family and caregivers are expecting the hoped-for outcome—recovery—and the technical aspects of care constitute milestones by which progress is measured toward that end. The readmission brings a different set of challenges. Although the management of septic shock has evolved to the point that immediate survival is now commonplace [1], long-term outcomes often involve chronic, high-dependency states that are inconsistent with explicit advance directives. Uncertainty about the outcome of individual patients compounds the ambiguities inherent in advance directives. Together, these often lead to conflicts among those caring for the patient. The conflicts arise not only from uncertainties about the outcome, but also from differing definitions of "success." In the technical world of clinical professional, success is often defined as survival to leave the ICU. In the moral world of families and friends, success often means returning to an independent life with resumption of previously enjoyable activities. Between these poles lies the purgatory of prolonged high-dependency care. Effective resolution of the conflict requires that all parties acknowledge and understand the others' perspectives.

The surgeon's perspective

The qualities that define a "surgical personality" are described by anthropologist Joan Cassell in three monographs that focus on surgeons [2], women surgeons [3], and SICUs [4]. She compares the temperament of surgeons to that of test pilots. Decisiveness, control, confidence, and certitude are qualities of successful surgeons. Surgeons perform operations that are spectacular and definitive, but are also often irreversible, and are always attributable. The surgeon typically views his relationship with the patient as a "covenant to cure." Actions and events that threaten the covenant—relinquishing responsibility for care of the patient to another practitioner, losing control over key decisions, and proposals to redirect care exclusively toward comfort with the expectation of death—are strongly rebuffed by the admitting surgeon. Such "ownership" of the patient and sense of responsibility to pursue an ideal outcome is valuable in ensuring that the patient has a strong advocate who can access all available tools to facilitate recovery; however, surgical intransigence with respect to sharing responsibility and refocusing efforts on comfort can confuse families and deny the dying patient both dignity and control.

The intensivist's perspective

In contrast to the surgeon's "cure at any cost" perspective, Cassell [4] describes the intensivist's perspective more holistically, with symptom relief and comfort included as core responsibilities. In particular, curative efforts without meaningful chances for success are generally viewed by intensivists as inappropriate, even harmful. From the surgeon's perspective, persistence in the face of overwhelming odds is viewed as a noble obligation. From the intensivist's perspective, persistence in the face of overwhelming odds is costly, often painful, and disrespectful if the patient has expressed any wish to avoid heroic measures under the circumstances.

This is not say that intensivists are any less goal-oriented than surgeons. Indeed, intensivists embrace evidence-based, goal-directed care.

Somewhat to the dismay of surgeons, intensivist-led critical care appears to improve overall outcomes. The efficacy of having a dedicated intensivist caring for ICU patients, whether in a medical, surgical, or pediatric ICU, has been shown in a recent review [5]. Survival is improved and complications decreased by having an intensivist making rounds, coordinating care and making decisions. The effect is not trivial. Depending on the specific patient subset looked at (septic, post-aneurysm surgery, severity of illness score), mortality can be decreased by up to 50%.

The reasons for this general improvement with intensivist involvement in patient care are incompletely known. The presence and participation of an intensivist-directed team can identify and treat problems before catastrophic complications occur. Knowledge of recent technical advances may be more accessible to intensivists than in the memory of surgeons. Definition of sepsis and its various manifestations, mechanical ventilatory support in acute lung injury [6], and description and treatment of endocrine dysfunction in the critically ill [7] have led to goal-directed protocols with improved survival. Evidence-based studies on transfusion triggers [8], oral care and ventilator-associated pneumonia [9], insertion, and care of central venous catheters [10] all appear to reduce adverse outcomes.

This is not to say that surgeons cannot master the knowledge and apply the technologies. But, more often than not, surgeons do not have the time to do so and to simultaneously meet the demands of operative practice. Both continuing education in critical care medicine and presence at the ICU bed-side are especially time-intensive. Surgeons are affected by the increasing de-mands on clinical time as much as any other specialist. As a consequence, they must spend progressively more time in the operating room and in the office, at the cost of less available time to see and manage patients in the ICU.

Economic issues relating to critical care

Independent of the wishes of the surgeon, there are also economic con-straints that are imposed by the institutions in which they practice.

In the United States, acute care accounts for greater than 90 billion dol-lars per year, making up greater than 20% of acute care hospital costs [11,12]. The Leapfrog Group [13] looked at the effect of having a intensivist directing patient care in the ICU, and showed not only improved outcomes but significant cost savings to the institution because of the decrease in length of stay and complications.

Because of the shortage of critical care physicians, at the present time only 10% to 20% of United States ICUs are units have dedicated intensivist staffing [11]. This has led to the proliferation of tele-ICU groups who help manage patients at a distance using sophisticated computer technology [12].

Ethical issues in the intensive care unit

A point of major controversy arises in the ICU when despite aggressive care for cure, the patient does not respond. As in the example given at the beginning of this article in the case of the elderly patient who has the anastomotic leak and sepsis, and who 2 weeks after readmission is still on the ventilator with deteriorating renal function. The next cure strategies would be tracheostomy, planning on a long-term weaning process and inser-tion of access for long-term nutritional support; and perhaps renal replace-ment therapy to manage fluid and electrolyte abnormalities. There is another option that includes changing the goal of therapy from cure to comfort.

This area is where the surgeon and intensivist often disagree. The surgeon sees a patient who may "take a while to recover" in a long-term care facility, but he has a benign colon lesion, and he could survive and go back to his former life. The intensivist sees an elderly man who has multisystem prob-lems and who has a minimal chance—even after a prolonged hospital and long-term, acute-care facility—of returning to his former life, which was already limited by his pre-existing medical problems.

When the discussion turns to end-of-life issues, who makes the decisions greatly determines the course [4]. When the surgeon makes the decision, the most important goal is often defeating death. When the intensivist has sole responsibility, quality of life is a significant variable. Because in most cases the patient is not able to participate in the discussions, major family unhappiness can occur when they view conflict between the professionals caring for their loved one [13].

Specific areas of conflict and possible solutions

Prediction, projection, and prognostication: why professionals differ in their approach to the patient and family, and the content of their discussions

When major differences occur, discussions should first occur between the intensivist and surgeon, and then with the family. In rare instances, a member of the hospital ethics committee may also participate. Part of the conflict also arises because, although specific interventions have been shown to be of benefit, there is not a nationwide registry of the outcome of subsets of critically ill patients [14].

Turf and referrals

A surgeon may consult, for example, a pulmonary physician on all patients who have asthma. While in the ICU, the need to involve another consultant should be discussed, because one or the other physician may have a preference. The intensivist is typically skilled at the management of most major common medical conditions as well as critical care issues, and often it is better to have one person orchestrating the total care rather than "breaking" the patient up into organ system, because there are interactions.

"ICU protocols are fine for someone else's patient, but give my patient two units of blood."

Often, the surgeon may not have been exposed to the evidence-based study on which a protocol is based [8]. This should be provided and transfusion triggers available. Even when the data are known, individual surgeon preferences based on personal experience or training experience may lead to a discussion of how the data applies to "my patient" and why he is different.

Rationing of the resources of the intensive care unit: who gets in, when does a patient get transferred?

The issues of admission and discharge criteria for the ICU for the most part are obvious, but in cases when a discharge is being blocked by an admitting surgeon, the intensivist may have to intervene. The needs of the system and whether a particular patient meets discharge criteria may occasionally override a specific surgeon's wish for "one extra day."

The surgeon's role in the "integrated team of dedicated experts"

This is where the surgeon can have the greatest impact in insuring that her patients receive the care that they wish them to have. Communication is the most important factor. The surgeon who communicates her wishes and expectations and who is responsive to evaluating a protocol that has been shown to have a better outcome in a large group of patients will be a desired participant in the critical care team. Surgeons should likewise be told by the team when an adverse event occurs, and areas of controversy should be discussed with them before involving the family. In this way, many problems can be averted.

Summary

Conflict between the surgeon and the intensivist caring for the patient in the SICU is easily understood. The intensivist is motivated by increasing evidence that a team approach, evidence-based medicine, and a compassionate approach to the relief of suffering are the goals of an ICU. This is substantiated by many studies showing that these approaches decrease length of stay, hospital costs, complications, and mortality.

The surgeon is motivated by wanting to cure the patient, and is used to being the one in charge—"the captain of the ship." Most are probably unaware of the studies showing the effect of a dedicated intensivist as far as patient outcome.

The key for both is communication. For the intensivist, this includes making sure that adverse events are reported in a timely fashion, that important decisions are discussed, and that the surgeon is included in the team. For the surgeon, this means being willing to discuss rather than dictate, and considering different approaches.

References

[1] Dellinger P, Carlet J, Ma The Tsur J, et al. Surviving Sepsis Campaign guidelines for management of severe sepsis and septic shock. Crit Care Med 2004;32(3):858–73.
[2] Cassell J. Expected miracles: surgeons at work. Philadelphia: Temple University Press; 1991.
[3] Cassell J. The woman in the surgeon's body. Cambridge (MA): Harvard University Press; 1998.
[4] Cassell J. Life and death in the intensive care unit. Philadelphia: Temple University Press; 2005.
[5] The Leapfrog Group. Leapfrog surgery summary. Available at: www.leapfroggroup.org. Accessed July 16, 2006.
[6] The Acute Respiratory Distress Syndrome Network. Ventilation with lower tidal volumes as compared with traditional tidal volumes for acute lung injury and the acute respiratory distress syndrome. N Engl J Med 2000;342:1301–8.
[7] Annane D, Sebille V, Charpentier C. Effect of treatment with low doses of hydrocortisone and fludrocortisone on mortality in patients with septic shock. JAMA 2002;288:862–7.

 [8] Hebert P, Wells G, Blajchman M. A multicenter, randomized, controlled clinical trial of transfusion requirements in critical care. N Engl J Med 1999;340:409–17.

 [9] Mori H, Hirasawah, Oda S, et al. Oral care reduces incidence of ventilator-associated pneumonia in ICU populations. Intensive Care Med 2006;32:230–6.

[10] Coopersmith C, Rebmann T, Zack J, et al. Effect of an education program on decreasing catheter-related bloodstream infections in the surgical intensive care unit. Crit Care Med 2002;30:59–64.

[11] Provost P, Needham D, Waters H, et al. Intensive care unit physician staffing: financial modeling of the Leapfrog standard. Crit Care Med 2004;32:1247–53.

[12] Celi L, Hassan E, Marquardt C. The eICU: it's not just telemedicine. Crit Care Med 2001;29: N183–9.

[13] Cassell J, Buchman T, Streat T, et al. Surgeons, intensivists, and the covenant of care: administrative models and values affecting care at the end of life—updated. Crit Care Med 2003; 31(5):1551–9.

[14] Buchman T. Critical care: On target. Crit Care Med 2003;31(4):1003–5.

ELSEVIER
SAUNDERS

SURGICAL
CLINICS OF
NORTH AMERICA

Surg Clin N Am 86 (2006) 1359–1387

Critical Care Issues in the Early Management of Severe Trauma

Alberto Garcia, MD[a,b,c,*]

[a]*Trauma Division, Hospital Universitario del Valle, Calle 5 No. 36–08, Cali, Columbia*
[b]*Emergencies Unit, Clinica Valle el Lili, Carrera, 98 No. 18–49, Cali, Columbia*
[c]*Department of Surgery, Universidad del Valle, Calle 48 No. 36–00, Cali, Columbia*

Violent trauma and road traffic injuries kill more than 2.5 million people in the world every year. It has been calculated by the World Health Organization that in 2002 there occurred 1.6 million violent deaths [1] and 1.2 million deaths from traffic injury [2], for a combined mortality of 48 deaths per 100,000 population per year.

Most trauma deaths occur at the scene or in the first hour after trauma, with a proportion from 34% to 50% occurring in hospitals [3]. These deaths could be prevented by optimization of trauma care. Preventability of trauma deaths has been reported as high as 76% [4] and as low as 1% in mature trauma systems [5,6].

Prehospitalization procedures, elapsed time to hospital arrival are, of course, vital to the whole trauma scenario, but errors made in the in-hospital phase of care are responsible for one third to two thirds of the reported by different authors [7,8]. Of these, intensive care unit (ICU) errors are among the most frequent and significant. Errors in the ICU management of trauma patients were studied by Duke and colleagues [9]. They reported 165 ICU trauma deaths. Two hundred fifty-eight errors occurred in 81 patients (52%), and 134 of them contributed to death in 52 patients (34%). ICU errors were classified as management errors (82%), diagnostic (9%), technique (5%), and system inadequacies (4%). Davis and colleagues [10] identified critical care errors in 30% of 125 trauma deaths with errors. These errors contributed to 48% of all preventable deaths.

Funded in part by Fogerty International Center NIH Grant No. 1 D43 TW007560-01.

* Carrera 4 Oeste #1-65, Apartamento 1303, Edificion San Antonio del Peñón Cali, Colombia.

E-mail address: agarciam@telesat.com.co

The most common critical care errors are related to airway and respiratory management, fluid resuscitation, neurotrauma diagnosis and support, and delayed diagnosis of critical lesions [9,10].

It is imperative for the general surgeon who takes care of trauma patients to know how to deal with these critical aspects, to reduce preventable morbidity and mortality. In the next segment, the situations in which the participation of the surgeon is crucial, during the initial phases of reanimation and stabilization of the critically traumatized patient will be discussed.

Airway and ventilation management

Airway and respiratory management errors are the most common of those identified by several authors [9–11]. The mechanically ventilated trauma patient may experience alterations in oxygenation as a result of the trauma itself or because of complications of therapeutic maneuvers. The source must be identified and treated expeditiously, to avoid additional injury, particularly in patients with encephalic trauma.

The cardinal manifestation is a sudden or a rapidly progressing desaturation, frequently accompanied by tachycardia and arrhytmias, and occasionally by agitation. Hypertension announces the cardiovascular collapse, and bradicardia appears immediately after the total collapse [12]. The symptoms should not be attributed to agitation when it is present, and other possible causes must be ruled out before. Diagnosing the complication involves a directed physical examination, the analysis of the airway pressures and ventilator volumes, chest radiographs, and sometimes the measurement of arterial blood gases (ABG), and the urinary bladder pressure (Table 1).

The emergency conditions in which the access to the airways must be gained, the displacement to diagnosis areas or operating room and the agitation, often present, make the critical trauma patient prone to airway complications [13–16]. Accidents of the airway cause preventable deaths and increase morbidity, length of stay, and costs [17–20]. Adequate staffing and protocolization could have avoided more than the half of them [20–22].

Disconnection, accidental extubation, and proximal orotracheal tube migration

Disconnection and extubation are easily recognized by the rapid deterioration of the patient, and the ventilator alarms of low pressure and gas leak. Reintubating the patient, after oxygenating him or her with mask-bag manual ventilation, is the treatment for the accidental extubation.

Migration of the tube to the pharynx produces a subtler clinical picture. The most remarkable physiopathologic alteration is alveolar hypoventilation due to gas leak. Occasionally, the loss of positive pressure produces hypoxemia in patients who need positive end expiratory pressure (PEEP). The appearance of saliva bubbles in the mouth must cause suspicion. The

Table 1
Differentiation of airway and ventilation crises

Condition	Peak pressure	Plateau pressure	Clinical finding
Low or normal peak inspiratory pressure			
Extubation/proximal tube migration	Low	Low	Noises and saliva bubbles in the mouth
Disconnection	Low	Low	Disconnection from the ventilatory circuits
Negative pressure	Low	Low	Agytation. Low pressures alternating with high pressures
High peak inspiratory pressure			
Artificial airway obstruction	High	Normal	Cuff deflation test: minimal change
Patient's airway obstruction	High	Normal	Cuff deflation test: scape and pressures reduction
Atelectasis	High	High	Asymmetry. Chest X-rays confirmation
Acute lung injury	High	High	Chest X-rays confirmation
Tension pneumothorax	High	High	Asymmetry. Needle confirmation
Massive diaphragmatic hernia	High	High	Asymmetry. Chest X-rays confirmation
Intraabdominal hypertension	High	High	Symmetric diminished breath sounds. Elevated intravesical pressure

ABG will show hypercarbia, and the ventilator will indicate low airways pressure and low expired gas volume. The diagnosis is confirmed by direct laryngoscopy, and the complication is treated by replacing the tube. Protocols of endotracheal tube securing and ventilator circuit checking should avoid these complications [21,23,24].

Airway obstruction

Acute airway obstruction can develop in the trauma mechanically ventilated patient at any level, from different causes: artificial airway may occlude by kinking, biting, impacted secretions, or clots; trachea and bronchii tubes by hematoma, clots, or secretions; and small airways by secretions or bronchospasm [25,26]. Foreign bodies can obstruct the airways at any level [27] (Fig. 1). Manifestations include inspiratory effort, elevated peak inspiratory pressure, low level of plateau pressure (this difference results from the increased resistance to airflow), and decreased tidal volume. Oxygenation is compromised as well as CO_2 excretion [28]. Chest radiographs may not reveal any acute abnormality, unless clots or secretions have caused an atelectasis.

Kinking and biting are easily detected and corrected. Differentiating obstruction in the artificial airway or distal to it is critical, and often difficult to do. Passing a suction catheter into the endotracheal tube may detect an

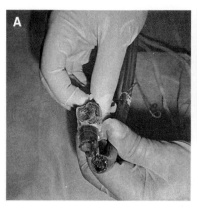
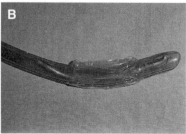

Fig. 1. (*A*) Orotracheal tube occluded by clots in a patient with lung contusion and hemoptysis. He developed sudden dyspnea, agitation, and desaturation. The peak airway pressure and plateau pressure was 38 and 28 cm H_2O, respectively. A suction catheter passed easily. The patient improved after changing the occluded tube. (*B*) Orotracheal tube occluded by a segment of a broken guide, in a BTI intubated in the emergency room. The mechanical ventilation was difficult and airway obstruction was suspected because of high peak airway pressure and normal plateau pressure. The patient improved after changing the tube.

obstruction in it. Nevertheless, the distal advance does not exclude the endotracheal tube occlusion by clots or impacted secretions. The cuff deflation test [28] may help to find the obstruction site: the cuff of the endotracheal tube is deflated while the patient continues being ventilated. When the obstruction locates distal to the tube a dramatic reduction in the peak inspiratory pressure and a marked leak are observed. On the other hand, when the endotracheal tube is occluded, high peak inspiratory pressure persists and there is minimal leakage. Occasionally, the only way to be sure of the obstruction of the tube is by changing it. Broncoscopy may be required.

Acute reduction of respiratory system compliance

A group of mechanically ventilated trauma patients exhibit a picture of rapidly progressive elevation of the peak inspiratory pressure, with a parallel increase of the plateau pressure, reduction of the tidal volume, and variable hypoxemia and hypercarbia. This complex may be attributed to acute lung injury or atelectasis. Nevertheless, it may correspond to an extrapulmonary cause, that is, tension pneumothorax [29,30], massive diaphragmatic hernia [31–34], or intraabdominal hypertension [35–37]. Clearly, diagnosing these entities has critical transcendence, as they cause rapid hemodynamic deterioration and are susceptible to specific surgical treatment (Fig. 2).

The elevation of the plateau pressure discards airway obstruction, and some clinical clues permit us to diagnose or to suspect specific entities: thorax asymmetry with an increase of chest volume on the compromised side, tracheal deviation to the opposite side, resonance, and diminished breath

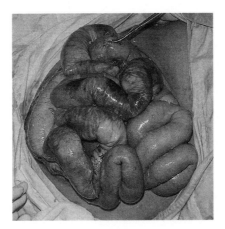

Fig. 2. Segmental intestine necrosis in a patient with peritonitis after penetrating abdominal trauma and late surgical decompression of the abdominal cavity. The respiratory manifestations were managed with oxygen 100% and high PEEP levels; the hemodynamic instability with IV fluids and norepinefrine infusion. As a consequence, the intraabdominal hypertension syndrome was diagnosed and treated late.

sounds of the compromised side in tension pneumothorax; tracheal deviation to the compromised side, decreased chest volume, dullness, and decreased breath sounds in massive atelectasis (Fig. 3), and increase of the chest volume of the compromise side, tracheal deviation to the opposite side, dullness, and diminished breath sounds of the compromised side in massive diaphragmatic hernia (Fig. 4).

Tension pneumothorax is confirmed by the insertion of a 12 Fr intravenous (IV) catheter in the second intercostal space. A chest radiograph gives clues to differentiate the other entities. Compartment abdominal syndrome diagnosis is confirmed by measurement of bladder pressure. Definitive treatment is made by surgery.

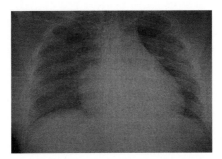

Fig. 3. Monobronchial intubation in a BTI patient. He was intubated in the emergency room and transported to the ICU. In the first evaluation there were desaturation, tracheal deviation to the left, and diminished breath sounds in the left hemythorax. Chest radiographs shows the tip of the tube in the main right bronchi, and signs of loss of volume in the left lung.

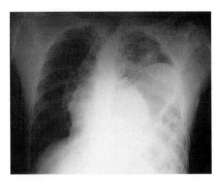

Fig. 4. Massive left diaphragmatic hernia. The patient was dyspneic, tachycardic, and had tracheal deviation to the right and diminished breath sounds of the left hemythorax. (Courtesy of Diego Rivera, MD, Hospital Universitario del Valle, Cali, Columbia.)

Evaluation and treatment of the circulatory state

The objectives of the circulatory assessment during the initial evaluation of the trauma patient (recognizing the state of circulatory shock, identifying the bleeding source, controlling the hemorrhage, and replacing IV fluids and eventually blood components), must be kept during critical care reanimation. Some of the most common errors reported during this phase of the treatment are related to the failure in the accomplishment of these principles [7,9,10].

Recognizing a state of shock

Relying exclusively on the vital signs to diagnose hypovolemic shock may be misleading. Supine tachycardia or hypotension are specific but not sensitive to detecting moderate bleedings. Sensitivity of supine hypotension (blood pressure <95 mm Hg) was only 33%, while specificity was 96%, to detect a blood loss of 630 to 1150 mL, in healthly volunteers. In other words, the presence of these signs confirm hypovolemia, but their absence do not discard it [38]. Celoria and colleagues [39] failed to predict a low wedge pressure or a low cardiac output, based on clinical parameters in one third of a group of surgical critical patients; additionally, most of the patients in whom they predicted low wedge pressure or cardiac output, had normal values. Shoemaker and colleagues [40] showed that vital signs were not able to differentiate survivors from nonsurvivors in a group of shock patients. Abou-Khalil and colleagues [41] found evidence of persistent hypoperfusion in 80% of critically traumatized patients under hemodynamic reanimation, despite the normalization of their vital signs.

Hypoperfusion, frequently resulting from a low cardiac output (compared with the required for that current physiological status) [42], causes cellular damage, activation of inflammatory response, and increases multiple organ dysfunction syndrome and death risks, if not corrected in a few hours [43–48].

The aforementioned arguments constitute the rational basis for perfusion monitoring and perfusion-based resuscitation in trauma patients, and for invasive monitoring when the hypovolemia or hypoperfusion do not correct themselves despite adequate volume substitution.

Volume reposition

There has been a lot of controversy about the fluid that must be employed in the resuscitation of hemorrhagic shock patients.

When compared with crystalloids, colloid solutions expand faster in the intravascular space, and remain there longer [49,50], which in turn, produces a quicker restoration of the cardiac output and oxygen transport variables, with less infused volume and less edema formation. When endpoints such as mortality and morbidity are examined, colloids and crystalloids are equally effective. Roberts and colleagues [51] found in a meta-analysis, a pooled relative risk from 1.02 (95% confidence interval, 0.93 to 1.11), in 42 analyzed controlled clinical trials, with a total of 7576 patients included. The same results were achieved when the analysis was performed for each different colloid. In a large randomized controlled clinical trial published recently, albumin 4% or normal saline were administered during the first 4 days of the treatment of critical care patients. The study included 6997 individuals. Mortality was the same in both groups, as well as the complications possibly attributable to the fluid regimes. The differences in the amount of fluid administered were small [52].

In view of the proven absence of benefits of colloids, the absence of harm of crystalloids, and the considerable expense difference favoring crystalloids, these solutions must be considered the first choice for the resuscitation of trauma patients [53].

The required volume to resuscitate a trauma patient exceeds the basal needs for several reasons: at least two thirds of the given crystalloids are redistributed to the interstitium, making it necessary to administer three times the lost volume; the shift of fluids to the interstitium will continue from a few hours to several days, in proportion to the depth and duration of the shock [54,55]. Additionally, the patient may still have some degree of active hemorrhage. In consequence, the needed volume cannot be predicted, and must be carefully titrated to reach specific goals to avoid persistent hypovolemia or excessive fluid supply.

Endpoints for the resuscitation

Correcting overt signs of hypovolemia (hypotension, tachycardia, altered mental status, and oliguria) constitutes the first step in the resuscitation of a trauma patient. However, achieving these goals cannot be considered satisfactory, because, as already mentioned, they fail to identify hidden hypoperfusion in the state of compensated shock. In consequence, resuscitation directed to the early identification and correction of perfusion deficit has been proposed.

Early monitoring with a pulmonary artery catheter has been advocated, and resuscitation toward supraphysiologic values of cardiac index, oxygen delivery, and oxygen consumption has been proposed, and several controlled clinical trials have been performed. Their results were consolidated in three meta-analyses. The first one found methodologic limitations of the primary studies, which made it difficult to reach solid conclusions [56]. The authors found a nonstatistically significant trend toward a reduced mortality, a shorter ICU stay, and a significant mortality reduction in the experimental group, when the analysis was limited to the studies in which the hemodynamic optimization started before the surgical procedure. Ivanov and coworkers [57] found in their meta-analysis a significant reduction in morbidity when the hemodynamic resuscitation of critically ill patients was guided by the pulmonary artery catheter. Kern and Shoemaker [58] reviewed the impact of hemodynamic optimization, directed to supranormal values, in high-risk patients. They concluded that the mortality was reduced in the studies in which the treatment was instituted before organ failure was established, and when the mortality of the control group exceeded 20%.

It seems that the hemodynamic optimization only can be beneficial if started early after the trauma and is directed to the correction of the underlying perfusion deficit. So, markers of anaerobic metabolism, such as lactate or base excess, must be evaluated and followed to trace the recovery of shock at the cellular level.

Lactic acidosis has been associated with alterations in oxygen supply for the past 50 years [59,60]. Its prognostic value in hemorrhagic shock was established in terms of identifying the risk of death as well as in predicting infectious complications and multiorgan failure [61,62]. Several authors have shown that the early clearance of the lactic acidosis correlates with a better chance of survival. All patients who corrected the acidosis in the first 24 hours survived. Mortality increased as the time elapsed to normalization was longer [63,64].

Other measurements of metabolic acidosis have shown a correlation with mortality [65,66]. The most extensively studied is base deficit. It has been shown in animal and clinical studies of hemorrhagic shock that the severity of metabolic acidosis determined by this method correlates with a higher probability of death [67–69], as well as with a higher risk of multiple organ dysfunction syndrome [43,48]. The velocity of normalization of the base deficit has not been related with the prognosis. Lactate and base deficit have been compared. They showed a good correlation in the first evaluation [65], but lactate showed a better performance after the resuscitation with IV fluids, and in the identification of compensated shock [64].

Regional analysis of perfusion could give the most sensitive approximation [70]. Preliminary reports regarding regional CO_2 measurement in sensible microvascular beds, as manifestation of hypoperfusion, are promising

[71–73]. Measurement of oxygen tension or saturation in certain tissues has permitted the identification of occult hypoperfusion in animal studies and in some limited clinical experiences published [71,74–78]. Unfortunately, these methods have not been fully evaluated, and none of them has reached widespread use.

Transfusion threshold and coagulopathy correction

The transfusion of red blood cells is a common practice in trauma patients. It was found in a multicenter trial that 55% of the trauma patients who were admitted to the ICU received transfusions during their stay [79].

The decision of transfusing red blood cells (RBCs) is, in part, motivated by the aim of improving the oxygen-carrying capacity of the blood and reducing the oxygen debt: "the higher hemoglobin level is the best." This concept has been challenged by the understanding of the tolerance of low levels of hemoglobin by the critically ill patient, and by the knowledge of the detrimental effects of transfusion in terms of immunosuppresion [80,81], increased risk of infection [82], increased risk of blood-borne infection acquisition [79], increased risk of multiorgan failure [43,48], and death [83], when compared with matched critically ill patients.

The threshold for RBC transfusion was examined in a randomized clinical trial, in which 838 euvolemic critically ill patients with hemoglobin levels below 9.0 g/dL within 72 hours after admission were assigned to receive RBC transfusions to maintain the Hb concentration between 10.0 and 12.0 g/dL (Liberal group), or to receive RBC transfusions only when Hb concentration fell below 7.0 to maintain the Hb concentration between 7.0 and 9.0 g/dL (Restrictive group). Overall 30-day mortality, length of stay, and morbidity were not different for either group [84]. Hill and co-workers [85], who undertook a meta-analysis comparing liberal and restrictive transfusion strategies, confirmed the conclusions reached by these researchers. They found an additionally 40% reduction in exposure to transfusions in the patients allocated in the restrictive groups.

The current recommendation for critical care patients younger than 55 years and without significant heart disease is to administer transfusions to maintain hemoglobin concentrations between 7.0 and 9.0 g/dL.

Coagulopathy is a common event in trauma patients. Its origin is multicausal, and the main etiologic factors are hypothermia, fibrinolysis activated by tissular trauma and by endothelial damage, and dilution of coagulation factors and platelets [86–91]. Occasionally, a traumatized patient has a preexisting condition such as liver or hematologic diseases or anticoagulant treatment that can predispose to bleeding [92], and must be identified in the anamnesis.

The entity is recognized by bleeding from different places such as intravenous sites, the nasogastric tube, the vesical catheter or the surgical drains, and nonmechanical bleeding in the surgical field. This complication as so many other things is better to prevent than to have to treat later. Prevention is accomplished by hypothermia prevention and treatment [93–97] (Box 1) and shock limitation, which in turn, is guaranteed by rapid interruption of the hemorrhage and aggressive hemodynamic resuscitation. Prophylactic administration of platelets or plasma usually do not prevent coagulopathy [98,99].

The characterization of coagulopathy is made in most of the cases by simple laboratory tests: platelet count, activated partial thromboplastin time, prothrombin time-international normalized ratio, and fibrinogen concentration, which guide the administration of fresh frozen plasma, platelets, and cryoprecipitate [87–91]. Damage control surgery is a powerful ancillary tool in the coagulopathic patient who is being operated on. It permits the expeditious control of the nonmechanical bleeding, limits the extension of the surgery, and stops the vicious circle of bleeding–hypothermia–coagulopathy.

The hypotense or hypoperfused trauma patient in the ICU

Frequently, a critically traumatized patient shows hypotension or persistence of the indicators of hypoperfusion. It often results from a mismatch between the fluids required and the fluids administered. This situation must be distinguished from occult bleeding and from intrathoracic hypertension that may result from a tension pneumothorax [29,30], a massive diaphragmatic hernia [31–34], or intra-abdominal hypertension [36,37]. On rare occasions cardiac tamponade will result from a missed cardiac wound or from liquid accumulation in the pericardial sac after a wound or an incision (Table 2) [100–102].

Persistent hemorrhage must be identified and treated immediately. It is easily recognized when there is external bleeding coming from the drains

---

Box 1. Hypothermia prevention and treatment

- Rationalize ICU temperature
- Keep the patient's skin dry
- Avoid unnecessary body exposition
- Limit cavities exposition
- Administer warmed fluids and blood
- Administer humidified gases
- Correct shock as early as possible
- Actively warm the patient.
  - Surface warming (forced warmed air and resistive warmers, better than circulating water mattresses)
  - Continuous arteriovenous rewarming (very effective)
  - Cardiopulmonary bypass (the most effective)
  - Cavities rewarming (not recommended)

Table 2
Differential diagnosis of the hypotense or hypoperfused trauma patient

Condition	Filling pressures	Airway pressures	Observations
Ongoing hemorrhage	Low	Low or normal	Hb drops Source of bleeding is found if looked for
Fluids shifts, or vasodilation	Low	Low or normal	Hb does not drop Source of bleeding is not found
Myocardial depression or contusion	High	Low or normal	Echocardiogram shows contractility alterations
Cardiac tamponade	High	Low or normal	Subxyphoid echo or subxyphoid pericardial window identify pericardial effusion
Tension pneumothorax or massive diaphragmatic hernia	High	High	Clinical diagnosis Radiologic confirmation if clinical signs are nor clear
Intraabdominal Hypertension	High	High	Oliguria Elevated intravesical pressure

or the surgical wound (Fig. 5). It is more difficult to recognize when the patient has not been operated on, or when the drains or the chest tube become occluded by clots. In these cases the reexamination of the patient, aided by a chest radiograph, an ultrasound directed to detect liquid in the cavities [103–105], and a high suspicion index will help to diagnose the complication. The treatment should not be delayed, and will consist of surgical exploration with the strong consideration of performing damage control procedures. Angiographic embolization may be employed in selected cases; which depends on the experience of the team in these cases and the resources available (Fig. 6) [106–112].

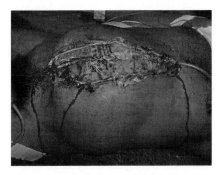

Fig. 5. Patient with massive bleeding due to a gunshot wound to the liver. It was controlled by a catheter with a balloon. The photography shows blood coming from the wound. The patient was reexplored and a wound of a diaphragmatic vein was found and treated.

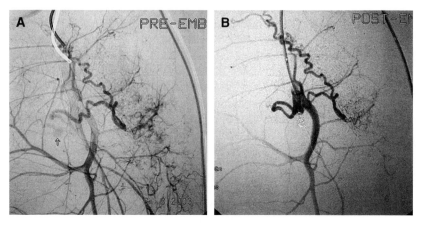

Fig. 6. Bleeding control in a patient with pelvic fracture. (Courtesy of Diego Rivera, MD, Hospital Universitario del Valle, Calle, Columbia.) (*A*) The arteriography identifies a torn artery bleeding. (*B*) The arteriography after coils embolization shows that the bleeding has stopped.

Conditions that course with elevation of the intrathoracic pressure decrease the venous return and the cardiac output, with potential disastrous consequences that will not subside unless the cause be removed. The hemodynamic profile includes low cardiac output, high filling pressures, and high peripheral vascular resistances. The elevated intrathoracic pressure hinders lung expansion and oxygenation. The mechanically ventilated patient shows elevated airway pressures, hypoxemia, and sometimes hypercarbia [31,36,37]. The physical examination can identify asymmetry in tension pneumothorax and diaphragmatic hernia. As the presence of a chest tube does not preclude the development of a pneumothorax (Fig. 7), the presence of a silo in the abdominal wall does not prevent abdominal hypertension (Fig. 8). The diagnosis is based on clinical grounds in some instances, but in the cases of diaphragmatic hernia and abdominal hypertension a chest radiograph and the urinary bladder pressure must be obtained. The correct treatment must be performed immediately, and sometimes, due to the enormous instability, the surgical procedure must be performed in the ICU [113,114].

Cardiac tamponade must be suspected in the presence of elevated filling pressures. Neck vein distension diminished heart sounds and paradoxal pulse are absent in most cases. Subxyphoid echo will confirm the diagnosis [115], and subxyphoid pericardial window will be diagnostic in traumatic hemopericardium and therapeutic in inflammatory pericardial effusion (Fig. 9) [100,101,116,117].

Independently of the cause of the hypotension or the hypoperfusion signs, the monitoring must be increased and include at least a radial artery catheter and a central venous catheter. The infused volume must be titrated to reach specific goals: the mean arterial blood pressure must be of 65 mmHg or more during the first 30 minutes, and the lactate and base deficit

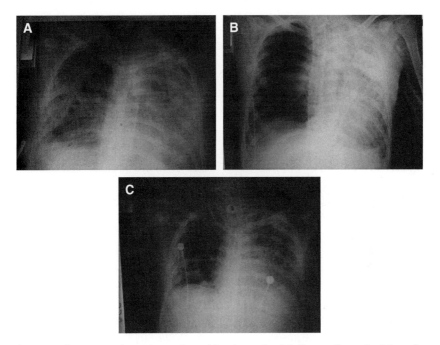

Fig. 7. Tension pneumothorax in a patient with a chest tube. (*A*) Chest radiographs 5 days after a right thoracotomy and tractotomy of the three lobes. (*B*) Chest radiographs 3 days later. A massive right pneumothorax with left deviation of the mediastinal structures, compression of the left lung, and a chest tube are seen. The patient looked restless and dyspneic. He had tachycardia and resonance of the right thorax, with diminished breath sounds. (*C*) Chest radiography after the insertion of a second chest tube.

must show a clear trend to normalize in the first 6 hours, with complete normalization at the end of the first day (Table 3).

To avoid infusing excessive amounts of IV solutions and its complications, the condition of responsiveness to volume must be identified [50,118–120]. The filling heart pressures have been used traditionally to accomplish this task, being that the pulmonary artery wedge pressure is considered as the standard. Other methods such as the right ventricular end-diastolic volume, measured with a specially designed pulmonary artery catheter or the aortic blood velocity, and left ventricle end-diastolic area determined by echocardiography have been tested [121]. The accuracy of all these static variables to determine the status of responsiveness is low, motivating the search of dynamic, more reliable measurements, of which the variations of the arterial pressure with the respiratory cycle have proven to be accurate and easy to obtain [122,123]. Other objectives to be accomplished in the initial hours is a hemoglobin concentration >7.0 g/dL and a pulse oximetry (SatP) >94%.

A pulmonary artery catheter must be considered in the first few hours if there is not a clear response. This is to facilitate the decisions about the

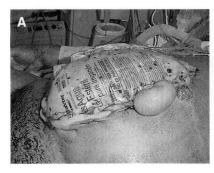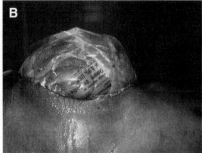

Fig. 8. A second episode of intraabdominal hypertension in a patient with intraabdominal hypertension after massive fluid resuscitation for an extraabdominal trauma. (*A*) Eighteen hours after a laparotomy and collocation of a Bogota Bag. The patient developed a scenario of difficult ventilatory support, with progressive elevation of the airway pressures, requirement of high oxygen concentrations, and high PEEP levels; hypotension despite IV fluids and high dose of norepinefrine. The urinary bladder pressure risen to 28 cm H_2O. (*B*) After the decompression the respiratory and hemodynamic changes reverted to normal. The patient requires a bigger silo than before.

amount of fluids to be given and the necessity of administering inotropes if the cardiac output is judged not to be enough despite an adequate status of intravascular volume or vasopressors if the cardiac output is good but hypotension persists, due to a very low peripheral vascular resistance.

Initial neurologic evaluation of the trauma patient

Errors in diagnosis, monitoring, and treatment of brain trauma patients are among the most frequently reported in the intensive care phase treatment of the trauma patient. Of the errors reported by Duke and colleagues

Table 3
Endpoints of the resuscitation

Parameter	Goal	Observations
MAP	>65 mm Hg in the first 30 minutes	TBI patients need MAP >70 mm Hg
Lactic Acidosis	<2.1 mmol/L	Trend to reduction in the first 6 hours Complete clearance in 24 hours
Base deficit	>−5.0 mEq/L	Trend to reduction in the first 6 hours Complete clearance in 24 hours
Hemoglobin	7.0–9.0 g/dL	Patients with significant heart disease or older than 55 years may need higher levels
SatP	>94%	With the lowest PEEP that permits keeping F_{IO_2} <0.6

Abbreviations: MAP, mean arterial pressure; PEEP, positive end expiratory pressure; TBI, traumatic brain injury.

[9], 54% contributed to death. In the publication by Davis and coworkers [10], 60% of the monitoring errors were classified as neurologic, while 12% of the management errors corresponded to this category. One fourth of the neurologic errors of this study contributed to death.

Usually the condition of severe brain trauma (Glasgow coma scale of 8 or less) has been diagnosed in the prehospital phase or in the emergency room. In these cases the tracheal intubation has been achieved previously and the patient is transferred to the ICU directly from the computed axial tomography (CT) suite if surgery is not indicated, or from the surgical theater when a surgical operation was required. Occasionally, the cause of the emergency intervention has been extracranial, and in such cases it is possible that the CT had not yet been done. Usually the possibility of an intracranial lesion has been ruled out with measurement of the intracranial pressure (ICP), completed by an air ventriculography [124]. If an intracranial lesion has not been ruled out, the arrangements to perform the CT must be made.

The optimal resuscitation constitutes the first step in the optimal treatment of the brain trauma patient, in virtue of the acknowledged deleterious role of secondary insults such as hypotension and hypoxia [125,126]. Maintaining SatP at a level >94%, the systolic blood pressure above 90 mm Hg, the mean arterial blood pressure above 70 mm Hg, and the $PaCO_2$ around 35 mm Hg seem reasonable goals [124].

The oxygenation goal must be rapidly obtained by manipulating FiO_2, while PEEP is titrated. Concerns about the worsening of ICP with PEEP have not been confirmed [127,128]. In any case, it must be titrated at the lowest possible level. Sedation must be used to permit ventilatory support, and contribute to lower ICP. Care must be taken to avoid hemodynamic instability due to an excessive dose of sedatives. Neuromuscular blockade should be used only if indispensable, as continuous protracted relaxation, used to facilitate the ICP management, does not improve the results, prolongs ICU stay, and increases complication risks [129].

Isotonic crystalloids (preferable normal saline), should be used to reach the blood pressure goal. Vasopressors should be used briefly to sustain blood pressure, while the volume resuscitation is performed. If continuous administration is necessary due to hypotension despite the absence of hypovolemia, then phenyleprine or noradrenaline are preferred [130,131].

The patient must be maintained normothermic, as deliberate hypothermia has failed in improve the prognosis of patients with traumatic brain injury [132,133]. The head must be elevated, after the normovolemia has been restituted, because under these circumstances it improves ICP and cerebral perfusion pressure (CPP). The torso must not be flexed until the spine has been cleared, so the head will be elevated by reversed Trendelenberg position [130].

The ICP measurement must be started as early as can be permitted by the patient's stabilization process. The ICP is managed with the goal of maintaining CPP above 50–60 mm Hg. The ICP threshold above which interventions are warranted is 20 mm Hg [124], and they are applied in a sequential fashion, with the addition of a new treatment when the present one is inadequate (Box 2).

When intracranial hypertension is diagnosed, ventricular drainage is the first intervention to be employed if available [124]. When other ICP measurement methods are employed, an intraventricular catheter must be inserted. Its safety and effectiveness have been proven: the risk of hemorrhage associated with its insertion is low, and the risk of infection less than 2% [134]. The drainage must be intermittent, with a maximum of five times per hour, with a duration of 2 minutes each. Continuous drainage makes the ICP measurement inaccurate. The ICP is continuously measured.

If intracranial hypertension persists despite the maximum of five drainages per hour, hyperventilation is indicated. The ventilator is set to drive the $PaCO_2$ to 30 mmHg. Monitoring the CO_2 expired makes this task easy, provided that the monitor is calibrated against the $PaCO_2$.

Box 2. Management of the traumatic brain injury patient

Basic management
SatP >94%
$Paco_2$ around 35 mm Hg
MAP >70 mm Hg
Normothermia
Head elevated to 30° (if normovolemic)

ICP management goals
ICP <20 mm Hg
CPP >50 mm Hg

First line measures to control ICP
Intermittent ventricular drainage[a]
Hyperventilation to $Paco_2$ 30–35 mm Hg
Mannitol bolus (0.25 g/Kg)[a]

Second tier therapies for intracranial hypertension
Barbiturates
Hypothermia
Optimized hyperventilation ($Paco_2$ to 25–30 mm Hg)
Decompresive craniotomy

CPP, cerebral pressure of perfusion; ICP, intracranial pressure; MAP, mean artery pressure; SatP. pulse-oximetry.

---

[a] Consider hypertonic saline

If hyperventilation does not control the ICP, mannitol must be administered in a bolus at a dose of 0.25 g/kg. Administering it in infusion or at higher doses do not improve the result [135]. Osmolarity and intravascular volume status must be monitored, because hyperosmolarity or hypovolemia may occur and negatively affect the prognosis.

Along the process, care must be taken to maintain adequate oxygenation and blood pressure. The persistence on intracranial hypertension despite the above-mentioned therapies must reach the suspicion of an intracranial mass. In this situation, a new CT must be obtained [130]. Additionally, a second tier therapy must be considered [124].

The first of the second tier therapies is optimized hyperventilation. There is a small group of patients who could benefit from lower the $PaCO_2$ below 30 mm Hg. It is undertaken if a method such as jugular venous saturation, which permits monitoring global brain ischemia, is being used [136]. The parameters of the ventilator are modified to increase slowly minute volume, until ICP controls or jugular venous saturation reaches its lower threshold (60–70%).

Barbirurates have long been used in the treatment of intracranial hypertension. Although their effect may be deleterious in the initial management compared with mannitol, barbiturates improve survival probability when used in patients with intracranial hypertension, refractory to other therapies [137]. The most commonly employed is pentobarbital sodium, at an IV load doses of 10 mg/kg over 30 minutes, followed by an infusion of 5 mg/kg/h, for 3 hours and then maintained at 1 to 3 mg/kg/h. The infusion is administered until ICP control for 24 hours; then is reduced by 50% per day. The aim is to induce profound coma, with burst suppression on electroencephalogram. Barbiturates can produce severe hypotension. Patients must be monitored carefully, to avoid potential disastrous consequences.

In recent years, decompressive craniectomy has emerged as a potential second tier therapy. It allows the brain to swell, without further ICP increasing. It has been used lately in intracranial hypertension refractory to other treatments [138]. The technique carries with it a high mortality that, in part, can be attributed to several secondary injuries previously suffered by the patients. It is strongly recommended in patients with complications from the other therapies. The results could be better if applied earlier in the course of intracranial hypertension [139].

Hypertonic saline has been used in the treatment of intracranial hypertension instead of mannitol [140–142]. In spite of the impressive support given by animal studies, the clinical evidence fails to show the expected benefits [143].

Prophylactic anticonvulsivants do not provide any protection against posttraumatic epilepsy, and should not be given prophylactically [124]. They are indicated when the patient has had seizures or when its detection will be impossible, such as when neuromuscular blockade is used.

Corticosteroids have been used for many years in the treatment of the traumatic brain injury. Literature evidence does not support its use.

A mega randomized controlled clinical trial showed that corticosteroids group had a higher mortality than the control group. In consequence, this group of drugs must not be used in patients with traumatic brain injury [144,145].

Missed injuries and tertiary survey

Delayed diagnosis of lesions has been reported to occur between 0.5% to 38%, in different trauma populations [146–152]. When the analysis concentrates on high energy trauma, the incidence exceeds 10%.The most common undiagnosed injuries in the primary and secondary surveys are fractures located on long bones, ribs, and clavicles [150,153]. Less frequent but not less important are fractures of the spine, face, and pelvis [154]; with a much lower reported frequency are intrathoracic and intraabdominal lesions. Visceral and vascular missed wounds are more frequent in series with penetrating trauma mechanisms [146,148,155].

The impact of delayed diagnosis has been determined: they cause a change in the treatment in one third to two thirds of the affected patients, with requirement of a surgical intervention in 20% of the cases [150,156–158]. Sharma and coworkers [159] found missed injuries in 58% of the analyzed autopsies, with negative impact on survival in 3% of them. Hollow viscus perforation is infrequent in blunt trauma [160], but delays in diagnosis and treatment result in a significant increase in morbidity and mortality [161]. Hemorrhage has been reported between 18% and 25% of all preventable deaths, some of them corresponding to an intracavital bleeding not timely recognized [8,155,162].

The reasons associated with delayed diagnosis have been investigated, and include trauma severity, conditions that alter the process of attention, conditions that complicate the clinical evaluation, and errors in the process (Box 3) [147,152,154,163,164].

To limit the number and the impact of the lesions diagnosed lately, a "tertiary survey" has been proposed [147,151,165]. It consists of a systematic review of the patient at the completion of the first day. The patient must be reexamined, and all the diagnostic investigations must be reevaluated. All the detected lesions must be cataloged. The participation of the trauma surgeons and the radiology team increases the probability of detecting undiagnosed lesions, and may reduce preventable deaths [166]. Missed lesions were reduced between 39% and 57% in prospective trials in which a tertiary survey was performed [147,150,167].

Of paramount importance is the diagnosis of occult bleeding and hollow viscera perforation. The first situation was discussed earlier. The second one requires experience to detect that the evolution moves away from the expected pattern: the fluids requirements are higher than the usual, there is no tolerance to the enteral feeding, there is no tolerance of the weaning from the ventilator, and there are new and unexpected organ dysfunctions.

Box 3. Causes of missed injuries

Trauma severity
Multiple systems
Severe brain injury

Conditions that complicate the complete clinical evaluation
Altered consciousness
- Brain trauma
- Early sedation-intubation
- Intoxication
Early surgical intervention

Altered process of attention
Referral
Workload excess

Error
Inadequate physical examination
Inaccurate interpretation of diagnostic investigations
Inadequate surgical sequence

In such cases a perforation of a hollow viscera must be considered. Endoscopy and esophagogram will permit the diagnosis of an esophageal wound (Fig. 10), and in some cases abdominal CT will help to diagnose an abdominal hollow viscus perforation. In these cases, diagnostic peritoneal lavage, a laparoscopy, or an exploratory laparotomy will identify an intestinal perforation missed by image methods. Surgical treatment must be performed without hesitation.

Other considerations during the first day

Critically traumatized patients pose significant infection risk. Antibiotic administration is indicated in abdominal penetrating trauma, and in open fractures. The indication is less clear previous to the insertion of a chest tube [168–173]. In any case, protracted administration is not indicated, provided that it does not confer additional protection and increases antibiotic-related complications, and in some instances the risk of nosocomial infections [174–176]. Randomized clinical trials and comparative nonrandomized studies have proven it [177–181]. Comprehensive guides have been developed, regarding short antibiotic courses [173,182]. Operative site infection is best prevented by early surgical treatment, when indicated: early control of bleeding, early measures to control spillage from bowel perforations, gentle manipulation of the tissues, avoidance of unnecessary maneuvers, and complete debridement of dead or severely contaminated tissues. Irrigating the cavities with warm normal saline, to remove all the contaminants and blood

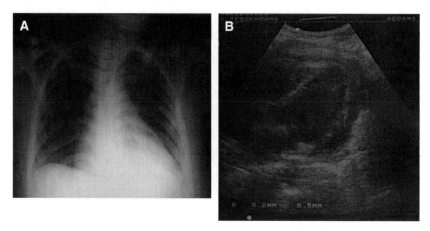

Fig. 9. Cardiac tamponade of late presentation. The patient had received a precordial stab-wound. A left chest tube was inserted because of hemothorax. A subxyphoid window did not show pericardial effusion. (*A*) The patient developed dyspnea 5 days later. The chest radiograph shown enlargement of the cardiac silhouette. (*B*) A new subxyphoid echo showed a pericardial effusion. The patient was treated with a subxyphoid pericardial window; 400 cc of sterile liquid were obtained.

remnants is a final complementary step. Nosocomial infections are prevented by avoiding unnecessary use of invasive dispositives. Adequate insertion technique, appropriated care, and removal of them as early as possible are recommended when they are indispensable [183–186].

An enteral access for nutrition must be gained from the first day, as early enteral feeding reduces infection risk [187–191].

Severely traumatized patients have increased risk of thromboembolic complications [192,193]. Prophylactic measures must be instituted from the first day. Pharmacologic prophylaxis with a low molecular weight heparin is the choice for the nonbleeding patient. When bleeding risk is considered to be increased, intermittent pneumatic compression is indicated [194–198].

Summary

Increasingly in an ever more violent society, trauma surgeons are going to be placed in stressful situations, calling for crucial split-second decisions. Then only their skill and that of their support staff can significantly reduce ICU mortality.

ICU trauma patients must be resuscitated toward specific goals. Ventilation must be directed to keep blood oxygenation at safe levels, hemodynamic support to the early correction of perfusion deficit, and neurologic support to avoid secondary insults and to maintain a cerebral perfusion pressure. All these with less intense support must be possible, to avoid complications attributable to treatment.

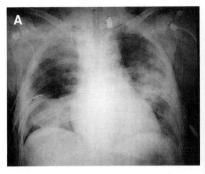
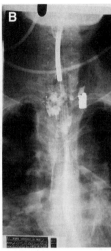

Fig. 10. Missed esophageal perforation. (*A*) The patient received a gunshot wound in the right periclavicular region. He was intubated and mechanically ventilated after massive subcutaneous emphysema and right pneumothorax. Bronchoscope, esophagoscope, and arteriography were performed. All negative. Three days later he continued on mechanical ventilation with right inferior lobe atelectasis and progressive lung infiltrates. (*B*) A missed esophageal perforation was suspected and a contrast esophagogram performed, which identifies the lesion.

Respiratory, hemodynamic or neurologic complications may arise, with catastrophic consequences if not treated in a timely and appropriate manner. A systematic and ordered approach by priorities will permit identifying the cause of the crisis. The solution will consist of adjustments in the treatment in some cases, but frequently a surgical intervention will be crucial in cases such as tension pneumothorax, massive diaphragmatic hernia, intraabdominal hypertension, and occult bleeding. Identifying its indication is a key determining factor and prompt and precise execution definitive.

References

[1] Krug EG, Dahlberg LL, Mercy JA, et al. World report on violence and health. Geneva: World Health Organization; 2002.

[2] Peden M, Scurfield R, Sleet D, et al. World report on road traffic injury prevention. Geneva: World Health Organization; 2004.

[3] Wayatt J, Beard D, Gray A, et al. The time of death after trauma. BMJ 1995;310:1502.

[4] Jatt A, Khan MR, Zafar H, et al. Peer review audit of trauma deaths in a developing country. Asian J Surg 2004;27:54–8.

[5] Stewart RM, Myers JG, Dent DL, et al. Seven hundred fifty-three consecutive deaths in a level I trauma center: the argument for injury prevent. J Trauma 2003;54:66–71.

[6] Durham R, Shapiro D, Flint L. In-house trauma attendings: is there a difference? Am J Surg 2005;190:960–6.

[7] Esposito TJ, Sandddal TL, Reynolds SA, et al. Effect of a voluntary trauma system on preventable death and inappropriate care in a rural state. J Trauma 2003;54:633–70.

[8] Maio MR, Burney RE, Gregor MA, et al. A study of preventable trauma mortality in rural Michigan. J Trauma 1996;41:83–90.

[9] Duke GJ, Morley PT, Cooper DJ, et al. Management of severe trauma in intensive care units and surgical wards. Med J Aust 1999;170:416–9.

[10] Davies JW, Hoyt DB, McArdle MS, et al. The significance of critical care errors in causing preventable death in trauma patients in a trauma system. J Trauma 1991;31:813–8.

[11] Quiroz F, Garcia A, Perez M. Análisis de mortalidad prevenible en 150 casos de trauma carotídeo. Panam J Trauma 1995;5:116.

[12] Nunn JF. Applied respiratory physiology. 4th edition. Cambridge, Butterworth-Heinemann; 1993.

[13] Chang DW. AARC clinical practice guideline in-hospital transport of the mechanically ventilated patient—2002 revision & update. Respir Care 2002;47:721–3.

[14] Mort T. Emergency tracheal intubation: complications associated with repeated laryngo-scopic attempts. Anest Analg 2004;99:607–13.

[15] Wong DT, Lai K, Chung FF, et al. Cannot Intubate–cannot ventilate and difficult intuba-tion strategies: results of a Canadian National Survey. Anesth Analg 2005;100:1439–46.

[16] Mort T. The incidence and risk factors for cardiac arrest during emergency tracheal intu-bation: a justification for incorporating the ASA guidelines in the remote location. J Clin Anesth 2004;16:508–16.

[17] Krinsley SJ, Barone JE. The drive to survive. Unplanned extubation in the ICU. Chest 2005;128:560–6.

[18] Epstein SK, Nevins ML, Chung J. Effect of unplanned extubation on outcome of mechan-ical ventilation. Am J Respir Crit Care Med 2001;163:1755–6.

[19] DeLassence A, Alberti C, Assoulay E, et al. Impact of unplanned extubation and reintuba-tion after weaning on nosocomial pneumonia risk in the intensive care unit. A prospective multicenter study. Anesthesiology 2002;97:148–56.

[20] Kapadia FN, Bajan K, Raje KV. Airway accidents in intubated intensive care unit patients: an epidemiological study. Crit Care Med 2000;28:659–64.

[21] Carrion MI, Ayuso D, Marcos M, et al. Accidental removal of endotracheal and nasogas-tric tubes and intravascular catheters. Crit Care Med 2000;28:63–6.

[22] Needham DM, Thompson DA, Holzmueller CG, et al. A system factors analysis of airway events from the Intensive Care Unit Safety Reporting System (ICUSRS). Crit Care Med 204;32:2227–33.

[23] Mort T. Unplanned tracheal extubation outside the operating room: a quality improve-ment audit of hemodynamic and tracheal airway complications associated with emergency tracheal reintubation. Anesth Analg 1998;86:1171–6.

[24] Pesiri AJ. Two-year study of the prevention of unintentional extubation. Crit Care Nurs Q 1994;17:35–9.

[25] Arney KL, Judson MA, Sahn SA. Airway obstruction arising from blood clot three reports and a review of the literature. Chest 1999;115:293–300.

[26] Collins KA, Presnell SE. Asphyxia by tracheobroncial trombus. Am J Forensic Med Pathol 2005;26:327–9.

[27] Shalmovitz GZ, Halpern P. Delated obstruction of endotracheal tubes by aspirated foreign bodies: report of two cases. Ann Emerg Med 2004;43:630–3.

[28] Sprung J, Bourke DL, Harrison G, et al. Endotracheal tube and tracheobronchial obstruc-tion as causes of hypoventilation with high inspiratory pressures. Chest 1994;105:550–2.

[29] DeLassence A, Timsit JF, Taflet M, et al. Pneumothorax in the intensive care unit inci-dence, risk factors, and outcome. Anesthesiology 2006;104:5–13.

[30] Chen KY, Jern JS, Liao WY, et al. Pneumothorax in the ICU. Patient outcomes and prog-nostic factors. Chest 2002;122:678–83.

[31] Burshell SA, Takiguchi SA, Myers SA, et al. Unilateral lung hyperinflation and auto-positive end-expiratory pressure due to a ruptured right hemidiaphragm. Crit Care Med 1996;24:1418–21.

[32] Guth AA, Pachler HL, Kim V. Pitfalls in the diagnosis of blunt diaphragmatic injury. Am J Surg 1995;170:5–9.

[33] Voeller GL, Reisser JR, Fabian TC, et al. Blunt diaphragmatic injuries: a five- year experience. Am Surg 1990;56:28–31.

[34] Lee WC, Chen RJ, Fang JF, et al. Rupture of the diaphragm after blunt trauma. Eur J Surg 1990;160:479–83.

[35] Balogh Z, McKinley B, Cocanour CS, et al. Secondary abdominal compartment syndrome is an elusive early complication of traumatic shock resuscitation. Am J Surg 2002;184: 538–44.

[36] Balogh Z, McKinley B, Holcomb JB, et al. Both primary and secondary abdominal compartment syndrome can be predicted early and are harbingers of multiple organ failure. J Trauma 2003;54:848–61.

[37] Ertel W, Oberholzer A, Platz A, et al. Incidence and clinical pattern of the abdominal compartment syndrome after "damage-control" laparotomy in 311 patients with severe abdominal and/or pelvic trauma. Crit Care Med 2000;28:1747–53.

[38] McGee S, Abernethy WB 3rd, Simel DL. The rational clinical examination. Is this patient hypovolemic? JAMA 1999;281:1022–9.

[39] Celoria G, Steingrub JS, Vickers-Lati M, et al. Clinical assessment of hemodynamic values in two surgical intensive care units. Effects on therapy. Arch Surg 1990;125:1036–9.

[40] Shoemaker WC, Appel PL, Kran H. Physiologic patterns in surviving and nonsurviving shock patients. Arch Surg 1973;106:630–6.

[41] Abou-Khalil B, Scalea TM, Trooskin SZ. Hemodynamic responses to shock in young trauma patients: need for invasive monitoring. Crit Care Med 1994;22:633–9.

[42] Dutton RP. Shock and trauma anesthesia. Anest Clin North Am 1999;17:83–95.

[43] Sauaia A, Moore FA, Moore EE, et al. Early predictors of postinjury multiple organ failure. Arch Surg 1994;129:1036–9.

[44] Moore FA, Haenel JB, Moore EE, et al. Incommensurate oxygen consumption in response to maximal oxygen availability predicts postinjury multiple organ failure. J Trauma 1992; 33:58–65.

[45] Shoemaker WC, Appel PL, Kran H. Hemodynamic and oxygen transport responses insurvivors and nonsurvivors of high risk surgery. Crit Care Med 1993;21:977–90.

[46] Kirton O, Windsor J, Wedderburn R, et al. Failure of splanchnic resuscitation in the acutely injured trauma patient correlates with multiple organ system failure and length of stay in the ICU. Chest 1998;113:1064–9.

[47] Garcia A. Resuscitación en trauma y cirugía mayor. Rev Col Cirug 2001;16:26–38.

[48] Losada HF, Garcia A. Riesgo de disfunción orgánica múltiple, después de toracotomía por trauma. Rev Med Sur (Chile) 2001;23:46–53.

[49] Griffel MI, Kauffman B. Pharmacology of colloids and crystalloids. Crit Care Clin 1992;8: 235–53.

[50] Grocott MPW, Mythen MC, Gan TJ. perioperative fluid management and clinical outcomes in adults. Anesth Analg 2005;100:1093–106.

[51] Roberts I, Alderson P, Bunn F, et al. Colloids versus crystalloids for fluid resuscitation in critically ill patients. Colloids versus crystalloids for fluid resuscitation in critically ill patients. Cochrane Database Syst Rev 2004;(1):CD000567.

[52] Investigators TSAFES. A comparison of albumin and saline for fluid resuscitation in the intensive care unit. N Engl J Med 2004;350:2247–56.

[53] Mora RRA, Alí A, Borráez O, et al. Reunión de consenso: terapia de fluídos en pacientes críticamente enfermos. Acta Col Cuidado Intensivo 2005;8:52.

[54] Shires GT, Cohn D, Carrico CT. Fluid therapy in hemorrhagic shock. Arch Surg 1964;88: 688–92.

[55] Riddez L, Hahn RG, Brismar B, et al. Central and regional hemodynamics during acute hypovolemia and volume substitution in volunteers. Crit Care Med 1997;25: 635–40.

[56] Heyland DK, Cook DJ, King D, et al. Maximizing oxygen delivery in critically ill patients: a methodologic appraisal of the evidence. Crit Care Med 1996;24:617–24.

[57] Ivanov R, Allen J, Calvin JE. The incidence of major morbidity in critically ill patients managed with pulmonary artery catheters: a meta-analysis. Crit Care Med 2000;28:615–9.

[58] Kern JW, Shoemaker WC. Meta-analysis of hemodynamic optimization in high-risk patients. Crit Care Med 2002;30:1686–92.

[59] Huckabee WE. Relationships of pyruvate and lactate during anaerobic metabolism: I. Effect of infusion of pyruvate or glucose and of hyperventilation. J Clin Invest 1958;37:244–54.

[60] Huckabee WE. Relationships of pyruvate and lactate during anaerobic metabolism: II. Exercise and formation of O-debt. J Clin Invest 1958;37:255–63.

[61] Broder G, Weil MH. Excess lactate—an index of reversibility of shock in human patients. Science 1964;143:1457–9.

[62] Crowl AC, Young JS, Kahler DM, et al. Occult hypoperfusion is associated with increased morbidity in patients undergoing early femur fracture fixation. J Trauma 2000;48:260–7.

[63] Abramson D, Scalea TM, Hitchcock R, et al. Lactate clearance and survival following injury. J Trauma 1993;35:548–9.

[64] Husain FA, Martin MJ, Mullenix PS, et al. Serum lactate and base deficit as predictors of mortality and morbidity. Am J Surg 2003;185:485–91.

[65] Kaplan LJ, Kellum JA. Initial pH, base deficit, lactate, anion gap, strong ion difference, and strong ion gap predict outcome from major vascular injury. Crit Care Med 2004;32:1120–4.

[66] FitzSullivan E, Salim A, Demetriades D, et al. Serum bicarbonate may replace the arterial base deficit in the trauma intensive care unit. Am J Surg 2005;190:941–6.

[67] Dunham CM, Siegel JH, Weireter L, et al. Oxygen debt and metabolic acidemia as quantitative predictors of mortality and the severity of the ischemic insult in hemorrhagic shock. Crit Care Med 1991;19:231–43.

[68] Davis JW, Shackford SR, Holbrook TL, et al. Base deficit as a sensitive indicator of compensated shock and tissue oxygen utilization. Surg Gynecol Obstet 1991;173:473–6.

[69] Rutherford EJ, Morris JA, Reed GW, et al. Base deficit stratifies mortality and determines therapy. J Trauma 1992;33:417–23.

[70] Porter J, Ivatury RR. In search of the optimal end points of resuscitation in trauma patients: a review. J Trauma 1998;88:908–14.

[71] Tatevossian RG, Wo CC, Velmahos GC, et al. Transcutaneous oxygen and CO_2 as early warning of tissue hypoxia and hemodynamic shock in critically ill emergency patients. Crit Care Med 2000;28:2248–53.

[72] Hameed SM, Cohn SM. Gastric tonometry. The role of mucosal pH measurement in the management of trauma. Chest 2003;123:475s–81s.

[73] Marik PE, Bankov A. Sublingual capnometry versus traditional markers of tissue oxygenation in critically ill patients. Crit Care Med 2003;31:818–22.

[74] Knudson MM, Bermudez KM, Doyle CA, et al. Use of tissue oxygen tension measurements during resuscitation from hemorrhagic shock. J Trauma 1997;42:608–14.

[75] McKinley BA, Butler BD. Comparison of skeletal muscle PO2, PCO2, and pH with gastric tonometric P(CO2) and pH in hemorrhagic shock. Crit Care Med 1999;27:1869–77.

[76] Venkatesh B, Meacher R, Muller MJ, et al. Monitoring tissue oxygenation during resuscitation of major burns. J Trauma 2001;50:485–94.

[77] Benaron DA, Parachikov IH, Friedland S, et al. Continuous, noninvasive, and localized microvascular tissue oximetry using visible light spectroscopy. Anesthesiology 2004;100:1469–75.

[78] Crookers BA, Cohn SM, Bloch S, et al. Can near-infrared spectroscopy identify the severity of shock in trauma patients? J Trauma 2005;58:806–16.

[79] Shapiro MJ, Gettinger A, Corwin HL, et al. Anemia and blood transfusion in trauma patients admitted to the intensive care unit. J Trauma 2003;55:269–74.

[80] van de Watering LM, Hermans J, Houbiers JGA, et al. Beneficial effects of leukocyte depletion of transfused blood on postoperative complications in patients undergoing cardiac surgery a randomized clinical trial. Circulation 1998;97:562–8.

[81] van Hilten JA, van de Watering LM, van Bockel JH, et al. Effects of transfusion with red cells filtered to remove leucocytes: randomised controlled trial in patients undergoing major surgery. BMJ 2004;328:1281–4.

[82] Claridge J, Sawyer RG, Schulman AW, et al. Blood transfusions correlate with infections in trauma patients in a dose-dependent manner. Am Surg 2002;68:556–72.

[83] Vincent JL, Baron JF, Reinhart K, et al. Anemia and blood transfusion in critically ill patients. JAMA 2002;288:1499–507.

[84] Hebert PC, Wells G, Blajchman MA, et al. A multicenter, randomized, controlled clinical trial of transfusion requirements in critical care. N Eng J Med 1999;340:409–17.

[85] Hill SR, Carless PA, Henry DA, et al. Transfusion thresholds and other strategies for guiding allogeneic red blood cell transfusion. The Cochrane Database of Systematic Reviews Cochrane Database Syst Rev 2002;(2):CD002042.

[86] Gubler KD, Gentilello LH, Hassantash SA, et al. The impact of hypothermia on dilutional coagulopathy. J Trauma 1994;36:847–51.

[87] Garcia A. Coagulopatía asociada al trauma. Rev Col Cirug 1996;11:17–23.

[88] DeLougery T. Coagulation defects in trauma patients: etiology, recognition, and therapy. Crit Care Clin 2004;20:13–24.

[89] Wolberg AS, Meng SH, Monroe DM III, et al. A systematic evaluation of the effect of temperature on coagulation enzyme activity and platelet function. J Trauma 2004;56: 1221–8.

[90] Hardy J-F, de Moerloose P, Samama M. Massive transfusion and coagulopathy: pathophysiology and implications for clinical management. Can J Anesth 2004;51:293–310.

[91] Spahn DR, Rossaint R. Coagulopathy and blood component transfusion in trauma. BJA 2005;95:130–9.

[92] McKenna R. Postoperative medical complications. Abnormal coagulation in the postoperative priod contributing to excessive bleeding. Med Clin North Am 2001;85: 1277–310.

[93] Gentilello L, Jurkovich G, Stark M, et al. Is hypothermia in the victim of major trauma protective or harmful?: A randomized, prospective study. Ann Surg 1997;226:439–49.

[94] Sessler DI. Complications and treatment of mild hypothermia. Anesthesiology 2001;95: 531–43.

[95] Kober A, Scheck T, Fulesdi B, et al. Effectiveness of resistive heating compared with passive warming in treating hypothermia associated with minor trauma: a randomized trial. Mayo Clin Proc 2001;76:369–75.

[96] Petrone P, Kuncir EJ, Asensio J. Surgical management and strategies in the treatment of hypothermia and cold injury. Emerg Med Clin North Am 2003;21:1165–78.

[97] Negishi C, Hasegawa K, Mukai S, et al. Resistive-heating and forced-air warming are comparably effective. Anest Analg 2003;96:1683–7.

[98] Counts RB, Haisch C, Simon TL, et al. Hemostasis in massively transfused trauma patients. Ann Surg 1979;190:91–9.

[99] Reed RL, Ciavarella D, Heimbach DM, et al. Prophylactic platelet administration during massive transfusion. A prospective, randomized, double-blind clinical study. Ann Surg 1986;203:48–58.

[100] Yugueros P, Sarmiento J, Ferrada R. Síndrome postpericardiotomía. Rev Col Cirug 1993; 8:90–100.

[101] Campbell NC, Thompson SR, Muckard DJJ, et al. Review of 1198 cases of penetrating cardiac trauma. Br J Surg 1997;84:1737–40.

[102] Orliaguet G, Ferjani M, Riuo B. The heart in blunt trauma. Anesthesiology 2001;95: 544–8.

[103] Tso P, Rodriguez A, Cooper C, et al. Sonography in blunt abdominal trauma: a preliminary progress report. J Trauma 1992;33:39–44.

[104] Rozicki GS, Ocshner MG, Jaffin JH, et al. Prospective evaluation of surgeons' use of ultrasound in the evaluation of trauma patients. J Trauma 1993;34:516–27.

[105] McKenney KL, McKenney MG, Cohn SM, et al. Hemoperitoneum score helps determine need for therapeutic laparotomy. J Trauma 2001;50:650–6.

[106] Sclafani SSJA, Shaftan GW, Scalea TM, et al. Nonoperative salvage of computed tomography—diagnosed splenic injuries: utilization of angiography for triage and embolization for hemostasis. J Trauma 1995;39:818–27.

[107] Velmahos G, Demetriades D, Chahwan S, et al. Angiographic embolization for arrest of bleeding after penetrating trauma to the abdomen. Am J Surg 1999;178:367–73.

[108] Velmahos G, Chahwan S, Falabella A, et al. Angiographic embolization for intraperitoneal and retroperitoneal injuries. World J Surg 2000;24:539–45.

[109] Velmahos GC, Toutoouzas K, Vassiliu P, et al. A prospective study on the safety and efficacy of angiographic embolization for pelvic and visceral injuries. J Trauma 2002;52: 3003–8.

[110] Kushimoto S, Arai M, Aiboshi J, et al. The role of interventional radiology in patients requiring damage control laparotomy. J Trauma 2003;54:171–6.

[111] Mohr A, Lavery RF, Barone A, et al. Angiographic embolization for liver injuries: low mortality, high morbidity. J Trauma 2005;55:1077–82.

[112] Yeh MW, Hom JK, Schecter WP, et al. Endovascular repair of an actively hemorrhaging gunshot injury to the abdominal aorta. J Vasc Surg 2005;42:1007–9.

[113] Barba CA. The intensive care unit as an operating room. Surg Clin North Am 2000;80: 957–73.

[114] Mayberry JC. Bedside open abdominal surgery. Utility and wound management. Crit Care Clin 2000;16:151–72.

[115] Rozicki GS, Feliciano DV, Ocshner MG, et al. The role of ultrasound in patients with possible penetrating cardiac wounds: a prospective multicenter study. J Trauma 1999;46: 543–52.

[116] Bar-Nathan M, Richardson D, Garcia A. Indicaciones de toracotomia en trauma. In: Rodriguez A, Ferrada R, editors. Texto de trauma. Sociedad Panamericana de Trauma. Cali: Feriva; 1997.

[117] Ferrada A, Rodriguez A. Trauma cardiaco. Tratamiento quirurgico. Rev Col Cirug 2001; 16:5–15.

[118] Lowell JA, Schifferdecker C, Driscoll DF, et al. Postoperative fluid overload: not a benign problem. Crit Care Med 1990;18:728–33.

[119] Venn R, Steela A, Richardson P, et al. Randomized controlled trial to investigate influence of the fluid challenge on duration of hospital stay and perioperative morbidity in patients with hip fractures. Br J Anaesth 2002;88:65–71.

[120] Balogh Z, McKinley B, Cocanour CS, et al. Supranormal trauma resuscitation causes more cases of intraabdominal compartment. Arch Surg 2003;138:637–43.

[121] Michard F, Teboul J-F. Predicting fluid responsiveness in ICU patients. A critical analysis of the evidence. Chest 2002;121:2000–8.

[122] Weiss YG, Oppenheim-Eden A, Gilon D, et al. Systolic pressure variation in hemodynamic monitoring after severe blast injury. J Clin Anesth 1999;11:132–5.

[123] Michard F, Boussat S, Chemla D, et al. Relation between respiratory changes in arterial pulse pressure and fluid responsiveness in septic patients with acute circulatory failure. Am J Respir Crit Care Med 2000;162:134–8.

[124] Bullock R, Chesnut RM, Clifton G, et al. Guidelines for the management of severe head injury—revision. J Neurotrauma 2000;17:457–627.

[125] Chesnut RM, Marshall LF, Klauber MR, et al. The role of secondary brain injury in determining outcome from severe head injury. J Trauma 1994;34:216–22.

[126] Jeremitsky E, Omert L, Dunham M, et al. Harbingers of poor outcome the day after severe brain injury: hypothermia, hypoxia, and hypoperfusion. J Trauma 2003;55:388–9.

[127] Huyhn T, Messer M, Sing RF, et al. Positive end-expiratory pressure alters intracranial and cerebral perfusion pressure in severe traumatic brain injury. J Trauma 2002;53: 488–92.

[128] Caricato A, Conti G, Della Corte F, et al. Effects of PEEP on the intracranial system of patients with head injury and subarachnoid hemorrhage: the role of respiratory system compliance. J Trauma 2005;58:571–6.
[129] Hsiang JK, Chesnut RM, Crisp CB, et al. Early, routine paralysis for intracranial pressure control in severe head. Crit Care Med 1994;22:1471–6.
[130] Chesnut RM. Management of brain and spine injuries. Crit Care Clin 2004;20:25–55.
[131] Feinstein AJ, Patel MB, Sanui M, et al. Resuscitation with pressors after traumatic brain injury. J Am Coll Surg 2005;201:536–45.
[132] Clifton GL, Miller ER, Choi SC, et al. Lack of effect of induction of hypothermia after acute brain injury. N Eng J Med 2001;344:556–63.
[133] Alderson P, Gadkary C, Signorini DF. Therapeutic hypothermia for head injury. Cochrane Database Syst Rev 2004;(4):CD001048.
[134] Ghajar R., Intracranial pressure monitoring techniques. New Horiz 1995;3:395–9.
[135] Marshall LF, Smith RW, Rausher LA, et al. Mannitol dose requirements in brain injured patients. J Neurosurg 1978;48:169–72.
[136] Cruz J. The first decade of continuous monitoring of jugular bulb oxyhemoglobinsaturation: management strategies and clinical outcome. Crit Care Med 1998;26:344–51.
[137] Eisenberg H, Frankiwski R, Contant C, et al. The comprehensive central nervous system trauma centers. High-dose barbiturate control of elevated intracranial pressure in patients with severe head injury. J Neurosurg 1988;69:15–23.
[138] Gaab MR, Rittierodt M, Lorenz M, et al. Traumatic brain swelling and operative decompression: a prospective investigation. Acta Neurochir 1990;51:s326–8.
[139] Bullock MR, Chesnut R, Ghajar R, et al. Surgical management of traumatic brain lesions. Neurosurgery 2006;58:s225–46.
[140] Berger S, Schurer L, Hartl R, et al. Reduction of post-traumatic intracranial hypertension by hypertonic/hyperoncotic saline/dextran and hypertonic mannitol. Neurosurgery 1995;37:87–107.
[141] Khanna S, Davis D, Peterson B, et al. Use of hypertonic saline in the treatment of severe refractory posttraumatic intracranial hypertension in pediatric traumatic brain injury. Crit Care Med 2000;28:1144–51.
[142] Peterson B, Khanna S, Fisher B, et al. Prolonged hypernatremia controls elevated intracranial pressure in head-injured pediatric patients. Crit Care Med 2000;28:1136–43.
[143] Cooper J, Myles P, McDermott F, et al. Prehospital hypertonic saline resuscitation of patients with hypotension and severe traumatic brain injury. JAMA 2004;291:1350–77.
[144] Roberts I, Yates D, Sandercock P, et al. Effect of Intravenous corticosteroids on death within 14 days in 10008 adults with clinically significant head injury (MRC CRASH trial). Lancet 2004;364:1321–8.
[145] Edwards P, Arango M, Balica L, et al. Final results of MRC CRASH, a randomised placebo-controlled trial of intravenous corticosteroid in adults with head injury-outcomes at 6 months. Lancet 2005;365:1957–9.
[146] Scalea TM, Phillips TF, Goldstein AS, et al. Injuries missed at operation: nemesis of the trauma surgeon. J Trauma 1988;28:962–6.
[147] Enderson BL, Reath DB, Meadors J, et al. The tertiary trauma survey: a prospective study of missed injury. J Trauma 1990;30:666–9.
[148] Hirshberg A, Wall MJ, Mattox KL, et al. Causes and patterns of missed injuries in trauma. Am J Surg 1994;168:299–303.
[149] Buduhan G, McRitchie DI. Missed injuries in patients with multiple trauma. J Trauma 2000;49:600–5.
[150] Vles WJ, Veen EJ, Roukema JD, et al. Consequences of delayed diagnoses in trauma patients: a prospective study. J Am Coll Surg 2003;197:596–602.
[151] Brooks A, Holroyd B, Riley B. Missed injury in major trauma patients. Injury 2004;35:407–10.

[152] Jimenez-Gomez LM, Amunategui I, Sanchez JM, et al. Missed injuries in patients with multiple trauma: analysis of a trauma registry. Cir Esp 2005;78:303–7.

[153] Sharma OP, Scala-Barnett DM, Oswanski MF, et al. Clinical and autopsy analysis of delayed diagnosis and missed injuries in trauma patients. Am Surg 2006;72:174–9.

[154] Born CT, Ross SE, Iannacone WM, et al. Delayed identification of skeletal injury in multisystem trauma: the "missed" fracture. J Trauma 1989;29:1643–6.

[155] Garcia A, Lalsie R, Paredes J, et al. Mortalidad prevenible por trauma en Cali. Colombia, 1998. Acta Col Cuidado Intensivo 2001;4:106–7.

[156] Rizoli SB, Boulanger BR, McLellan BA, et al. Injuries missed during initial assessment of blunt trauma patients. Accid Anal Prev 1994;26:681–6.

[157] Furnival RA, Woodward GA, Schunk JE. Delayed diagnosis of injury in pediatric trauma. Pediatrics 1996;98:56–62.

[158] Meijer JMR, Janssens M, Hammacher ER. Injuries missed in dealing with severely wounded accident victims in the emergency room. Ned Tijdschr Geneeskd 1999;40:1742–5.

[159] Sharma BR, Gupta M, Harish D, et al. Missed diagnoses in trauma patients vis-a-vis significance of autopsy. Injury 2005;36:976–83.

[160] Watts DD, Fahkhry S, and the EAST Multi-institutional HVI Research Group. Incidence of hollow viscus injury in blunt trauma: an analysis from 275,557 trauma admissions from the EAST Multi-Institutional Trial. J Trauma 2003;54:289–94.

[161] Fakhry SM, Brownstein M, Watts DD, et al. Relatively short diagnostic delays (< 8 hours) produce morbidity and mortality in blunt small bowel injury: an analysis of time to operative intervention in 198 patients from a multicenter experience. J Trauma 2000;48:408–14.

[162] Sirlin CB, Brown MA, Andrade-Barreto O, et al. Abdominal trauma: clinical value of negative screening US scans. Radiology 2004;230:661–8.

[163] Ball CG, Kirkpatrick AW, Laupland KB, et al. Factors related to the failure of radiographic recognition of occult posttraumatic pneumothoraces. Am J Surg 2005;189:541–6.

[164] Ball CG. Are occult pneumothoraces truly occult or simply missed? J Trauma 2006;60:294–8.

[165] Grossman MD, Born C. Tertiary survey of the trauma patient in the intensive care unit. Surg Clin North Am 2000;80:805–24.

[166] Hoff WS, Sicoutris CP, Lee SY, et al. Formalized radiology rounds: the final component of the tertiary survey. J Trauma 2004;56:291–5.

[167] Bifl WL, Harrington DT, Cioffi WC, et al. Implementation of a tertiary trauma survey decreases missed injuries. J Trauma 2003;54:38–44.

[168] Maxwell RA, Campbell DJ, Fabian TC, et al. Use of presumptive antibiotics following tube thoracostomy for traumatic hemopneumothorax in the prevention of empyema and pneumonia—a multi-center trial. J Trauma 2004;57:742–9.

[169] Grover FL, Richardson JD, Fewel JG, et al. Prophylactic antibiotics in the treatment of penetrating chest wounds. A prospective double-blind study. J Thorac Cardiovasc Surg 1977;74:528–36.

[170] LeBlanc KA, Tucker WY. Prophylactic antibiotics and closed tube thoracostomy. Surg Gynecol Obstet 1985;160:259–63.

[171] Nichols RL, Smith JW, Muzic AC, et al. Preventive antibiotic usage in traumatic thoracic injuries requiring closed tube thoracostomy. Chest 1994;106:1493–8.

[172] Gonzalez RP, Holevar MR. Role of prophylactic antibiotics for tube thoracostomy in chest trauma. Am Surg 1998;64:617–20.

[173] Luchette FA, Barrie PS, Oswanski MF, et al. Practice management guidelines for prophylactic antibiotic use in tube thoracostomy for traumatic hemopneumothorax: the EAST practice management guidelines work group. J Trauma 2000;48:753–7.

[174] Namias N, Harvill S, Ball S, et al. Cost and morbidity associate with antibiotic prophylaxis in the ICU. J Am Coll Surg 2000;190:503–4.

[175] Velmahos G, Toutzas KG, Sarkisyan G, et al. Severe trauma is not an excuse for prolonged antibiotic prophylaxis. Arch Surg 2002;137:537–42.

[176] Hoth JJ, Franklin GA, Stassen NA, et al. Prophylactic antibiotics adversely affect nosocomial pneumonia i trauma patients. J Trauma 2000;55:549–54.

[177] Dellinger EP, Wertz HJ, Lennard ES, et al. Efficacy of short-course antibiotic prophylaxis after penetrating intestinal injury. Arch Surg 1986;121:23–30.

[178] Demetriades D, Lakhoo M, Pezikis A, et al. Short-course antibiotic prophylaxis in penetrating abdominal injuries: ceftriaxone versus cefoxitin. Injury 1991;22:20–4.

[179] Fabian TC, Croce MA, Payne LW, et al. Duration of antibiotic therapy for penetrating abdominal trauma: a prospective trial. Surgery 1992;112:788–95.

[180] Sarmiento JM, Aristizabal G, Rubiano J, et al. Prophylactic antibiotics in abdominal trauma. J Trauma 1994;37:803–6.

[181] Kirton O, O'Neill PA, Ketsner M, et al. Perioperative antibiotic use in high-risk penetrating hollow viscus injury: a prospective randomized, double-blind, placebo-control trial of 24 hours versus 5 days. J Trauma 2000;49:822–32.

[182] Luchette FA, Borzotta AP, Croce MA, et al. Practice management guidelines for prophylactic antibiotic use in penetrating abdominal trauma: the EAST practice management guidelines work group. J Trauma 2000;48:508–18.

[183] Eggimann P, Pittet D. Infection control in the ICU. Chest 2001;120:2059–93.

[184] Mollitt DL. Infection control: avoiding the inavitable. Surg Clin North Am 2002;82: 365–78.

[185] Coffin SE, Zaoutis KE. Infection control, hospital epidemiology, and patient safety. Infect Dis Clin North Am 2005;19:647–65.

[186] Garcia A, Duque P, Urrutia L, et al. Factores de Riesgo de la UTI Asociada a la sonda vesical. Rev Col Cirug 2005;20:135–43.

[187] Moore EE, Jones TN. Benefits of immediate jejunostomy feeding after major abdominal trauma—a prospective, randomized study. J Trauma 1986;26:874–81.

[188] Moore FA, Moore EE, Jones TN, et al. TEN versus TPN following major abdominal trauma–reduced septic morbidity. J Trauma 1989;29:916–22.

[189] Kudsk KA, Croce MA, Fabian TC, et al. enteral versus parenteral feeding effects on septic morbidity after blunt and penetrating abdominal trauma. Ann Surg 1992;215: 503–11.

[190] Marik PE, Zaloga GP. Early enteral nutrition in acutely ill patients: a systematic review. Crit Care Med 2001;29:2264–70.

[191] Jacobs DG, Jacobs DO, Kudsk K, et al. Practice management guidelines for nutritional support of the trauma patient. J Trauma 2004;57:660–79.

[192] Geerts WH, Code KI, Jay RM, et al. A prospective study of venous thromboembolism after major trauma. N Eng J Med 1994;331:1601–6.

[193] Knudson MM, Ikossi DG, Khaw L, et al. Thromboembolism after trauma an analysis of 1602 episodes from the American College of Surgeons National Trauma Data Bank. Ann Surg 2004;240:490–8.

[194] Rogers FB, Cipolle MD, Velmahos G, et al. Practice management guidelines for the prevention of venous thromboembolism in trauma patients: The EAST Practice Management Guidelines Work Group. J Trauma 2002;53:142–64.

[195] Kirn J, Gearheart MM, Zurick A, et al. Preliminary report on the safety of heparin for deep venous thrombosis prophylaxis after severe head injury. J Trauma 2002;53: 38–433.

[196] Garcia A. Enfermedad tromboembólica en trauma. Panam J Trauma 2003;10:25–39.

[197] Alejandro KV, Acosta JA, Rodriguez PA. Bleeding manifestations after early use of low-molecular-weight heparins in blunt splenic injuries. Am Surg 2003;69:1006–9.

[198] Geerts WH, Pinneo GF, Heith JA, et al. Prevention of venous thromboembolism: The Seventh ACCP Conference on Antithrombotic and Thrombolytic Therapy. Chest 2004; 126:338s–400s.

ELSEVIER
SAUNDERS

SURGICAL
CLINICS OF
NORTH AMERICA

Surg Clin N Am 86 (2006) 1389–1408

Basic Ventilator Management:
Lung Protective Strategies

Michael Donahoe, MD

*Division of Pulmonary, Allergy, and Critical Care Medicine, University of Pittsburgh
School of Medicine, 3459 Fifth Avenue, 628 NW, Pittsburgh, PA 15213, USA*

Acute respiratory failure is manifested clinically as a patient with variable degrees of respiratory distress, but characteristically an abnormal arterial blood partial pressure of oxygen or carbon dioxide. The application of mechanical ventilation in this setting can be life saving. An emerging body of clinical and basic research, however, has highlighted the potential adverse effects of positive pressure ventilation. Direct injury to the lung, specifically attributable to mechanical ventilatory support, is now appreciated from diverse pathogenic mechanisms. Clinicians involved with the care of critically ill patients must recognize and seek to prevent these complications using lung protective ventilation strategies. This article discusses the basic concepts of mechanical ventilation, reviews the categories of ventilator-associated lung injury, and discusses current strategies for the recognition and prevention of these adverse effects in the application of mechanical ventilation.

Physiologic concepts of ventilator support

Lung inflation during mechanical ventilation occurs when pressure and airflow are applied to the airway opening. Incremental airway opening pressure equilibrates with alveolar pressure producing a transpulmonary pressure gradient between the alveoli and the pleural space. The transpulmonary pressure gradient interacts with respiratory system mechanics (primarily lung–chest wall compliance and airways resistance) to achieve a volume change in the lung parenchyma. Exhalation occurs passively when the airway opening pressure returns to atmospheric pressure (or end-expiratory pressure). The primary determinants of expiratory airflow

E-mail address: donahoem@upmc.edu

become the respiratory system elastic recoil pressure acquired during inflation and expiratory airflow resistance.

The interaction of the ventilator delivery mode, patient mechanics, and patient effort result in variable parameters of ventilatory function. For pressure-targeted modes of breath delivery, the airway opening pressure remains constant (set variable), and tidal volume varies with changes in patient lung compliance or airways resistance. Incremental patient effort in this mode favors a reduction in airway pressure, signaling the ventilator to provide additional airflow (and volume) to achieve the prescribed pressure target. In contrast, for volume-targeted modes, changes in lung mechanics do not alter the volume delivered but rather serve to modify the airway opening pressure. Likewise, incremental patient effort in this mode of breath delivery does not produce changes in tidal volume or flow but only serves to modify the measured circuit pressure.

If the transpulmonary pressure at end-expiration remains positive, this is termed "positive end-expiratory pressure" (PEEP). PEEP can result from either the use of expiratory circuit valves in applied modes of ventilation (applied PEEP), or result from incomplete alveolar equilibration with the airway opening pressure at end-expiration (intrinsic PEEP [PEEPi]).

PEEPi may develop within the alveoli because of inadequate expiratory time, premature collapse of the airways during expiration, or by both mechanisms. Minute ventilation, expiratory time fraction, and the expiratory time constant for each alveolar unit (the product of resistance and compliance) interact to determine the presence or absence of PEEPi. An increase in minute ventilation (increase in tidal volume or respiratory frequency), prolongation of the expiratory time fraction, or an increase in the expiratory time constant favors the development of PEEPi.

The presence of PEEPi produces an additional interaction variable in the relationship of delivery mode, patient respiratory system mechanics, and patient effort. In volume-targeted modes of ventilation, the presence of PEEPi leads to increments in the peak airway opening pressure and the end-inspiratory plateau pressure for a given tidal volume delivery. For pressure-targeted modes, the presence of PEEPi with a constant airway opening pressure target leads to a decrease in the transpulmonary pressure gradient and a reduction in the delivered tidal volume.

The breath delivered during mechanical ventilation is distributed to the individual alveolar units within the lung. In most clinical lung conditions, this distribution is not uniform. Patients with lung disease are often characterized by a heterogeneous distribution of lung air and edema fluid [1]. Variable airways resistance, compliance, and residual capacity characterize each alveolar unit, and the degree of heterogeneity between alveolar units advances with disease. In both pressure and volume-targeted modes of breath delivery, the delivered tidal volume is preferentially distributed to alveolar units with low airways resistance, high compliance, or both. This heterogeneity of alveolar unit physiology and tidal volume distribution, best characterized for the patient with acute lung injury (ALI) or adult respiratory distress syndrome (ARDS), leads to a risk of injury from mechanical forces not encountered in normal lung physiology.

The heterogeneity of the injured lung produces three variants of alveoli units: (1) normal alveoli ventilated throughout the respiratory cycle but prone to overdistention, (2) fluid-filled or collapsed alveoli that are never inflated during the respiratory cycle, and (3) fluid-filled or collapsed alveoli that are inflated during the inspiratory portion of the respiratory cycle only to collapse again at end-expiration. These latter units may be "recruitable," meaning a return to normal ventilation throughout the respiratory cycle, with the use of specific ventilatory techniques.

The most common technique to recover recruitable lung units is the application of PEEP. PEEP, when successful, acts to maintain alveolar volume, improving ventilation-perfusion relationships, and improves indices of oxygenation. In addition, by stabilizing alveolar volume throughout the respiratory cycle, PEEP can limit the cycle of recruitment-derecruitment in susceptible alveoli that can occur with tidal breathing. This recruitment-derecruitment process from tidal breath cycling can lead to sheer stress within the alveoli, which contributes to ventilator-induced lung injury (VILI) [2]. Stabilization of alveolar volume is also believed to limit surfactant breakdown in susceptible alveoli [3].

Similar to tidal volume, PEEP is also limited by the presence of heterogeneity in lung units in a given disease state. The selection of the appropriate level of PEEP is a balance of recruiting alveoli at risk for collapse or derecruitment injury without producing overdistention of normal alveolar units. Further, PEEP-mediated increases in airway pressure may serve to redirect blood flow to less compliant, less well-aerated lung regions, leading to increased physiologic dead space. Overexpansion of open alveoli units with PEEP can lead to further compression of nearby ventilated airspaces that are less compliant.

Alveoli recruitment can also be achieved by a technique of periodically, but briefly, raising transpulmonary pressure to higher levels than are associated with tidal ventilation, termed "recruitment maneuvers" [4–6]. Recruitment maneuvers are used to establish initial alveolar patency, which is then maintained at lower tidal pressures and PEEP levels than are needed to open the same collapsed units. High airway pressures may be required transiently to open refractory but recruitable lung units or collapsed airways [7,8]. Numerous methods for recruitment have been explored in the literature including intermittent sighs, episodic increases in PEEP, and sustained application of pressure to achieve total lung capacity [4,6,9]. Alternatively, alterations in the timing of breath delivery may be used to produce a more sustained inspiratory elevation in mean airway pressure (prolonged inspiratory time) or intrinsic PEEP (inverse inspiratory/expiratory ratio).

Adverse effects of mechanical ventilation

The improvements in gas exchange achieved with positive pressure ventilation and alveolar recruitment must be weighed against the potential injurious effects of positive pressure, volume, and supplemental oxygen on the lung. The major components of ventilator-associated lung injury are outlined in Table 1.

Oxygen toxicity

Both normal human and animal investigations suggest a spectrum of airway and parenchymal injury occurs in association with the administration of supplemental oxygen [10–12]. Attributed to the generation of reactive oxygen species, excess oxygen administration is associated with an early inflammatory response in the normal human lung, and a pathologic picture consistent with diffuse alveolar damage in animal models. From these investigations, it is inferred that supplemental oxygen is potentially injurious in the setting of respiratory failure. The specific role oxygen toxicity plays in the diseased human lung, such as ARDS, however, has been most problematic to determine because of the presence of confounding variables. A recent clinical trial in ARDS has compared a higher fraction of inspired oxygen (F_{IO_2})– lower PEEP management with a lower F_{IO_2}–higher PEEP management with no appreciable difference in patient outcome [13]. In addition to direct lung injury, additional physiologic complications of supplemental oxygen administration include absorption atelectasis and accentuation of hypercapnia.

Ventilator-induced lung injury

Early in the common use of ventilator support for respiratory failure, clinicians recognized that lungs inflated with high inspiratory pressures had

Table 1
Types of lung injury associated with the application of mechanical ventilation

Oxygen toxicity	Lung injury attributable to the use of high inspired oxygen concentrations
Ventilator induced lung injury	
Volutrauma	An overexpansion of alveolar units most often attributed to high tidal volume ventilation
Atelectrauma	Sheer stress-induced injury caused by unstable alveoli recruiting and derecruiting with each tidal breath most often attributed to low end-expiratory airway pressures in a heterogeneously injured lung
Biotrauma	A local and systemic inflammatory response of the lung to the tissue damage produced by *volutrauma* and *atelectrauma*
Barotrauma	The development of extra-alveolar air most commonly attributed to high airway pressure ventilation

a propensity to develop extra-alveolar air leaks termed "barotrauma." More recent investigation has identified additional forms of VILI: volutrauma, resulting from an overexpansion of alveolar units; atelectrauma, resulting from sheer stress-induced injury caused by unstable alveoli recruiting and derecruiting with each tidal breath; and biotrauma, which is a local and systemic inflammatory response of the lung to the tissue damage produced by volutrauma and atelectrauma [14]. Although significant human clinical trials now exist to confirm aspects of VILI in ALI-ARDS, the relative contribution of the various forms of VILI and the specific methods to control their emergence remain speculative. This fact has prompted some investigators to favor the term "ventilator-associated lung injury" when discussing clinical studies.

The strongest evidence for ventilator-associated lung injury in humans was demonstrated by the ARDS Network (ARDSNet) tidal volume trial for patients with ALI-ARDS [15]. In this trial, patients with ALI-ARDS from varying causes were randomly assigned to a ventilation protocol characterized by a tidal volume of 6 mL/kg predicted ideal body weight with a plateau pressure maintained ≤ 30 cm H_2O, or to a tidal volume of 12 mL/kg predicted body weight with a plateau pressure ≤ 50 cm H_2O. The study was stopped after the randomization of 861 patients because of a marked reduction in mortality in the low tidal volume population (31% versus 40%, $P = .007$). A secondary analysis of the dataset confirmed the relative benefit of low tidal volume ventilation extended to patients with different risk factors for the ARDS [16]. Subsequent to the publication of this trial, debate has ensued as to whether the trial establishes a standard for the use of a 6 mL/kg predicted ideal body weight tidal volume in ARDS, or more specifically, a standard for the use of the actual ARDSNet ventilation protocol in all patients with ARDS [17]. Independent of this debate, the ARDSNet tidal volume trial clearly establishes the negative effect of high tidal volume and airway pressures on patient outcome. From this landmark study, lung protective strategies have evolved as a standard of care for patients with ALI-ARDS on mechanical ventilation, although clinicians may modify the specifics of the ARDSNet protocol in their practice.

The results of the ARDSNet tidal volume are supported by an extensive dataset gathered in animal models of ALI-ARDS. In these models, mechanical ventilation leads to histologic changes characterized by high permeability edema in previously uninjured lungs and exacerbated injury in the diseased lung [18–21]. Isolation of the effect of pressure versus volume (stretch) mediated injury using high airway pressure ventilation with restricted chest and abdominal excursion has suggested that overdistention, rather than pressure-related injury, is most problematic (volutrauma) [22]. The magnitude of injury is reduced with the presence of end-expiratory pressure, further suggesting that repeated opening and closing of damaged lung units may extend the injury (atelectrauma) [23]. Unlike the normal lung, where the transalveolar pressure is uniformly distributed across the alveolar units during lung inflation, in the heterogeneously injured lung the strain of alveolar unit inflation is also heterogeneously distributed. The traction forces exerted on collapsed alveoli by surrounding expanded lung units are increased and applied to a smaller region [24]. This principle of alveolar interdependence can produce greatly increased and potentially harmful stress at the interface between collapsed and expanded lung units. These data collectively suggest that avoiding the risks of volutrauma and atelectrauma favors a combination of low tidal volume, high end-expiratory pressure ventilation. This approach has been termed the "open-lung approach."

Additional evidence for the entity of VILI in patients has been demonstrated by Ranieri and coworkers [25] who confirmed a relative reduction in proinflammatory bronchoalveolar lavage and peripheral blood cytokines in ALI-ARDS patients who underwent low tidal volume ventilation (mean tidal volume 7.6 mL/kg, mean plateau pressure 24.6 cm H_2O, mean PEEP 14.8 cm H_2O) compared with patients who underwent a more conventional ventilation strategy (mean tidal volume 11.1 mL/kg, mean plateau pressure 31 cm H_2O). Over the first 36 hours of monitoring, bronchoalveolar lavage neutrophils, tumor necrosis factor-α, interleukin (IL)-1β, IL-6, and IL-8 were reduced in the low tidal volume ventilation population. Plasma levels of IL-6 were also significantly reduced. This relationship of low tidal volume ventilation to reduced IL-6 levels compares favorably with similar findings in the low tidal volume ARDSNet population [15,26].

This relationship between mechanical stress from ventilator support and the release of inflammatory mediators has been termed "biotrauma." Experimental lung injury models, ranging from mechanically stressed cellular systems, to isolated lung preparations, and intact animals have shown that injurious ventilatory strategies are associated with the release of proinflammatory mediators [3,27–32]. This inflammatory response seems to precede evidence for histologic damage and is mediated by stretch-activated pathways. The specific mediators and magnitude of the inflammatory response, however, has been debated [33–35]. The reported variability in specific mediators may represent conflict in the models or alternatively reflect variable pathophysiologic processes of VILI in the models explored.

The second component of the biotrauma hypothesis holds that spillover of lung-generated inflammatory mediators from VILI propagates the host systemic inflammatory response and contributes to secondary pulmonary and additional organ dysfunction. Pretreatment with anti– tumor necrosis factor-α and IL-1 receptor antagonist antibodies in VILI models is protective for VILI, providing some experimental support for a sustaining role of the biotrauma response in VILI [36,37]. Further evidence for a systemic role of biotrauma in VILI comes from an experimental model of acid aspiration that has demonstrated that high tidal volume, low PEEP ventilation strategies are associated with changes in nonpulmonary organs including epithelial cell apoptosis in the kidney and small intestine [38]. VILI has been associated with altered gut permeability, which is reversed with the administration of anti–tumor necrosis factor-α antibody [39]. The use of high tidal volume, low PEEP ventilation strategies in animal models has also been associated with increased rates of bacteremia and endotoxemia providing further evidence for a systemic component to the VILI biotrauma hypothesis [40,41]. From a clinical perspective, high tidal volume ventilation (12 mL/kg) in the ARDSNet tidal volume trial was associated with elevated IL-6 levels, and a greater number of days with nonpulmonary organ failure including circulatory, coagulation, and renal failure [15].

Whether VILI is a significant entity in patients without evidence for existing lung injury remains controversial and is only suggested by indirect evidence. A retrospective analysis of a multicenter patient cohort of mechanical ventilation subjects identified 205 patients who developed ARDS >48 hours following the initiation of mechanical ventilation [42]. Multivariate logistic regression analysis identified components of the initial ventilator management including the initial tidal volume, peak airway pressure, and PEEP as important predictors of the evolution to ALI-ARDS. Patients who developed ARDS were more likely to be ventilated with larger tidal volumes (>700 mL) and higher peak airway pressures (>30 cm H_2O) than patients who did not develop ARDS. These data confirmed similar results from a previous single center analysis and provide a confirmatory association between baseline ventilator characteristics and evolution to subsequent lung injury.

In randomized trials, short-term mechanical ventilation with high tidal volumes in adult patients with healthy lungs does not seem to induce a systemic inflammatory response [43]. Further, ventilation strategies do not seem to modify pulmonary or systemic inflammatory markers characteristic of major surgical procedures [44,45]. These data suggest that VILI may be dependent on a two-hit model wherein pulmonary inflammation (first hit) must be present for injurious mechanical ventilation (second hit) to aggravate the inflammatory response. This lack of a clearly demonstrable biotrauma response in normal lungs provides support for the important role of a heterogeneously injured lung in contributing to the pathogenesis of VILI.

Barotrauma

Pulmonary barotrauma refers to the development of extra-alveolar air and includes the clinical entities of pneumothorax, pneumomediastinum, subcutaneous emphysema, and pneumoperitoneum. Pulmonary barotrauma results from the rupture of alveolar air into the lung interstitium and subsequent dissection along fascial planes leading to the clinical entities described. Additional clinical manifestations of barotrauma include bronchopleural fistula, tension pneumothorax, tension lung cysts, systemic gas embolism, and subpleural air cysts.

Although generally accepted that higher inflation pressure or volume contributes to the development of barotrauma, the evidence to support this association has been inconsistent. Although some observational studies have found an association between high inspiratory airway pressures and PEEP and the development of barotrauma, others have not [46]. Amato and coworkers [4] reported that the use of high tidal volumes of 12 mL/kg and high airway pressures produced a 42% rate of pneumothorax compared with a 7% rate in patients where tidal volume and plateau pressures were restricted. In contrast, the ARDSNet tidal volume trial, despite showing a dramatic reduction in mortality with lower tidal volumes and plateau pressures, failed to show a difference in the incidence of barotrauma in the two study populations [15].

A retrospective review of 718 patients with ALI-ARDS from the ARDS-Net data set examined airway pressures at baseline, 1 day before the onset of barotrauma, and concurrent with the onset of barotrauma [46]. During the first 4 days of patient enrollment the cumulative incidence of barotrauma was 13%. Using multivariate analysis, a higher PEEP level at baseline and 24 hours before the onset of barotrauma was the only airway pressure measurement associated with the development of barotrauma. Although often reported that barotrauma occurs late in the course of ARDS, these investigators found most of the barotrauma events occurred in the first 4 days of ARDS [46].

In a more diverse clinical population of mechanically ventilated patients with various forms of lung disease, the overall incidence of barotrauma was 2.9%, varying with specific underlying lung disease from 2.9% in patients with chronic obstructive pulmonary disease to 10% in patients with chronic interstitial lung disease. Barotrauma was diagnosed a mean of 3.4 ± 4.2 days following the initiation of mechanical ventilation. Ventilator parameters, specifically tidal volume, airway pressures (peak and plateau), and PEEP were not significantly different between patients with and without the development of barotrauma [47].

In a literature review of 14 clinical studies, the reported incidence of barotrauma varied from 14% to 49% [48]. In this review, maintenance of an inspiratory plateau pressure ≤ 35 cm H_2O produced no relationship between ventilatory parameters and the development of barotrauma. In contrast, a plateau pressure > 35 cm H_2O was associated with an increased rate of barotrauma.

The existing data demonstrate an inconsistent relationship between airway pressures, tidal volume, and the development of barotrauma. Collectively, the data suggest that barotrauma can be minimized with factors that also regulate VILI, specifically restriction of tidal volume and management of plateau pressures ≤ 35 cm H_2O.

Disease-specific concepts in ventilator support

The emerging body of basic and clinical research in VILI has placed a renewed focus on important physiologic and bioinflammatory concepts in the ventilator management of critically ill patients. The translation of these concepts to the daily management of patients in the ICU is still limited, however, by the lack of important clinical studies. Current knowledge of important management concepts for two common forms of respiratory failure in the ICU and a review of noninvasive mechanical ventilation as an alternative respiratory support strategy are discussed.

Adult respiratory distress syndrome and acute lung injury

Patients with ARDS-ALI can be supported with either pressure-limited or volume-limited modes of ventilation, with the provision that appropriate focus is placed on the specific goals of mechanical ventilation [49]. Volume-limited modes offer a predictable tidal volume and minute ventilation with variable airway pressures based on changing lung mechanics. Pressure-limited modes offer predictable airway pressures yet provide variable lung volumes with changing lung mechanics. The attention of the clinician to these distinct differences and prompt recognition and explanation of changing physiologic variables is most important. In general, full-support modes are favored over partial-support modes early in the disease course because of variable lung mechanics and patient comfort.

Prospective clinical studies in patients with ARDS-ALI have suggested that lung protective ventilation strategies that incorporate lower tidal volume–plateau pressure strategies are associated with a reduced mortality rate in comparison with higher tidal volume–higher plateau pressure ventilation strategies [4,15,50–53]. In the largest clinical trial published, the beneficial effect of a relative tidal volume–plateau pressure reduction seemed to be independent of ARDS etiology and severity [16,54]. The physiologic targets in this trial were a tidal volume ≤ 6 mL/kg ideal body weight and a plateau pressure ≤ 30 cm H_2O (Table 2). The degree of hypercapnia experienced with low tidal volume ventilation seems to be modest and well tolerated. These trials establish a focus for the clinician on the prevention of mechanical trauma as a primary treatment goal rather than achieving normocapnia or avoiding oxygen toxicity.

In addition to the restriction of tidal volume, the other common feature to lung protection strategies is a relatively high level of PEEP (≥ 12–15 cm H_2O). Although the contribution of atelectrauma to VILI in ARDS-ALI is certain from animal models, the best method to select PEEP for a given patient with ARDS remains problematic. Both arbitrary scales and careful titration to a set PEEP above the lower inflection point (Pflex) of the pressure-volume curve have been used successfully in clinical trials as part of an overall lung protective ventilation strategy [4,15]. A recent clinical trial that provided uniform regulation of tidal volume (6 mL/kg ideal body weight) and compared a scale incorporating higher PEEP levels with lower PEEP levels showed no difference in ARDS patient outcome [13]. Although this might suggest atelectrauma has a minor role in VILI, this trial targeted PEEP to optimal oxygenation rather than minization of VILI. Clinicians remain limited

Table 2
ARDSNet lung protective (6 mL/kg predicted body weight) strategy

Mode	AC mode
Tidal volume	Set at 8 mL/kg predicted IBW and titrate to 6 mL/kg over 6 h
	May titrate up to 8 mL/kg IBW if plateau pressure ≤30 cm H_2O and evidence for breath stacking (>3 per min) or airway pressure<PEEP
	Titrate down to 4 mL/kg IBW if plateau pressure >30 cm H_2O
Inspiratory flow	Target: inspiratory:expiratory ratio at 1:1 to 1:3
Plateau pressure	Target: ≤30 cm H_2O.
	Measurement using a 0.5-s plateau q 4 hours and with each PEEP or tidal volume change
Arterial pH goal	Target: 7.30<pH ≤7.45 (if possible)
	Increase ventilator rate to 35 to maintain pH≥7.30
	If ventilator rate = 35 and pH <7.30, bicarb may be given
	If ventilator rate = 35, bicarb has been considered, and pH <7.15, tidal volume may be increased (Pplat may rise>30 cm H_2O)
PEEP and FiO_2	Target: PaO_2 = 55–80 mm Hg or SaO_2 = 88%–95%
	Measurement q 4 hours; adjustments for values outside the range following the combination scale outlined below
	PEEP 5 5 8 8 10 10 10 12 14 14 14 16 18 18 20–24
	FiO_2 0.3 0.4 0.4 0.5 0.5 0.6 0.7 0.7 0.7 0.8 0.9 0.9 0.9 1.0 1.0

Complete protocol available at www.ardsnet.org

Abbreviations: AC, assist control; FiO_2, fraction of inspired oxygen; IBW, ideal body weight; PaO_2, partial pressure of oxygen, arterial; PEEP, positive end-expiratory pressure; Pplat, plateau pressure; SaO_2, oxygen saturation, arterial.

Adapted from data in The Acute Respiratory Distress Syndrome Network. Ventilation with lower tidal volumes as compared with traditional tidal volumes for acute lung injury and the acute respiratory distress syndrome. N Engl J Med 2000;342:1301–8.

in selecting an appropriate PEEP level to minimize lung injury because of poor assessment tools for this parameter in the clinical setting.

Pressure-volume curves in patients with early ARDS often demonstrate an initial flat portion at low lung volumes, during which increases in pressure produce only small changes in volume. This early portion of the pressure-volume curve transitions to a curve with an increased slope with progressive lung inflation suggesting more physiologic compliance. The point at which compliance increases is called the Pflex. With continued lung inflation to total lung capacity, the slope of the pressure-volume curve again flattens, at a point called the upper inflection point. Inflation beyond this point can result in alveolar overdistention, decreased cardiac filling, and impaired oxygen delivery [55]. The open lung approach advocates that PEEP be applied to allow delivery of tidal volume above Pflex, but below the upper inflection point. Theoretically, this approach should limit the repeated opening and closing of lung units (cyclical atelectasis), while minimizing alveolar overdistention and the potential for VILI.

The open lung approach, as described by Amato and coworkers [4], incorporates a low tidal volume (<6 mL/kg) with the targeting of PEEP at 2 cm H_2O >Pflex of the pressure-volume curve. If a PEEP level cannot be determined, then a level of 16 cm H_2O is used. Driving pressure, defined as plateau pressure minus PEEP, is kept below 20 cm H_2O, and peak pressure is limited to 40 cm H_2O. Recruiting maneuvers are used, especially after inadvertent disconnections from the ventilator. In a randomized, unblinded trial involving 53 patients, the open lung protective ventilation approach resulted in an improved 28-day survival and a higher rate of weaning than did conventional treatment. The high mortality (71%) in the conventionally treated group raised doubt, however, about the improved 28-day survival seen in the protective ventilation group. In addition, most of the survival benefit in the open lung group occurred within the first 3 days of randomization, a finding that is difficult to explain if the usefulness of the technique is caused by the prevention of VILI. Although benefits of modified variations of this open lung ventilator strategy have been described, the open lung approach remains untested in a large patient clinical trial.

The use of Pflex as a target point in setting PEEP has significant limitations. The measurement is subject to significant interobserver variability, which can range from 5% to 9% [56]. Alterations in chest wall or abdominal compliance may suggest values of Pflex that do not accurately predict a parenchymal response to PEEP titration [57]. A significant fraction of patients may not demonstrate a clear Pflex in the pressure-volume curve [58]. Finally, the distribution of recruitment varies across lung regions and continues throughout the respiratory cycle raising questions as to the significance of Pflex as a marker for optimal lung recruitment [59].

Ideally, optimal PEEP prevents recruitment-derecruitment injury without placing additional stress of inflation on lung units that are already open. Gattinoni and coworkers [60] have demonstrated that the capacity for opening (or recruiting) collapsed alveolar units varies greatly among patients with ARDS. Recruitable lung in ALI-ARDS was defined as the proportion of lung weight newly aerated in transitioning from 5 to 45 cm H_2O airway pressure on CT scans of the chest. These investigators found approximately 24% of the lung could not be recruited even at a high level of airway pressure in the study subjects. They identified a tight correlation between the percentage of recruitable lung at 45 cm H_2O and the lung that remained recruited at a fixed level of PEEP equal to 15 cm H_2O ($r^2 = 0.72$, $P < .001$). The mode of injury (pulmonary-direct or extrapulmonary-indirect) was not helpful in predicting the potential recruitability of the injured lung, nor were specific physiologic variables. The combination of variables that yielded the best results for predicting recruitable lung was the presence of two of the following: a Pao_2:Fio_2 ratio of <150 at a PEEP of 5 cm H_2O; any decrease in alveolar dead space; and an increase in respiratory system compliance when PEEP was increased from 5 to 15 cm H_2O (sensitivity, 79%; specificity 81%).

These data emphasize the current limitation for clinicians in prescribing the appropriate level of PEEP to minimize VILI. A titration to higher levels of PEEP strictly to minimize oxygen toxicity is not supported by clinical trials [13]. Clinical trials that selectively compare PEEP titration with mechanical targets (ie, recruitable lung) are required to explore further the issue of optimal PEEP to prevent VILI.

The use of recruitment maneuvers has been advocated by some investigators to define PEEP responsiveness, assess cardiovascular interactions, manage ventilator disconnects, and stabilize recruited lung volume before individual PEEP titrations [61]. Two methods have been commonly advocated. The first uses a sustained elevation in airway pressure using a continuous positive airway pressure of 35 to 40 cm H_2O for 40 seconds before reinstituting the previous level of PEEP [4,62]. Alternatively, a high level of pressure-controlled ventilation (PEEP of 15–20 cm H_2O, driving pressure of 30 cm H_2O, plateau pressure of 50 cm H_2O) is provided for 1 to 2 minutes as tolerated [61]. These pressures may be titrated upward for patients with a markedly reduced extrathoracic compliance. Patients who demonstrate an improvement in oxygenation indices during these maneuvers are labeled PEEP responsive and likely to benefit from upward titration of the PEEP settings. The benefit to gas exchange from recruitment maneuvers is limited in duration and may be dependent on pre-existing PEEP levels [62]. The routine application of recruitment maneuvers seems to offer little benefit over appropriate PEEP titration [63].

The selection of mechanical ventilation variables in ALI-ARDS cannot be considered without attention to hemodynamic interactions. Positive pressure ventilation is frequently associated with the development of hypotension and reduced cardiac output. The increase in mean intrathoracic pressure associated with mechanical ventilation increases right atrial pressure reducing the gradient for systemic venous return. Further elevations in mean intrathoracic pressure with PEEP or auto-PEEP can additionally compromise venous return and this effect is most evident in patients with intravascular volume contraction. PEEP-related increases in alveolar volume could increase pulmonary vascular resistance leading to increased right ventricular afterload. Increased right ventricular afterload can shift the intraventricular septum leading to impaired left ventricular filling. If not titrated carefully, beneficial outcomes of PEEP on oxygenation indices (Pao_2:Fio_2 ratios) can be significantly offset by marked reductions in cardiac output and tissue oxygenation. The monitoring of arterial pulse pressure during PEEP titration can be a useful noninvasive tool to assess the impact of PEEP changes on cardiac output [64].

The safe application of mechanical ventilation to the patient with ARDS-ALI focuses on both the correction of abnormal gas exchange indices and limiting mechanically induced VILI. Further basic and clinical research into the mechanisms and protective strategies for VILI are needed especially in the area of optimal lung recruitment. ARDS patients must currently be recognized as a mixture of individual components of a heterogeneously injured lung, with variable extrathoracic compliance disorders, and wide-ranging hemodynamic interactions. No single formula or guideline for safe mechanical ventilation can be outlined in this setting. A few guiding principles can be outlined based on the current knowledge and existing clinical trials (Box 1).

Obstructive lung disease

The principles outlined to minimize the risk of VILI in severe ARDS-ALI presumably also apply to the patient with severe obstructive lung disease; however, little clinical data exist to confirm this hypothesis. In addition, the combination of high minute ventilation, expiratory flow limitation, and expiratory airflow resistance characteristic of patients with obstructive lung disease places them at risk for PEEPi. Because patients with obstructive lung disease have a significant degree of heterogeneity focused around the emptying of lung units, they can develop PEEPi even at relatively low minute ventilations.

PEEPi commonly goes undetected, because it is not registered on the pressure manometer of the ventilator, which equilibrates to the atmosphere. Physical examination, including palpation and auscultation of the chest for

---

Box 1. Guidelines for lung protective ventilation in adult respiratory distress syndrome and acute lung injury

Pressure and volume targeted modes seem to have equal efficacy in this population. The experience of the clinician and correct interpretation of changing physiologic indices is most important.

Reduction of tidal volume to ranges approaching 6 mL/kg predicted ideal body weight to maintain end-inspiratory plateau airway pressures ≤30 cm H_2O is strongly favored over higher tidal volume (>10 mL/kg) strategies.

Modification of target airway pressures is required in the setting of markedly altered chest wall or abdominal compliance.

Higher PEEP titration (12–5 cm H_2O) strictly to reduce inspired oxygen concentration is not favored by current studies. Higher PEEP titration to minimize recurrent lung derecruitment is suggested by animal models but specific reproducible clinical targets for titration are lacking. Recruitment maneuvers may have a role in identifying patients who are PEEP responsive and guide titration but are not routinely indicated.

Careful monitoring of hemodynamic indices is indicated with positive pressure airway titration to minimize the risk of impaired tissue perfusion with lung protective ventilation.

Hypercapnia is generally well tolerated and is acceptable in preference to higher tidal volume or plateau pressure ventilation or cardiovascular compromise.

the presence of persistent exhalation at the time of the initiation of the next breath, can confirm that PEEPi is present but is less useful in confirming its absence [65]. Inspection of expiratory flow-time curves in appropriately configured ventilators provides a similar assessment to careful physical examination. Occlusion of the expiratory port at end-expiration to allow equilibration across the entire lung, either manually or by a specially configured ventilator, allows an appropriate quantification of intrinsic PEEP. This method can still underestimate PEEPi in the setting of widespread airway closure where equilibration of airway pressure and alveolar pressure is not present [66].

Recognition of PEEPi is critical to the management of the obstructive lung disease population because it can impact both respiratory and hemodynamic assessments. PEEPi results in the underestimation of mean alveolar pressure as measured by mean airway pressure and produces erroneous calculations of static lung compliance if extrinsic PEEP is the assumed end-expiratory alveolar pressure. The increase in mean alveolar pressure, associated with PEEPi, exacerbates the hemodynamic effects of positive pressure ventilation and may increase the likelihood of barotrauma. PEEPi can produce hemodynamic instability, often manifested by hypotension in an obstructive lung disease patient, simply because of an increased respiratory rate (short cycle length) or increased expiratory airflow resistance. These hemodynamic changes can be misinterpreted as shock states caused by sepsis or cardiogenic failure if PEEPi is not appreciated. PEEPi can also produce difficulty triggering the ventilator for obstructive lung disease patients. This can "lock out" the patient from triggering the ventilator entirely.

Prevention of PEEPi is not always possible but limitation is achieved by a focus on increasing expiratory duration. Reducing minute ventilation by decreasing the respiratory rate (longer cycle length) or decreasing tidal volume (reduced inspiratory time fraction) is the most efficacious method to reduce PEEPi. In addition, efforts to relieve expiratory airflow obstruction are critical to the management of these patients.

Noninvasive mechanical ventilation

For patients with milder degrees of respiratory failure, the application of noninvasive mechanical ventilation offers an alternative that may correct milder abnormalities of gas exchange without exposure to the risks of endotracheal intubation. Theoretically, this form of assisted ventilation could significantly reduce the risk of VILI. Noninvasive mechanical ventilation refers to positive pressure ventilation delivered through a nasal or full-face mask with different levels of pressure support set for inspiration (10–15 cm H_2O) and expiration (5–8 cm H_2O). Noninvasive mechanical ventilation has shown efficacy in a number of patient populations in comparison with conventional management without noninvasive mechanical ventilation. The use of noninvasive mechanical ventilation is contraindicated in the patient with impending cardiovascular collapse or respiratory arrest; upper airway obstruction; excessive upper airway secretions; massive gastrointestinal bleeding; recent surgery of the upper airway or gastrointestinal tract; or in the setting of an altered mental status (inability to protect the airway). In the absence of these contraindications, however, noninvasive mechanical ventilation may offer a significant advantage to minimize the risk of ventilator support in specific patient populations.

The most investigated population for noninvasive mechanical ventilation has been patients experiencing chronic obstructive pulmonary disease exacerbations. Multiple clinical trials in this setting have suggested noninvasive mechanical ventilation reduces the requirement for intubation and may reduce hospital mortality in comparison with conventional management without noninvasive mechanical ventilation [67,68]. In general, the response to noninvasive mechanical ventilation in the first 2 hours is predictive of subsequent success or failure of this form of respiratory support [69].

Noninvasive mechanical ventilation has also shown efficacy in immunocompromised patients with acute respiratory failure. Clinical trials in patients following solid organ transplantation and with hematologic malignancies have suggested noninvasive mechanical ventilation is associated with decreased rates of intubation and intensive care unit mortality [70,71].

A benefit to the use of continuous positive airway pressure has been demonstrated for patients with cardiogenic pulmonary edema with a reduction in the rates of intubation and a trend toward a reduction in mortality [72]. Similar benefits on the rate of intubation have also been suggested for the use of noninvasive mechanical ventilation in this patient population especially for patients presenting with hypercapnia [73–75]. Comparative trials of these two modes of ventilatory support are lacking.

Finally, in acute hypoxemic respiratory failure of mixed etiologies, the results for noninvasive mechanical ventilation are also favorable. Early clinical trials had suggested that noninvasive mechanical ventilation in acute hypoxemic respiratory failure was associated with a reduction in the rates of endotracheal intubation with a more clear benefit to patients who also have hypercapnia [76,77]. The largest clinical trial of 105 patients with acute hypoxemic respiratory failure without hypercapnia demonstrated clear benefits to noninvasive mechanical ventilation in rates of endotracheal intubation, intensive care unit length of stay, and 90-day mortality [77].

The use of noninvasive mechanical ventilation provides an alternative to endotracheal intubation for patients with a variety of etiologies of acute respiratory failure. For patients with chronic obstructive pulmonary disease and cardiogenic pulmonary edema this mode of support is favored based on multiple clinical trials. For patients with acute hypoxemic respiratory failure and respiratory failure in the setting of immunosuppression, positive clinical trials also exist to consider the use of this modality as a further tool to minimize the risks associated with mechanical ventilation and endotracheal intubation.

Summary

Although positive pressure mechanical ventilation is a cornerstone in the management of patients with acute respiratory failure, a growing body of clinical and basic research has established direct injury to the lung as a possible consequence of this modality. Diverse pathogenic mechanisms have been identified and current clinical studies have provided some direction for clinicians involved with the management of patients, especially the patient with ALI-ARDS. Further clinical studies are needed to address specific issues especially in the area of end-expiratory pressure and lung recruitment strategies for the diverse patient population that is ARDS. Further basic and clinical research is needed to unravel the biochemical basis of stress-mediated lung inflammation and re-expansion injury. Understanding the basic mechanisms of VILI may provide pharmacologic directions to limit this complication in critically ill patients.

References

[1] Gattinoni L, Caironi P, Pelosi P, et al. What has computed tomography taught us about the acute respiratory distress syndrome? Am J Respir Crit Care Med 2001;164:1701–11.

[2] Muscedere JG, Mullen JB, Gan K, et al. Tidal ventilation at low airway pressures can augment lung injury. Am J Respir Crit Care Med 1994;149:1327–34.

[3] Nakamura T, Malloy J, McCaig L, et al. Mechanical ventilation of isolated septic rat lungs: effects on surfactant and inflammatory cytokines. J Appl Physiol 2001;91:811–20.

[4] Amato MB, Barbas CS, Medeiros DM, et al. Effect of a protective-ventilation strategy on mortality in the acute respiratory distress syndrome. N Engl J Med 1998;338:347–54.

[5] Lapinsky SE, Aubin M, Mehta S, et al. Safety and efficacy of a sustained inflation for alveolar recruitment in adults with respiratory failure. Intensive Care Med 1999;25:1297–301.

[6] Foti G, Cereda M, Sparacino ME, et al. Effects of periodic lung recruitment maneuvers on gas exchange and respiratory mechanics in mechanically ventilated acute respiratory distress syndrome (ARDS) patients. Intensive Care Med 2000;26:501–7.

[7] Crotti S, Mascheroni D, Caironi P, et al. Recruitment and derecruitment during acute respiratory failure: a clinical study. Am J Respir Crit Care Med 2001;164:131–40.

[8] Gaver DP III, Samsel RW, Solway J. Effects of surface tension and viscosity on airway reopening. J Appl Physiol 1990;69:74–85.

[9] Pelosi P, Cadringher P, Bottino N, et al. Sigh in acute respiratory distress syndrome. Am J Respir Crit Care Med 1999;159:872–80.

[10] Davis WB, Rennard SI, Bitterman PB, et al. Pulmonary oxygen toxicity: early reversible changes in human alveolar structures induced by hyperoxia. N Engl J Med 1983;309:878–83.

[11] Freeman BA, Crapo JD. Hyperoxia increases oxygen radical production in rat lungs and lung mitochondria. J Biol Chem 1981;256:10986–92.

[12] Sackner MA, Landa J, Hirsch J, et al. Pulmonary effects of oxygen breathing: a 6-hour study in normal men. Ann Intern Med 1975;82:40–3.

[13] Brower RG, Lanken PN, MacIntyre N, et al. Higher versus lower positive end-expiratory pressures in patients with the acute respiratory distress syndrome. N Engl J Med 2004;351:327–36.

[14] Pinhu L, Whitehead T, Evans T, et al. Ventilator-associated lung injury. Lancet 2003;361:332–40.

[15] Ventilation with lower tidal volumes as compared with traditional tidal volumes for acute lung injury and the acute respiratory distress syndrome. The Acute Respiratory Distress Syndrome Network. N Engl J Med 2000;342:1301–8.

[16] Eisner MD, Thompson T, Hudson LD, et al. Efficacy of low tidal volume ventilation in patients with different clinical risk factors for acute lung injury and the acute respiratory distress syndrome. Am J Respir Crit Care Med 2001;164:231–6.

[17] Eichacker PQ, Gerstenberger EP, Banks SM, et al. Meta-analysis of acute lung injury and acute respiratory distress syndrome trials testing low tidal volumes. Am J Respir Crit Care Med 2002;166:1510–4.

[18] Dreyfuss D, Basset G, Soler P, et al. Intermittent positive-pressure hyperventilation with high inflation pressures produces pulmonary microvascular injury in rats. Am Rev Respir Dis 1985;132:880–4.

[19] Corbridge TC, Wood LD, Crawford GP, et al. Adverse effects of large tidal volume and low PEEP in canine acid aspiration. Am Rev Respir Dis 1990;142:311–5.

[20] Webb HH, Tierney DF. Experimental pulmonary edema due to intermittent positive pressure ventilation with high inflation pressures: protection by positive end-expiratory pressure. Am Rev Respir Dis 1974;110:556–65.

[21] Parker JC, Townsley MI, Rippe B, et al. Increased microvascular permeability in dog lungs due to high peak airway pressures. J Appl Physiol 1984;57:1809–16.

[22] Hernandez LA, Peevy KJ, Moise AA, et al. Chest wall restriction limits high airway pressure-induced lung injury in young rabbits. J Appl Physiol 1989;66:2364–8.

[23] Dreyfuss D, Soler P, Basset G, et al. High inflation pressure pulmonary edema: respective effects of high airway pressure, high tidal volume, and positive end-expiratory pressure. Am Rev Respir Dis 1988;137:1159–64.

[24] Mead J, Takishima T, Leith D. Stress distribution in lungs: a model of pulmonary elasticity. J Appl Physiol 1970;28:596–608.

[25] Ranieri VM, Suter PM, Tortorella C, et al. Effect of mechanical ventilation on inflammatory mediators in patients with acute respiratory distress syndrome: a randomized controlled trial. JAMA 1999;282:54–61.

[26] Parsons PE, Eisner MD, Thompson BT, et al. Lower tidal volume ventilation and plasma cytokine markers of inflammation in patients with acute lung injury. Crit Care Med 2005; 33:1–6 [discussion: 230–2].

[27] Haitsma JJ, Uhlig S, Goggel R, et al. Ventilator-induced lung injury leads to loss of alveolar and systemic compartmentalization of tumor necrosis factor-alpha. Intensive Care Med 2000;26:1515–22.

[28] Tremblay L, Valenza F, Ribeiro SP, et al. Injurious ventilatory strategies increase cytokines and c-fos m-RNA expression in an isolated rat lung model. J Clin Invest 1997;99:944–52.

[29] Chiumello D, Pristine G, Slutsky AS. Mechanical ventilation affects local and systemic cytokines in an animal model of acute respiratory distress syndrome. Am J Respir Crit Care Med 1999;160:109–16.

[30] Vlahakis NE, Schroeder MA, Limper AH, et al. Stretch induces cytokine release by alveolar epithelial cells in vitro. Am J Physiol 1999;277(1 pt 1):L167–73.

[31] Vreugdenhil HA, Haitsma JJ, Jansen KJ, et al. Ventilator-induced heat shock protein 70 and cytokine mRNA expression in a model of lipopolysaccharide-induced lung inflammation. Intensive Care Med 2003;29:915–22.

[32] Held HD, Boettcher S, Hamann L, et al. Ventilation-induced chemokine and cytokine release is associated with activation of nuclear factor-kappaB and is blocked by steroids. Am J Respir Crit Care Med 2001;163(3 pt 1):711–6.

[33] Ricard JD, Dreyfuss D, Saumon G. Production of inflammatory cytokines in ventilator-induced lung injury: a reappraisal. Am J Respir Crit Care Med 2001;163:1176–80.

[34] Verbrugge SJ, Uhlig S, Neggers SJ, et al. Different ventilation strategies affect lung function but do not increase tumor necrosis factor-alpha and prostacyclin production in lavaged rat lungs in vivo. Anesthesiology 1999;91:1834–43.

[35] D'Angelo E, Pecchiari M, Della Valle P, et al. Effects of mechanical ventilation at low lung volume on respiratory mechanics and nitric oxide exhalation in normal rabbits. J Appl Physiol 2005;99:433–44.

[36] Imai Y, Kawano T, Iwamoto S, et al. Intratracheal anti-tumor necrosis factor-alpha antibody attenuates ventilator-induced lung injury in rabbits. J Appl Physiol 1999;87: 510–5.

[37] Narimanbekov IO, Rozycki HJ. Effect of IL-1 blockade on inflammatory manifestations of acute ventilator-induced lung injury in a rabbit model. Exp Lung Res 1995;21:239–54.

[38] Imai Y, Parodo J, Kajikawa O, et al. Injurious mechanical ventilation and end-organ epithelial cell apoptosis and organ dysfunction in an experimental model of acute respiratory distress syndrome. JAMA 2003;289:2104–12.

[39] Guery BP, Welsh DA, Viget NB, et al. Ventilation-induced lung injury is associated with an increase in gut permeability. Shock 2003;19:559–63.

[40] Murphy DB, Cregg N, Tremblay L, et al. Adverse ventilatory strategy causes pulmonary-to-systemic translocation of endotoxin. Am J Respir Crit Care Med 2000;162:27–33.

[41] Nahum A, Hoyt J, Schmitz L, et al. Effect of mechanical ventilation strategy on dissemination of intratracheally instilled *Escherichia coli* in dogs. Crit Care Med 1997;25:1733–43.

[42] Gajic O, Frutos-Vivar F, Esteban A, et al. Ventilator settings as a risk factor for acute respiratory distress syndrome in mechanically ventilated patients. Intensive Care Med 2005;31: 922–6.

[43] Wrigge H, Zinserling J, Stuber F, et al. Effects of mechanical ventilation on release of cytokines into systemic circulation in patients with normal pulmonary function. Anesthesiology 2000;93:1413–7.

[44] Wrigge H, Uhlig U, Zinserling J, et al. The effects of different ventilatory settings on pulmonary and systemic inflammatory responses during major surgery. Anesth Analg 2004;98: 775–81.

[45] Wrigge H, Uhlig U, Baumgarten G, et al. Mechanical ventilation strategies and inflammatory responses to cardiac surgery: a prospective randomized clinical trial. Intensive Care Med 2005;31:1379–87.

[46] Eisner MD, Thompson BT, Schoenfeld D, et al. Airway pressures and early barotrauma in patients with acute lung injury and acute respiratory distress syndrome. Am J Respir Crit Care Med 2002;165:978–82.

[47] Anzueto A, Frutos-Vivar F, Esteban A, et al. Incidence, risk factors and outcome of barotrauma in mechanically ventilated patients. Intensive Care Med 2004;30:612–9.

[48] Boussarsar M, Thierry G, Jaber S, et al. Relationship between ventilatory settings and barotrauma in the acute respiratory distress syndrome. Intensive Care Med 2002;28:406–13.

[49] Esteban A, Alia I, Gordo F, et al. Prospective randomized trial comparing pressure-controlled ventilation and volume-controlled ventilation in ARDS. For the Spanish Lung Failure Collaborative Group. Chest 2000;117:1690–6.

[50] Petrucci N, Iacovelli W. Ventilation with lower tidal volumes versus traditional tidal volumes in adults for acute lung injury and acute respiratory distress syndrome. Cochrane Database Syst Rev 2004;2:CD003844.

[51] Hickling KG, Walsh J, Henderson S, et al. Low mortality rate in adult respiratory distress syndrome using low-volume, pressure-limited ventilation with permissive hypercapnia: a prospective study. Crit Care Med 1994;22:1568–78.

[52] Villar J, Kacmarek RM, Perez-Mendez L, et al. A high positive end-expiratory pressure, low tidal volume ventilatory strategy improves outcome in persistent acute respiratory distress syndrome: a randomized, controlled trial. Crit Care Med 2006;34:1311–8.

[53] Kallet RH, Jasmer RM, Pittet JF, et al. Clinical implementation of the ARDS network protocol is associated with reduced hospital mortality compared with historical controls. Crit Care Med 2005;33:925–9.

[54] Brower R, Thompson BT. Tidal volumes in acute respiratory distress syndrome: one size does not fit all. Crit Care Med 2006;34:263–4 [author reply: 264–7].

[55] Dambrosio M, Roupie E, Mollet JJ, et al. Effects of positive end-expiratory pressure and different tidal volumes on alveolar recruitment and hyperinflation. Anesthesiology 1997;87: 495–503.
[56] O'Keefe GE, Gentilello LM, Erford S, et al. Imprecision in lower inflection point estimation from static pressure-volume curves in patients at risk for acute respiratory distress syndrome. J Trauma 1998;44:1064–8.
[57] Mergoni M, Martelli A, Volpi A, et al. Impact of positive end-expiratory pressure on chest wall and lung pressure-volume curve in acute respiratory failure. Am J Respir Crit Care Med 1997;156(3 pt 1):846–54.
[58] Ward NS, Lin DY, Nelson DL, et al. Successful determination of lower inflection point and maximal compliance in a population of patients with acute respiratory distress syndrome. Crit Care Med 2002;30:963–8.
[59] Gattinoni L, D'Andrea L, Pelosi P, et al. Regional effects and mechanism of positive end-expiratory pressure in early adult respiratory distress syndrome. JAMA 1993;269: 2122–7.
[60] Gattinoni L, Caironi P, Cressoni M, et al. Lung recruitment in patients with the acute respiratory distress syndrome. N Engl J Med 2006;354:1775–86.
[61] Marini JJ, Gattinoni L. Ventilatory management of acute respiratory distress syndrome: a consensus of two. Crit Care Med 2004;32:250–5.
[62] Brower RG, Morris A, MacIntyre N, et al. Effects of recruitment maneuvers in patients with acute lung injury and acute respiratory distress syndrome ventilated with high positive end-expiratory pressure. Crit Care Med 2003;31:2592–7.
[63] Villagra A, Ochagavia A, Vatua S, et al. Recruitment maneuvers during lung protective ventilation in acute respiratory distress syndrome. Am J Respir Crit Care Med 2002; 165:165–70.
[64] Michard F, Chemla D, Richard C, et al. Clinical use of respiratory changes in arterial pulse pressure to monitor the hemodynamic effects of PEEP. Am J Respir Crit Care Med 1999;159: 935–9.
[65] Kress JP, O'Connor MF, Schmidt GA. Clinical examination reliably detects intrinsic positive end-expiratory pressure in critically ill, mechanically ventilated patients. Am J Respir Crit Care Med 1999;159:290–4.
[66] Leatherman JW, Ravenscraft SA. Low measured auto-positive end-expiratory pressure during mechanical ventilation of patients with severe asthma: hidden auto-positive end-expiratory pressure. Crit Care Med 1996;24:541–6.
[67] Keenan SP, Sinuff T, Cook DJ, et al. Which patients with acute exacerbation of chronic obstructive pulmonary disease benefit from noninvasive positive-pressure ventilation? A systematic review of the literature. Ann Intern Med 2003;138:861–70.
[68] Ram FS, Picot J, Lightowler J, et al. Non-invasive positive pressure ventilation for treatment of respiratory failure due to exacerbations of chronic obstructive pulmonary disease. Cochrane Database Syst Rev 2004;1:CD004104.
[69] Anton A, Guell R, Gomez J, et al. Predicting the result of noninvasive ventilation in severe acute exacerbations of patients with chronic airflow limitation. Chest 2000;117:828–33.
[70] Antonelli M, Conti G, Bufi M, et al. Noninvasive ventilation for treatment of acute respiratory failure in patients undergoing solid organ transplantation: a randomized trial. JAMA 2000;283:235–41.
[71] Hilbert G, Gruson D, Vargas F, et al. Noninvasive ventilation in immunosuppressed patients with pulmonary infiltrates, fever, and acute respiratory failure. N Engl J Med 2001; 344:481–7.
[72] Pang D, Keenan SP, Cook DJ, et al. The effect of positive pressure airway support on mortality and the need for intubation in cardiogenic pulmonary edema: a systematic review. Chest 1998;114:1185–92.
[73] Levitt MA. A prospective, randomized trial of BiPAP in severe acute congestive heart failure. J Emerg Med 2001;21:363–9.

[74] Masip J, Betbese AJ, Paez J, et al. Non-invasive pressure support ventilation versus conventional oxygen therapy in acute cardiogenic pulmonary edema: a randomized trial. Lancet 2000;356:2126–32.

[75] Nava S, Carbone G, DiBattista N, et al. Noninvasive ventilation in cardiogenic pulmonary edema: a multicenter randomized trial. Am J Respir Crit Care Med 2003;168:1432–7.

[76] Martin TJ, Hovis JD, Costantino JP, et al. A randomized, prospective evaluation of noninvasive ventilation for acute respiratory failure. Am J Respir Crit Care Med 2000;161(3 pt 1): 807–13.

[77] Ferrer M, Esquinas A, Leon M, et al. Noninvasive ventilation in severe hypoxemic respiratory failure: a randomized clinical trial. Am J Respir Crit Care Med 2003;168:1438–44.

SURGICAL
CLINICS OF
NORTH AMERICA

Surg Clin N Am 86 (2006) 1409–1429

Ventilator-Associated Pneumonia

Jason R. Leong, DO[a],*, David T. Huang, MD, MPH[b]

[a]Department of Critical Care Medicine, University of Pittsburgh,
3550 Terrace Street, 655 Scaife Hall, Pittsburgh, PA 15261, USA
[b]Department of Emergency Medicine, University of Pittsburgh,
Pittsburgh, PA, USA

Ventilator-associated pneumonia (VAP) is a clinically and economically important hospital-acquired infection complicating the course of up to 28% of patients receiving mechanical ventilation and associated with an increase in over $40,000 in mean hospital charges per patient [1,2]. VAP is defined by the Centers for Disease Control and Prevention as pneumonia in persons who had a device to assist or control respiration continuously through a tracheostomy or by endotracheal intubation within the 48-hour period before the onset of the infection [3]. There has been difficulty defining the exact incidence of VAP primarily because of variability in diagnosis of VAP. Studies over the past 20 years estimate VAP frequencies range from 8% to 28% [1]. In one large study, Cook and colleagues [4] validated their diagnoses of VAP using five definitions of VAP and a blinded adjudication committee to determine the final outcome status of all patients with clinically suspected VAP. In this prospective cohort study of 1014 patients, 17.5% developed VAP, with an overall incidence of 14.8 cases per 1000 ventilator days. More recently, the National Nosocomial Infections Surveillance System of the Centers for Disease Control and Prevention reported that between January 2002 and June 2004, the rate of VAP in the United States ranged from 5.4 per 1000 ventilator days in major teaching medical-surgical ICUs to 15.2 per 1000 ventilator days in trauma ICUs [5]. Trauma victims may have a higher incidence of burns, severe head and neck injury, and aspiration. Each of these have been established as independent predictors of VAP, and may account for the significantly higher incidence of VAP reported in trauma ICUs [4,6]. Rello and colleagues [2] used a retrospective, matched cohort study of over 9000 patients to conclude

* Corresponding author. Legacy Health System, 1015 NW 22nd Avenue, R200, Portland, OR 97210.
   E-mail address: leongjr@yahoo.com (J.R. Leong).

0039-6109/06/$ - see front matter © 2006 Elsevier Inc. All rights reserved.
doi:10.1016/j.suc.2006.08.004   *surgical.theclinics.com*

that VAP occurred in 9.3% of patients (N = 842). Of these, more than 63% developed VAP during the first 48 hours of mechanical ventilation, 16% occurred between 48 and 96 hours, and approximately 21% were diagnosed after 96 hours of mechanical ventilation. The mean interval between intubation and identification of VAP was 3.3 ± 6.6 days.

Interestingly, the daily risk for developing VAP has been shown to decrease following the first week of mechanical ventilation. In the study by Cook and coworkers [4], VAP occurred at a rate of approximately 3% per day in the first week of mechanical ventilation, 2% per day in the second week, and 1% per day in the third week and beyond. Independent risk factors for VAP include respiratory disease (eg, chronic obstructive pulmonary disease, acute respiratory distress syndrome); cardiovascular disease; mechanical ventilation lasting ≥ 7 days; reintubation; witnessed aspiration; intrahospital patient transport; supine positioning; use of paralytic agents; burns; trauma; and central nervous system disease (eg, Glasgow Coma Score <9, head trauma) [4,7–9]. More recently, a high Abbreviated Injury Score for head and neck above >4 [10,11] was identified as an independent predictor of VAP in trauma patients with a specificity of 97% and positive predictive value of 90%. The authors noted that the need for supine positioning in patients with cervical fracture may have influenced this association [6].

Studies analyzing mortality attributed to VAP have reported conflicting results. At least four matched, cohort studies did not find any increase in mortality caused by VAP [2,12–14]. Other investigations, however, have conversely reported increased risk of death of up to 33% in patients with VAP varying based on the patient population and infecting organism [15,16]. Discrepancy between study findings may be caused by differences between factors, such as study design, affected patient populations, time elapsed to onset of pneumonia, diagnostic strategies, causative organisms, and adequacy of initial antibiotic therapy. For example, mortality associated with VAP may be higher in medical patients (perhaps because of underlying chronic disease) than in surgical patients [15]. Patients developing early onset VAP are less likely to be infected with multidrug-resistant (MDR) organisms (ie, *Pseudomonas*, *Acinetobacter*, methicillin-resistant *Staphylococcus aureus* [MRSA]) than those developing late-onset VAP. Furthermore, the prognosis for patients infected with MDR bacteria is significantly worse than those infected with fully susceptible pathogens [1,17,18]. In addition, the timely initiation of an appropriate antibiotic treatment regimen most certainly plays a significant role in survival outcome and may not have been analyzed in some trials [2,19–21].

Although debate surrounds mortality attributable to VAP, it has been consistently shown that patients with VAP are subject to increased morbidity. VAP has been associated with significant increases in length of ICU (11.7 ± 11 versus 5.6 ± 6.1 days) and hospital stay (25.5 ± 22.8 versus 14 ± 14.6 days) and increased number of days requiring mechanical ventilation (14 ± 15.5 versus 4.7 ± 7 days) [2,15,22]. Understandably, this has also translated into increased attributable costs of VAP with estimates ranging from \$12,000 to \$57,000 [2,22,23].

Pathogenesis

Pneumonia occurs when pathogens are able to invade and persist in the normally sterile lower respiratory tract and lung parenchyma. The source of the invading organism may be either endogenous (nasal carrier, sinusitis, oropharynx, trachea, gastric juice) or exogenous (health care personnel, ventilator circuit, nebulizers, endotracheal tube coated with biofilm) [24]. In patients developing VAP, the host's natural, anatomic barriers (glottis, larynx, ciliated epithelium, and mucus) are compromised by endotracheal intubation. Subglottic pooling with subsequent leakage of bacteria around the endotracheal tube cuff is the recognized primary route of bacterial entry into the lower respiratory tract [1,25]. Several factors including the patient's underlying comorbidities (eg, prior surgery, burns, immune suppression), exposure to antibiotics, medications delaying gastric emptying or increasing pH, and exposure to health care devices and personnel play a role in the bacterial colonization of the respiratory and digestive tracts [7,25]. Other potential routes of bacterial entry into the lungs, such as inoculation of ventilator circuit condensate, tracheal suctioning, fiberoptic bronchoscopy, and inhalation of contaminated aerosols, such as in-line nebulizers, are less frequently implicated. Hematogenous spread from infected catheters or bacterial translocation from the gastrointestinal tract is rare [1,24,25].

Etiology

The pathogens responsible for VAP vary according to duration of mechanical ventilation, local patterns of microorganism distribution, prior antibiotic exposure, patient comorbid conditions, and length of stay in the hospital and ICU [26–28]. Common pathogens include gram-negative bacilli, such as *Pseudomonas aeruginosa*, *Escherichia coli*, *Klebsiella pneumoniae*, *Enterobacter* species, and *Acinetobacter* species. Several studies report that approximately 35% to 60% of episodes of VAP were found to be caused by gram-negative bacilli. Gram-positive cocci have been found to play an increasingly important role in causing VAP. Kollef and coworkers [29] recently analyzed more than 4500 hospitalized patients from a large United States database with culture-positive pneumonia and found that *S aureus* was the dominant pathogen among all types of nosocomial pneumonia, and accounted for 42.5% of episodes of VAP. MRSA was found in 34.4% of the latter. Anaerobes, viruses, and fungi are not considered common causes of VAP [25].

Different microorganism patterns have been previously identified based on the time of onset of VAP. The American Thoracic Society consensus statement of 1996 classified patients developing nosocomial pneumonia as "early onset" (infection began within the first 4 days of hospitalization) or "late onset" (infection began after first 4 days of hospitalization) [30]. Designating VAP within these time frames allows clinicians to choose empiric antibiotic therapy based on epidemiologic bacterial patterns. Pathogens causing early onset VAP are most likely to include *Haemophilus influenzae*, *S pneumoniae*, methicillin-sensitive *S aureus*, or susceptible Enterobacteriaceae. Likewise, pathogens causing late-onset VAP include *P aeruginosa*, MRSA, *Acinetobacter* species, and other MDR gram-negative bacilli. In a single center study, Trouillet and coworkers [28] found that duration of mechanical ventilation ≥7 days (odds ratio = 6), antibiotic use within 15 days (odds ratio = 13.5), or use of broad-spectrum antibiotics (odds ratio = 4.1) correlated with a 57% incidence of VAP caused by potentially drug-resistant bacteria (MRSA, *P aeruginosa*, *Acinetobacter baumani*, *Stenotrophomonas maltophilia*). In contrast, in the subset of patients not mechanically ventilated for ≥7 days or not having received prior antibiotics, MRSA and *A baumani* were very rarely found, and *S maltophilia* was never found. Based on these findings, the investigators concluded that a rational approach to initial antibiotic choice could be made targeting particular pathogens based on time frame. Rello and coworkers [27] subsequently conducted a retrospective, comparative study of the microorganisms causing VAP in the ICUs of three different institutions, and contrasted their results with those of Trouillet and coworkers [28]. They found marked variability in the bacterial epidemiology of VAP across the four treatment sites. For instance, in Trouillet's ICU, most VAP caused by *A baumani* (90.9%) was found in those exposed to ≥7 days of mechanical ventilation and prior antibiotics. In contrast, Rello and coworkers [27] found that *A baumani* was the bacterial etiology in ≥50% of cases of VAP in those exposed to ≤7 days of mechanical ventilation or prior antibiotics. Rello and coworkers [27] concluded that treatment protocols based on another institution's pattern of pathogen distribution are not likely to be successful. Indeed, the causative agents for pneumonia may even differ from ICU to ICU within a single hospital [31,32].

In addition to recognizing time of onset and local bacterial epidemiologic and resistance patterns, the most recent joint consensus statement on nosocomial pneumonia from the American Thoracic Society and the Infectious Disease Society of America published in 2005 recommends patients be evaluated for being at risk for MDR organisms [25]. This latest concept recognizes that many patients are indeed at risk for MDR pathogens irrespective of elapsed time from admission to onset of infection. These patients may be classified as having "health-care associated pneumonia" if they have been admitted from a health care-associated facility (ie, nursing home, dialysis center, and so forth); recently hospitalized for greater than 2 days in the past 3 months; or received home infusion therapy [25,29].

Clinicians must also consider patient comorbidities when choosing appropriate antibiotic therapy for VAP. For instance, *S aureus* has been found to be more common in comatose or neurosurgical patients, trauma victims, and patients being treated with steroids. Patients with chronic obstructive pulmonary disease are at increased risk for *H influenzae*, *Moraxella catarrhalis*, or *Streptococcus pneumoniae* infection. Immune-compromised or immune-suppressed patients are at increased risk for opportunistic infections, such as *Candida* species and *Aspergillus fumigatus* [26].

Modifiable risk factors

Nosocomial infections are the most common complication affecting hospitalized patients. One fourth of these infections involve ICU patients, and VAP specifically has been associated as the cause of between 25% and 60% of the deaths attributed to nosocomial infections overall [7,33]. Effective strategies to prevent any nosocomial infection include appropriate hand washing or use of waterless antiseptic hand rubs; monitoring and timely removal of invasive devices (including endotracheal tubes); and microbiologic surveillance [25,33]. More specific to the prevention of VAP, identification and optimization of modifiable risk factors for VAP represents an important opportunity to reduce its development. Modifiable risk factors may be classified as nonpharmacologic and pharmacologic approaches to prevention of VAP [7,34]:

Nonpharmacologic approaches
Consider noninvasive positive pressure ventilation in select patients
Consider modified endotracheal tubes (ie, continuous aspiration of subglottic secretions, low volume/pressure cuff)
Oral preferred over nasal intubation
Minimize duration of mechanical ventilation
Minimize ventilator circuit changes
Consider early tracheotomy (risk-benefit ratio must be considered and care individualized pending further definitive investigations)
Semirecumbent body positioning
Avoid unnecessary blood transfusion (risk-benefit ratio must be considered and care individualized pending further definitive investigations)
Pharmacologic approaches
Avoid unnecessary selective digestive tract decontamination
Avoid unnecessary stress ulcer prophylaxis
Optimize glucose control

Nonpharmacologic approaches to preventing ventilator-associated pneumonia

Intubation

By definition, intubation and duration of mechanical ventilation are the primary risk factors for developing VAP. Early initiation of noninvasive positive pressure ventilation in select patients with chronic obstructive pulmonary disease and hypercapnic respiratory failure, cardiogenic pulmonary edema, or immune-compromised patients with pulmonary infiltrates and respiratory compromise can result in significant reduction in the rate of endotracheal intubation [35,36]. In a prospective, randomized trial of 64 patients with acute respiratory failure, Antonelli and coworkers [35] found more patients in the conventional ventilation group had pneumonia or sinusitis related to the endotracheal tube compared with the noninvasive positive pressure ventilation group (31% versus 3%). If intubation is required, oral intubation is encouraged over nasal intubation to reduce the incidence of sinusitis and potential for aspiration of infected nasal secretions into the lungs [7].

Endotracheal tube

Specific types of endotracheal tubes have been studied that may have a beneficial effect on the development of VAP. Efforts to reduce the volume of oropharyngeal secretions pooling and leaking around the endotracheal tube cuff into the lower respiratory tract using a specialized endotracheal tube with a dorsal lumen for intermittent drainage of subglottic secretions have shown a decrease in the incidence of VAP. There was no beneficial effect, however, on duration of mechanical ventilation, ICU length of stay, or mortality [37,38]. Other types of endotracheal tubes have been studied in a limited fashion and may have future promise in reducing the incidence of VAP. Recently, Young and coworkers [39] reported use of an endotracheal tube equipped with a low-volume, low-pressure cuff that resulted in a significant reduction in pulmonary aspiration in anesthetized and critically ill patients. Silver-coated endotracheal tubes have been shown in animal studies to inhibit the growth of *P aeruginosa* in the oropharynx-larynx and endotracheal tube [40].

Duration of mechanical ventilation

In patients that are subject to conventional mechanical ventilation, strategies should be implemented to decrease the number of days spent on the ventilator. Daily interruption of sedation has been shown to reduce the median duration of mechanical ventilation (4.9 versus 7.3 days, $P = .004$) and median ICU length of stay (6.4 versus 9.9 days, $P = .02$) [41,42]. Protocol-driven ventilator weaning strategies have been shown to reduce the use of mechanical ventilation, the rate of early reintubation, and VAP [43]. A recent survey revealed, however, that only 40% of Canadian intensivists practice daily interruption of continuous sedative or analgesic infusions [44]. Clearly, there is room for improvement.

Ventilator circuit changes

Several trials have shown that increasing the frequency of ventilator circuit changes does not affect the incidence of VAP. Condensate gathering within the circuit can, however, become contaminated and serves as bacterial reservoir that may be inadvertently inoculated into the lower respiratory tract when the patient turns or the ventilator circuit is manipulated. Use of heat and moisture exchangers coupled with monitoring and drainage of the ventilator circuit may be important measures to prevent VAP [7].

Early tracheostomy

Over the past several years, there has been controversy about the timing and role of tracheostomy in the ICU in reducing the development of VAP. The debate persists with recent findings of lower rates of VAP with early tracheostomy [45,46] and others finding no difference [47,48]. One prospective, randomized trial found the cumulative frequency of pneumonia was fivefold less common in severely ill medical ICU patients undergoing early percutaneous dilational tracheostomy (within 48 hours of intubation) versus those subject to delayed tracheostomy (at day 14–16) [45]. Improved lung mechanics and patient comfort necessitating less sedation or analgesics may have played an important role in the positive outcome. In addition, decreased number of days in the ICU (4.8 ± 1.4 versus 16.2 ± 3.8), and days requiring mechanical ventilation (7.6 ± 2 versus 17.4 ± 5.3), in conjunction with daily change of the tracheal tube inner cannula to prevent bacterial biofilm buildup, were likely significant factors in reducing the development of VAP. At the opposite end of the spectrum, Barquist and coworkers' [47] study of trauma patients undergoing tracheostomy at 8 days versus 28 days after intubation was stopped early citing no difference between the groups in any outcome variable including pneumonia rate. Comparison of these investigations is ineffectual because of the variability in defining "early" tracheostomy (2 days versus 8 days postintubation), and the vastly different patient populations that were studied. The disparities between the results of previous studies and the more recent analyses contribute to the lack of consensus of the impact of early tracheostomy on VAP [1]. Currently, further investigation is needed to define predictors of prolonged mechanical ventilation and to determine if the reported advantages [45] are applicable to less severely ill patients or patients in other ICU populations (ie, trauma, neurosurgical, and so forth) [49].

Body position

Placing mechanically ventilated patients in a semirecumbent body position (45 degrees) has been demonstrated to reduce the incidence of VAP more than 75% compared with those placed in a completely horizontal position (0 degrees) [8]. The placement of mechanically ventilated patients receiving enteral nutrition at 0 degrees of backrest elevation has been criticized as not being the standard of care, and may have played a significant role in the high rate of VAP seen in these patients (50%) [50]. Moreover, maintaining 45 degrees of semirecumbency was neither rigorously controlled for (ie, measured only once daily) nor analyzed for practicality [51]. A recent prospective, multicenter trial was conducted to assess the feasibility and effectiveness of semirecumbency in the prevention of VAP. The investigators found that the average position achieved among study centers ranged from 23 to 32 degrees, and that maintaining 45 degrees of semirecumbency was not feasible. The authors were unable to explain why the goal position of 45 degrees was not achieved; however, these data are consistent with other findings [52]. Furthermore, comparing the achieved level of elevation with 10 degrees of semirecumbency (rather than 0 degrees), there was no difference in the incidence of VAP [51].

Enteral nutrition, route of delivery

Nutritional support in the mechanically ventilated, critically ill patient is an accepted standard of care. Early enteral nutrition (within 48 hours of ICU admission) is generally regarded as beneficial in this setting with an associated 8% to 12% reduction in hospital discharge mortality [1,53]. Enteral nutrition has also been implicated as a risk factor for the development of nosocomial pneumonia, however, because of an increased risk of aspiration [8,25]. Feeding mechanically ventilated patients with a nasogastric tube in the supine position is clearly a risk factor for VAP [1,8]. In addition, the presence of a nasogastric tube has been identified as an independent risk factor for nosocomial pneumonia [54]. Studies investigating alternatives routes of enteral feeding, such as using a nasoenteric tube, have found no decrease in the incidence of VAP compared with feeding into the stomach by nasogastric tube [55]. The authors of a recent, small, preliminary investigation postulated that the presence of any type of tube may result in upper and lower esophageal sphincter dysfunction leading to an increased risk of aspiration. The investigators compared early percutaneous endoscopic gastrostomy placement ($\leq$24 hours of intubation) with feeding by nasogastric tube in patients mechanically ventilated for stroke or head injury, and showed a lower frequency of VAP (12.5% versus 44.4%) [56].

Transfusion

Transfusion practice in the ICU as it relates to VAP has received little attention [57,58]. Accumulating evidence has shown that transfusion of non-leukocyte depleted red blood cells may have an immunosuppressive effect on the recipient. Shorr and coworkers [57] conducted a secondary analysis of a large, prospective observational trial of transfusion practice in United States ICUs and found that transfusion was independently associated with VAP. Patients receiving 1 to 2 units of packed red blood cells had a nearly twofold increase in the risk of developing VAP. Indeed, fewer transfusions of packed red blood cells have been proved unharmful, and perhaps beneficial in select patient populations. Hebert and coworkers [59] conducted a randomized, prospective trial comparing a "restricted transfusion" policy that maintained hemoglobin levels between 7 and 9 g/dL compared with > 10 g/dL in patients without active bleeding or underlying cardiac disease. Patients randomized to the restricted transfusion arm received fewer packed red blood cells transfusions and experienced no adverse effect on outcome. In less severely ill patients (APACHE II scores <20, or age <55 years), mortality was improved. Although further investigation is warranted, restricting transfusion of red blood cells in select patient populations does not seem to be harmful, and may decrease the occurrence of VAP [57,58,60].

Pharmacologic approaches to preventing ventilator-associated pneumonia

Selective decontamination of the digestive tract

Attempts to prevent bacterial colonization of the oropharynx and stomach using topical or systemic antibiotics have been studied, and been a point of contention for more than 20 years [61]. Results from a prospective, controlled, randomized, unblinded trial demonstrated that selective decontamination of the digestive tract can decrease ICU and hospital mortality and colonization with resistant gram-negative bacteria. In the selective decontamination of the digestive tract group 69 (15%) patients died in the ICU compared with 107 (23%) in the control group (P = .002). Hospital mortality was lower in the selective decontamination of the digestive tract groups than in the control group (113 [24%] versus 146 [31%], P = .02) [62]. Conclusions from meta-analysis of selective decontamination of the digestive tract stated that using topical and systemic antibiotics could result in significant reductions in the incidence of VAP and reductions in mortality in critically ill surgical patients [63]. Despite this evidence, however, selective decontamination of the digestive tract has not been incorporated routinely in North America. Concerns include the quality of the available data on selective decontamination of the digestive tract; the lack of one single, best selective decontamination of the digestive tract regimen; and the inherently increased risk of promoting antibiotic resistance [25,64]. At this time, absent further definitive evidence, routine selective decontamination of the digestive tract is discouraged, but may benefit certain patient populations more than others (ie, surgical and trauma patients may benefit more than medical ICU patients who are more likely to enter the ICU already colonized) [7,25,64].

Stress ulcer prophylaxis

Patients requiring mechanical ventilation are at increased risk for developing stress ulcers, and clinically significant bleeding may ensue. Prophylaxis with histamine H_2-blockers has been shown to prevent such bleeding, however, perhaps at the expense of increased gastric bacterial colonization because of alkalinization of the gastric pH. Cook and coworkers [65] random-ized 1200 mechanically ventilated patients to either ranitidine or the cytopro-tective agent, sucralfate. Sucralfate does not alter gastric pH, and has been reported to be associated with lower incidence of VAP. The investigators found patients given ranitidine had a significantly lower risk of gastrointesti-nal bleeding, and no significant difference in the incidence of pneumonia. No-tably, although statistically insignificant, sucralfate did seem to have a small protective effect against pneumonia. As with all clinical decision making, if stress ulcer prophylaxis is indicated, the risk-to-benefit ratio of either medica-tion should be considered before treatment.

Intensive insulin therapy

Intensive insulin therapy in critically ill patients has received a great deal of attention in recent years. Van den Berghe and coworkers [66] titrated in-sulin therapy to achieve and maintain blood glucose levels ≤110 mg/dL and showed a significant reduction in morbidity and mortality in SICU patients. Intensive insulin therapy reduced antibiotic use, episodes of septicemia, and length of mechanical ventilation and stay in the ICU. The same primary in-vestigators recently published data on intensive insulin therapy in MICU patients. For those remaining in the ICU >3 days, there was decreased mor-bidity including less newly acquired renal injury, and earlier weaning from mechanical ventilation [67]. Aggressive treatment of hyperglycemia, with attention toward avoiding hypoglycemia, is recommended in critically ill patients to reduce antibiotic use, septic episodes, ICU length of stay, and duration of mechanical ventilation.

Approach to diagnosis

VAP is a common infection in the ICU. Despite this, the diagnosis of VAP remains challenging and there is a lack of diagnostic standardization. One of the major stumbling blocks to improving diagnosis of VAP is that there is no diagnostic gold standard for diagnostic techniques against which to compare [25]. Traditionally, postmortem histopathologic examination of lung tissue has been considered the gold standard used to confirm the pres-ence of pneumonia. A recent review of postmortem studies used to evaluate diagnostic techniques for VAP concluded, however, that comparison between techniques is complicated because the studies may have failed to recognize several important factors, such as presence of underlying lung dis-ease, duration of mechanical ventilation, prior use of antibiotics, and timing of postmortem analysis, which may have affected the relationship between histology and bacteriology in VAP [68].

Numerous studies evaluating two diagnostic strategies, a clinical and an invasive-quantitative approach, have been done. Although a standard diagnostic approach has yet to be agreed on, the optimal diagnostic algorithm should take into account certain factors (Box 1) [25].

Clinically, a presumptive diagnosis of VAP is often made when a patient develops a new radiographic infiltrate in the setting of fever, leukocytosis, and purulent tracheal secretions. Gram staining and nonquantitative cultures of endotracheal aspirate or sputum are often used to define the bacterial etiology and direct initial antibiotic therapy. Use of semiquantitative cultures (reported as light, moderate, or heavy growth) of endotracheal aspirates can be used, but are not as reliable as quantitative cultures to define the presence of pneumonia and the need for antibiotics [69]. Use of clinical criteria alone to diagnose pneumonia in the mechanically ventilated patient has been criticized as being overly sensitive and poorly specific [25,69] leading to overestimation of the incidence of VAP because noninfectious processes mimicking it are included [70]. For instance, pulmonary infiltrates on chest radiograph, such as atelectasis, alveolar hemorrhage, pulmonary infarction, congestive heart failure, and the fibroproliferative phase of acute respiratory distress syndrome, may all be misinterpreted as pneumonia [68]. Further, the nonspecific systemic signs of infection, such as fever, tachycardia, or leukocytosis, can be caused by any inflammatory condition leading to a release of cytokines, such as trauma or recent surgery. Although the clinical strategy places weight on prompt antibiotic therapy to minimize mortality, antibiotic use can be significantly greater than when using an invasive-quantitative strategy [70]. Singh and coworkers [71] conducted a randomized, controlled trial of an antibiotic management strategy that incorporated a modified clinical pulmonary infections score (CPIS) to minimize unnecessary antibiotic use in patients at low risk for VAP (CPIS ≤6). All patients clinically suspected of having VAP were given at least 3 days of empiric antibiotic (ciprofloxacin). In patients randomized to the experimental arm, the antibiotic was discontinued if the CPIS remained ≤6 at Day 3. In the control arm, antibiotic use in patients with a CPIS ≤6 on Day 3 was left to the discretion of the treating physician. Antibiotics were continued an average of 9.8 days in the latter. There was no adverse effect on length of stay or mortality in the experimental group. This approach demonstrated that discontinuing antibiotics at Day 3 in those with a low

---

Box 1. Criteria for optimal diagnostic algorithm

- Accurately identifying patients with pulmonary infection
- Timely collection of appropriate cultures
- Promoting early initiation of effective antibiotic therapy while allowing for appropriate streamlining or de-escalation of therapy
- Identifying patients with extrapulmonary sources of infection

likelihood of VAP (as determined by a CPIS ≤6) safely led to substantially lower antimicrobial therapy costs ($6482 versus $16,004); antimicrobial resistance; and superinfections (13% versus 33%).

Fabregas and coworkers [72] used the diagnostic standard of histology plus positive microbiologic cultures of immediate postmortem lung samples to compare a clinical approach to invasive sampling techniques, and found that combining the presence of new or worsening infiltrates on chest radiograph with at least two of three clinical signs of infection (fever, leukocytosis or leukopenia, and purulent secretions) led to a "reasonable" diagnosis of VAP (sensitivity 69%, specificity 75%). In addition, clinical criteria had comparable diagnostic value with invasive sampling techniques. Still, this approach is associated with a high rate of false-negative (30%–35%) and false-positive (20%–25%) diagnoses [1]. As such, the suboptimal sensitivity and specificity of the clinical approach has led some to favor a quantitative bacteriologic strategy.

To minimize antibiotic overtreatment of VAP and guide management, the quantitative approach uses quantitative cultures of lower respiratory tract secretions. Specimens are gathered by bronchoalveolar lavage (BAL) or protected specimen brush (PSB) with or without fiberoptic bronchoscopy (FOB) to define the presence of pneumonia and the microbiologic etiology. A culture growth threshold must be met to diagnose VAP using this technique (BAL $>10^4$ cfu/mL, PSB $>10^3$ cfu/mL) [25,70]. Growth below the threshold is generally considered colonization or contamination. This approach seems more objective and is a potentially attractive alternative to the more subjective clinical approach. The quantitative information can be used to identify the bacterial etiology, and to tailor or discontinue antibiotics based on culture and sensitivity results. Fagon and coworkers [70] compared an invasive management strategy (quantitative) with a noninvasive (clinical) strategy. The invasive, quantitative strategy used FOB to gather BAL and PSB samples for direct microscopic examination and used the quantitative culture results to adjust therapy (treatment was discontinued when results were negative, and use of antibiotics with narrower spectra of activity was based on identification of and susceptibility-test results for pathogens cultured at significant concentrations). Decisions made using the noninvasive, clinical strategy were based on clinical evaluation; immediate Gram staining of sputum; and results of qualitative endotracheal aspirate culture (treatment was withheld when culture was negative). The investigators concluded that compared with the clinical (noninvasive) strategy, the invasive (quantitative) management strategy improved early survival at 14 days (16.2% versus 25.8%) and resulted in fewer early organ failures and more antibiotic-free days at 28 days (11.5 ± 9 versus 7.5 ± 7.6) [70]. In addition, the authors postulated a negative BAL or PSB specimen (in the absence of antibiotic use within the past 72 hours) may help to direct attention toward timely identification of extrapulmonary sites of infection.

A recently conducted meta-analysis of the randomized, controlled trials of invasive diagnostic strategies (including the study by Fagon and coworkers [70]) in suspected VAP confirmed that use of invasive cultures did indeed consistently result in decreased antibiotic use [73]. Invasive strategies did not result in a reduction in mortality, however, as Fagon and coworkers [70] had found. The authors of the meta-analysis reasoned that invasive, quantitative sampling seems to have a significant impact on subsequent antibiotic therapy and use. It does not directly affect the initial antibiotic prescription, however, which if inadequate or delayed has been shown to increase the risk for death up to twofold [19,21,74]. Although the impact of quantitative cultures on patient outcome remains controversial, the best available evidence demonstrates that this strategy results in less antibiotic use thereby minimizing the emergence of resistant pathogens [1].

The major disadvantages of the invasive, quantitative approach using FOB to obtain a BAL or PSB specimen include the potential for false-negative results [72] and the difficulty and cost associated with performing routine bronchoscopy in patients suspected of having VAP. Strict use of the quantitative approach may lead to failure to treat a particular patient or a specific pathogen based on a false-negative culture result. To decrease the number of false-negative culture results (for both invasive and noninvasively collected specimens), samples should be obtained before administration of antibiotics. When a patient is unstable and cultures cannot readily be obtained or are negative, however, empiric antibiotics should not be withheld or discontinued.

Both endotracheal aspirate and nonbronchoscopic protected specimens from the lower respiratory tract obtained using blinded protected telescopic catheters (or mini-BAL) are less expensive and labor intensive alternatives to FOB (because nurses and respiratory therapists can be trained to use the protected telescopic catheters to obtain quantitative cultures). Brun-Buisson and coworkers [69] conducted a prospective observational study that examined the diagnostic accuracy of these techniques when compared with BAL collected by FOB. The authors concluded that despite widespread use and high sensitivity, qualitative cultures gathered by endotracheal aspirate are nonspecific for VAP when compared with bronchoscopic BAL. Semiquantitative cultures by endotracheal aspirate significantly improved the specificity (82%) but decreased sensitivity (77%). By comparison, blinded protected telescopic catheter quantitative specimens demonstrated suboptimal sensitivity (77%) and high specificity (97%). Mentec and colleagues [75] similarly evaluated these techniques in a prospective, multicenter study and also found the specificity of blinded protected telescopic catheters to be high (90%–100%). Interestingly, the authors also found that the sensitivity could be increased (84%–86%) when visible secretions were expelled from the catheter at the time of collection. Further, when visible secretions were expelled, the performance of this technique closely approximated that of bronchoscopic BAL. Although there is a lack of a universally accepted diagnostic reference test, current evidence suggests that quantitative or semiquantitative cultures of lower respiratory tract specimens should be obtained. Non-bronchoscopic techniques, such as the blinded protected telescopic catheters, are less costly, more readily available, and have been shown to be practical alternatives to bronchoscopic BAL [69,75].

Using elements of both the clinical and quantitative diagnostic approaches to VAP in a complementary fashion may achieve the goals of consistently identifying patients with VAP and promoting early and effective antibiotic treatment while limiting overuse (Fig. 1).

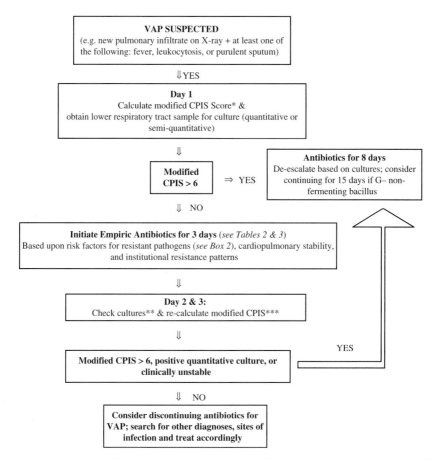

Fig. 1. Proposed algorithm summarizing approach to diagnosis and antibiotic treatment of ventilator-associated pneumonia. May not apply to immune-suppressed or -compromised patients. CPIS, clinical pulmonary infection score; VAP, ventilator-associated pneumonia.*Modified CPIS [71]. **If using quantitative cultures, growth threshold is bronchoalveolar lavage or mini bronchoalveolar lavage $> 10^4$ cfu/mL, PSB $> 10^3$ cfu/mL. Growth below the threshold is generally considered colonization or contamination [25,70]. ***If using semiquantitative cultures, the results are incorporated into the CPIS score.

Initial treatment

The choice of initial empiric antibiotics for clinically suspected VAP is influenced by the patient's risk factors for being infected with MDR pathogens (Box 2) [25], cardiopulmonary stability, institutional bacterial resistance patterns, and which if any antibiotics the patient has received recently (Tables 1 and 2) [1,25,27,28].

If a patient has been recently exposed to an antibiotic for another infection and subsequently develops VAP, the initial empiric therapy should include an agent from another antibiotic class [74,76]. Most treatment failures have been associated with inadequate initial antibiotics that fail to cover MDR pathogens adequately [19]. Once the appropriate empiric antibiotic regimen has been chosen, it is imperative to administer the antibiotics without delay [21,74]. Iregui and coworkers [19] found that delayed administration (>24 hours) of appropriate antibiotics has been associated with excess mortality. With this in mind, antibiotics must not be delayed for the sake of gathering culture specimens particularly if the patient is unstable.

De-escalation and duration of treatment

De-escalation of initial empiric, broad-spectrum antibiotic treatment involves streamlining or narrowing antibiotic therapy based on results of lower respiratory tract culture and sensitivity. For example, if initial therapy was directed at MDR pathogens, and a properly obtained culture (gathered in the absence of antibiotic use within the 72 hours prior) reveals no evidence of these pathogens, then therapy can be de-escalated to target the cultured organism. A de-escalation strategy was recently evaluated in a prospective, observational trial [20]. Culture specimens were gathered using either FOB with PSB or BAL or quantitative tracheal aspirate in 115 patients clinically suspected of having VAP. Prescription of initial

---

Box 2. Risk factors for multidrug-resistant pathogens

- Subject to antibiotics in the preceding 90 days
- Currently hospitalized for 5 or more days, or have been hospitalized >2 days in past 90 days
- There is high degree of community or institutional antibiotic resistance
- Resident of a nursing home or extended care facility
- Receiving home infusion therapy or wound care
- Receiving chronic dialysis within 30 days
- Family member known to be infected with MDR pathogen
- Immune suppressed or compromised

Table 1
Initial empiric antibiotic therapy for ventilator-associated pneumonia in patients without
known risk factors for multidrug-resistant pathogens, early onset, and any disease severity

Potential pathogen	Recommended antibiotic
Streptococcus pneumoniae[a]	Ceftriaxone
Haemophilus influenzae	or
Methicillin-sensitive Staphylococcus aureus	Levofloxacin, moxifloxacin, or ciprofloxacin
Antibiotic-sensitive enteric gram-negative bacilli	or
Escherichia coli	Ampicillin-sulbactam
Klebsiella pneumoniae	or
Enterobacter species	Ertapenem
Proteus species	
Serratia marcescens	

[a] Penicillin and multidrug-resistant S pneumoniae is increasing in frequency; levofloxacin
and moxifloxacin are preferred agents over ciprofloxacin.

Modified from Guidelines for the management of adults with hospital-acquired, ventilator-
associated, and healthcare-associated pneumonia. Am J Respir Crit Care Med 2005;171:388–
416; with permission.

empiric antibiotics was based on an established protocol. De-escalation was
performed in 40.7% of patients with early onset VAP (developed within 7
days of intubation) compared with 12.5% of patients with late-onset VAP
(developed after 7 days of intubation). De-escalation was implemented in
2.7% of episodes with potentially MDR pathogens (ie, nonfermenting
gram-negative bacilli or MRSA) compared with 49.3% among remaining
pathogens. The investigators concluded that de-escalation is less likely to
occur or be possible in the presence of nonfermenting gram-negative bacilli
or late-onset VAP.

Ongoing clinical and radiographic assessment is important while awaiting
culture results that typically take 2 to 3 days to result. For those with negative
cultures, de-escalation may not be possible. If these patients are unstable and
continue to display signs of infection, attention should be directed at extrapulmonary sites of infection with antibiotics accordingly adjusted. Clinically
improving or stable patients with negative cultures may have antibiotics
safely discontinued. Those considered at low risk for VAP (CPIS ≤6) may
be able to have antibiotics safely stopped at Day 3 with the benefit of substantially reducing antibiotic use, cost, and antibiotic resistance [71].

VAP carries a substantial cost in terms of morbidity and mortality. As
such, clinicians are justifiably unwilling to miss or undertreat such a threat-
ening infection. The traditional recommended duration of antibiotic therapy
for VAP has been 14 to 21 days [30]. The rationale behind this recommendation has been based on the risk of relapse after shorter courses of antibiotics. In recent years, this standard duration of therapy has been challenged
[71,77]. Chastre and colleagues [77] conducted a large (N = 401), prospective, randomized, multicenter study to determine whether 8 days of

Table 2
Initial empiric therapy for ventilator-associated pneumonia in patients with risk factors for multidrug-resistant pathogens, late-onset, and all disease severity

Potential pathogens	Recommended combination antibiotic therapy
Pathogens listed in Table 1, and MDR pathogens *Pseudomonas aeruginosa* *Klebsiella pneumoniae (ESBL)*[a] *Acinetobacter* species	Antipseudomonal cephalosporin (cefepime or ceftazidime) or Antipseudomonal carbapenem (imipenem or meropenem) or β-lactam/β-lactamase inhibitor (piperacillin-tazobactam) plus Antipseudomonal fluoroquinolone[a] (ciprofloxacin or levofloxacin) or Aminoglycoside (amikacin, gentamycin or tobramycin) plus
Methicillin-resistant *Staphylococcus aureus*[b] *Legionella pneumophila*[a]	Linezolid or vancomycin[b]

Abbreviations: ESBL, extended-spectrum β-lactamase; MDR, multidrug resistant.

[a] A carbapenem is recommended if an ESBL-producing strain, such as *K pneumoniae*, or an *Acinetobacter* species is suspected. A fluoroquinolone or macrolide (eg, azithromycin) should be included in the combination regimen instead of an aminoglycoside if *L pneumophila* is suspected.

[b] If methicillin-resistant *s aureus* is suspected or there is a high local incidence.

Modified from Guidelines for the management of adults with hospital-acquired, ventilator-associated, and healthcare-associated pneumonia. Am J Respir Crit Care Med 2005;171:388–416; with permission.

treatment is as effective as 15 days in patients with microbiologically (quantitatively) proved VAP. The primary outcome measures included death from any cause, pulmonary infection recurrence, and antibiotic-free days. The authors found that there was no significant difference in 60-day mortality, and those in the experimental arm enjoyed 50% more antibiotic-free days. The pulmonary infection recurrence rate in patients with VAP caused by nonfermenting gram-negative bacilli (eg, *P aeruginosa*, *Acinetobacter* sp, *Stenotrophomonas*) was higher, however, for those in the experimental arm than in those treated for 15 days (40.6% versus 25.4%). Despite this, the authors maintain that an 8-day regimen is safe for all patients because mortality and other unfavorable outcomes were unaffected by this increased recurrence rate. Further, they advocate ongoing clinical suspicion for recurrence of infection be maintained after antibiotics are discontinued. The investigators concluded that in non–immune-suppressed or -compromised patients with VAP, 8 days were not inferior to 15 days of antibiotic therapy in terms of 60-day mortality, and resulted in significantly more antibiotic-free days.

In addition, MDR pathogens emerged more frequently in those treated for 15 days, providing more evidence that indiscriminate antibiotic use leads to increased resistance (see Fig. 1).

Summary

VAP is a significant nosocomial infection affecting up to one third of patients requiring mechanical ventilation, and is associated with significant attributable morbidity and mortality. Several simple and effective preventive measures (ie, daily interruption of sedation, body positioning, and so forth) have been identified, but are suboptimally implemented. Clinicians should have a heightened clinical suspicion for VAP with diagnostic goals focusing on accuracy, gathering of lower respiratory tract (quantitative or semiquantitative) culture, and appropriate and timely initial antibiotic therapy.

As with all significant infections, early and adequate antibiotic therapy is important to optimize the management of patients with VAP. The incidence and etiologic patterns of the major pathogens (especially MDR bacteria) causing VAP must be taken into account when making empiric antibiotic therapy choices. Subsequent de-escalation and prescription of an appropriate duration of therapy guided by clinical response and culture results may lead to decreased morbidity and future antibiotic resistance.

References

[1] Chastre J, Fagon JY. Ventilator-associated pneumonia. Am J Respir Crit Care Med 2002; 165:867–903.

[2] Rello J, Ollendorf DA, Oster G, et al. Epidemiology and outcomes of ventilator-associated pneumonia in a large US database. Chest 2002;122:2115–21.

[3] Mayhall CG. Ventilator-associated pneumonia or not? Contemporary diagnosis. Emerg Infect Dis 2006;200–4.

[4] Cook DJ, Walter SD, Cook RJ, et al. Incidence of and risk factors for ventilator-associated pneumonia in critically ill patients. Ann Intern Med 1998;129:433–40.

[5] NNIS System. National Nosocomial Infections Surveillance (NNIS) Systems Report. Data summary from January 1992 through June 2004.

[6] Cavalcanti M, Ferrer M, Ferrer R, et al. Risk and prognostic factors of ventilator-associated pneumonia in trauma patients. Crit Care Med 2006;34:1067–72.

[7] Kollef MH. Prevention of hospital-associated pneumonia and ventilator-associated pneumonia. Crit Care Med 2004;32:1396–405.

[8] Drakulovic MB, Torres A, Bauer TT, et al. Supine body position as a risk factor for nosocomial pneumonia in mechanically ventilated patients: a randomised trial. Lancet 1999;354: 1851–8.

[9] Bercault N, Wolf M, Runge I, et al. Intrahospital transport of critically ill ventilated patients: a risk factor for ventilator-associated pneumonia–a matched cohort study. Crit Care Med 2005;33:2471–8.

[10] Cooke RS, McNicholl BP, Byrnes DP. Use of the Injury Severity Score in head injury. Injury 1995;26:399–400.

[11] Baker SP, O'Neill B, Haddon W Jr, et al. The injury severity score: a method for describing patients with multiple injuries and evaluating emergency care. J Trauma 1974;14:187–96.

[12] Bregeon F, Ciais V, Carret V, et al. Is ventilator-associated pneumonia an independent risk factor for death? Anesthesiology 2001;94:554–60.

[13] Papazian L, Bregeon F, Thirion X, et al. Effect of ventilator-associated pneumonia on mortality and morbidity. Am J Respir Crit Care Med 1996;154:91–7.

[14] Baker AM, Meredith JW, Haponik EF. Pneumonia in intubated trauma patients: microbiology and outcomes. Am J Respir Crit Care Med 1996;153:343–9.

[15] Heyland DK, Cook DJ, Griffith L, et al. The attributable morbidity and mortality of ventilator-associated pneumonia in the critically ill patient. The Canadian Critical Trials Group. Am J Respir Crit Care Med 1999;159(4 Pt 1):1249–56.

[16] Fagon JY, Chastre J, Vuagnat A, et al. Nosocomial pneumonia and mortality among patients in intensive care units. JAMA 1996;275:866–9.

[17] Rello J, Jubert P, Valles J, et al. Evaluation of outcome for intubated patients with pneumonia due to Pseudomonas aeruginosa. Clin Infect Dis 1996;23:973–8.

[18] Rello J, Torres A, Ricart M, et al. Ventilator-associated pneumonia by Staphylococcus aureus. Comparison of methicillin-resistant and methicillin-sensitive episodes. Am J Respir Crit Care Med 1994;150(6 Pt 1):1545–9.

[19] Iregui M, Ward S, Sherman G, et al. Clinical importance of delays in the initiation of appropriate antibiotic treatment for ventilator-associated pneumonia. Chest 2002;122:262–8.

[20] Rello J, Vidaur L, Sandiumenge A, et al. De-escalation therapy in ventilator-associated pneumonia. Crit Care Med 2004;32:2183–90.

[21] Luna CM, Aruj P, Niederman MS, et al. Appropriateness and delay to initiate therapy in ventilator-associated pneumonia. Eur Respir J 2006;27:158–64.

[22] Warren DK, Shukla SJ, Olsen MA, et al. Outcome and attributable cost of ventilator-associated pneumonia among intensive care unit patients in a suburban medical center. Crit Care Med 2003;31:1312–7.

[23] Cocanour CS, Ostrosky-Zeichner L, Peninger M, et al. Cost of a ventilator-associated pneumonia in a shock trauma intensive care unit. Surg Infect (Larchmt) 2005;6:65–72.

[24] Alcon A, Fabregas N, Torres A. Hospital-acquired pneumonia: etiologic considerations. Infect Dis Clin North Am 2003;17:679–95.

[25] Guidelines for the management of adults with hospital-acquired, ventilator-associated, and healthcare-associated pneumonia. Am J Respir Crit Care Med 2005;171:388–416.

[26] Rello J, Diaz E, Rodriguez A. Etiology of ventilator-associated pneumonia. Clin Chest Med 2005;26:87–95.

[27] Rello J, Sa-Borges M, Correa H, et al. Variations in etiology of ventilator-associated pneumonia across four treatment sites: implications for antimicrobial prescribing practices. Am J Respir Crit Care Med 1999;160:608–13.

[28] Trouillet JL, Chastre J, Vuagnat A, et al. Ventilator-associated pneumonia caused by potentially drug-resistant bacteria. Am J Respir Crit Care Med 1998;157:531–9.

[29] Kollef MH, Shorr A, Tabak YP, et al. Epidemiology and outcomes of health-care-associated pneumonia: results from a large US database of culture-positive pneumonia. Chest 2005;128: 3854–62.

[30] Hospital-acquired pneumonia in adults: diagnosis, assessment of severity, initial antimicrobial therapy, and preventive strategies. A consensus statement, American Thoracic Society, November 1995. Am J Respir Crit Care Med 1996;153:1711–25.

[31] Namias N, Samiian L, Nino D, et al. Incidence and susceptibility of pathogenic bacteria vary between intensive care units within a single hospital: implications for empiric antibiotic strategies. J Trauma 2000;49:638–45.

[32] White RL, Friedrich LV, Mihm LB, et al. Assessment of the relationship between antimicrobial usage and susceptibility: differences between the hospital and specific patient-care areas. Clin Infect Dis 2000;31:16–23.

[33] Burke JP. Infection control: a problem for patient safety. N Engl J Med 2003;348:651–6.

[34] Kollef MH. The prevention of ventilator-associated pneumonia. N Engl J Med 1999;340: 627–34.

[35] Antonelli M, Conti G, Rocco M, et al. A comparison of noninvasive positive-pressure ventilation and conventional mechanical ventilation in patients with acute respiratory failure. N Engl J Med 1998;339:429–35.

[36] Hilbert G, Gruson D, Vargas F, et al. Noninvasive ventilation in immunosuppressed patients with pulmonary infiltrates, fever, and acute respiratory failure. N Engl J Med 2001; 344:481–7.

[37] Kollef MH, Skubas NJ, Sundt TM. A randomized clinical trial of continuous aspiration of subglottic secretions in cardiac surgery patients. Chest 1999;116:1339–46.

[38] Smulders K, van der HH, Weers-Pothoff I, et al. A randomized clinical trial of intermittent subglottic secretion drainage in patients receiving mechanical ventilation. Chest 2002;121: 858–62.

[39] Young PJ, Pakeerathan S, Blunt MC, et al. A low-volume, low-pressure tracheal tube cuff reduces pulmonary aspiration. Crit Care Med 2006;34:632–9.

[40] Berra L, De Marchi L, Yu ZX, et al. Endotracheal tubes coated with antiseptics decrease bacterial colonization of the ventilator circuits, lungs, and endotracheal tube. Anesthesiology 2004;100:1446–56.

[41] Kress JP, Pohlman AS, O'Connor MF, et al. Daily interruption of sedative infusions in critically ill patients undergoing mechanical ventilation. N Engl J Med 2000;342:1471–7.

[42] Schweickert WD, Gehlbach BK, Pohlman AS, et al. Daily interruption of sedative infusions and complications of critical illness in mechanically ventilated patients. Crit Care Med 2004; 32:1272–6.

[43] Dries DJ, McGonigal MD, Malian MS, et al. Protocol-driven ventilator weaning reduces use of mechanical ventilation, rate of early reintubation, and ventilator-associated pneumonia. J Trauma 2004;56:943–51.

[44] Mehta S, Burry L, Fischer S, et al. Canadian survey of the use of sedatives, analgesics, and neuromuscular blocking agents in critically ill patients. Crit Care Med 2006;34:374–80.

[45] Rumbak MJ, Newton M, Truncale T, et al. A prospective, randomized, study comparing early percutaneous dilational tracheostomy to prolonged translaryngeal intubation (delayed tracheostomy) in critically ill medical patients. Crit Care Med 2004;32:1689–94.

[46] Moller MG, Slaikeu JD, Bonelli P, et al. Early tracheostomy versus late tracheostomy in the surgical intensive care unit. Am J Surg 2005;189:293–6.

[47] Barquist ES, Amortegui J, Hallal A, et al. Tracheostomy in ventilator dependent trauma patients: a prospective, randomized intention-to-treat study. J Trauma 2006;60:91–7.

[48] Bouderka MA, Fakhir B, Bouaggad A, et al. Early tracheostomy versus prolonged endotracheal intubation in severe head injury. J Trauma 2004;57:251–4.

[49] Lee JC, Fink MP. Early percutaneous dilatational tracheostomy leads to improved outcomes in critically ill medical patients as compared to delayed tracheostomy. Crit Care 2005;9:E12.

[50] Combes A. Backrest elevation for the prevention of ventilator-associated pneumonia: back to the real world? Crit Care Med 2006;34:559–61.

[51] van Nieuwenhoven CA, Vandenbroucke-Grauls C, van Tiel FH, et al. Feasibility and effects of the semirecumbent position to prevent ventilator-associated pneumonia: a randomized study. Crit Care Med 2006;34:396–402.

[52] Heyland DK, Cook DJ, Dodek PM. Prevention of ventilator-associated pneumonia: current practice in Canadian intensive care units. J Crit Care 2002;17:161–7.

[53] Doig GS, Simpson F. Early enteral nutrition in the critically ill: do we need more evidence or better evidence? Curr Opin Crit Care 2006;12:126–30.

[54] Joshi N, Localio AR, Hamory BH. A predictive risk index for nosocomial pneumonia in the intensive care unit. Am J Med 1992;93:135–42.

[55] Kearns PJ, Chin D, Mueller L, et al. The incidence of ventilator-associated pneumonia and success in nutrient delivery with gastric versus small intestinal feeding: a randomized clinical trial. Crit Care Med 2000;28:1742–6.

[56] Kostadima E, Kaditis AG, Alexopoulos EI, et al. Early gastrostomy reduces the rate of ventilator-associated pneumonia in stroke or head injury patients. Eur Respir J 2005;26:106–11.

[57] Shorr AF, Duh MS, Kelly KM, et al. Red blood cell transfusion and ventilator-associated pneumonia: a potential link? Crit Care Med 2004;32:666–74.

[58] Shorr AF, Kollef MH. Ventilator-associated pneumonia: insights from recent clinical trials. Chest 2005;128(Suppl 2):583S–91S.

[59] Hebert PC, Wells G, Blajchman MA, et al. A multicenter, randomized, controlled clinical trial of transfusion requirements in critical care. Transfusion Requirements in Critical Care Investigators, Canadian Critical Care Trials Group. N Engl J Med 1999;340:409–17.

[60] Croce MA, Tolley EA, Claridge JA, et al. Transfusions result in pulmonary morbidity and death after a moderate degree of injury. J Trauma 2005;59:19–23.

[61] Bonten MJ, Krueger WA. Selective decontamination of the digestive tract: cumulating evidence, at last? Semin Respir Crit Care Med 2006;27:18–22.

[62] de Jonge E, Schultz MJ, Spanjaard L, et al. Effects of selective decontamination of digestive tract on mortality and acquisition of resistant bacteria in intensive care: a randomised controlled trial. Lancet 2003;362:1011–6.

[63] Nathens AB, Marshall JC. Selective decontamination of the digestive tract in surgical patients: a systematic review of the evidence. Arch Surg 1999;134:170–6.

[64] Vincent JL. Selective digestive decontamination: for everyone, everywhere? Lancet 2003;362:1006–7.

[65] Cook D, Guyatt G, Marshall J, et al. A comparison of sucralfate and ranitidine for the prevention of upper gastrointestinal bleeding in patients requiring mechanical ventilation. Canadian Critical Care Trials Group. N Engl J Med 1998;338:791–7.

[66] Van den Berghe BG, Wouters P, Weekers F, et al. Intensive insulin therapy in the critically ill patients. N Engl J Med 2001;345:1359–67.

[67] Van den Berghe BG, Wilmer A, Hermans G, et al. Intensive insulin therapy in the medical ICU. N Engl J Med 2006;354:449–61.

[68] Nseir S, Marquette CH. Diagnosis of hospital-acquired pneumonia: postmortem studies. Infect Dis Clin North Am 2003;17:707–16.

[69] Brun-Buisson C, Fartoukh M, Lechapt E, et al. Contribution of blinded, protected quantitative specimens to the diagnostic and therapeutic management of ventilator-associated pneumonia. Chest 2005;128:533–44.

[70] Fagon JY, Chastre J, Wolff M, et al. Invasive and noninvasive strategies for management of suspected ventilator-associated pneumonia: a randomized trial. Ann Intern Med 2000;132:621–30.

[71] Singh N, Rogers P, Atwood CW, et al. Short-course empiric antibiotic therapy for patients with pulmonary infiltrates in the intensive care unit: a proposed solution for indiscriminate antibiotic prescription. Am J Respir Crit Care Med 2000;162(2 Pt 1):505–11.

[72] Fabregas N, Ewig S, Torres A, et al. Clinical diagnosis of ventilator associated pneumonia revisited: comparative validation using immediate post-mortem lung biopsies. Thorax 1999;54:867–73.

[73] Shorr AF, Sherner JH, Jackson WL, et al. Invasive approaches to the diagnosis of ventilator-associated pneumonia: a meta-analysis. Crit Care Med 2005;33:46–53.

[74] Kollef MH, Ward S. The influence of mini-BAL cultures on patient outcomes: implications for the antibiotic management of ventilator-associated pneumonia. Chest 1998;113:412–20.

[75] Mentec H, May-Michelangeli L, Rabbat A, et al. Blind and bronchoscopic sampling methods in suspected ventilator-associated pneumonia: a multicentre prospective study. Intensive Care Med 2004;30:1319–26.

[76] Rello J, Ausina V, Ricart M, et al. Impact of previous antimicrobial therapy on the etiology and outcome of ventilator-associated pneumonia. Chest 1993;104:1230–5.

[77] Chastre J, Wolff M, Fagon JY, et al. Comparison of 8 vs 15 days of antibiotic therapy for ventilator-associated pneumonia in adults: a randomized trial. JAMA 2003;290:2588–98.

ELSEVIER
SAUNDERS

SURGICAL
CLINICS OF
NORTH AMERICA

Surg Clin N Am 86 (2006) 1431–1456

Practical Issues of Hemodynamic Monitoring at the Bedside

Patricio M. Polanco, MD[a],
Michael R. Pinsky, MD, CM, Dr hc[b],*

[a]*Division of Trauma, Department of Surgery, University of Pittsburgh School of Medicine, F1275 Scaife Hall, 3550 Terrace Street, Pittsburgh, PA 15261, USA*
[b]*Department of Critical Care Medicine, University of Pittsburgh School of Medicine, 606 Scaife Hall, 3550 Terrace Street, Pittsburgh, PA 15261, USA*

The hemodynamic monitoring of a surgical patient acquires a major relevance in high-risk patients and those suffering from surgical diseases associated with hemodynamic instability, such as hemorrhagic or septic shock; however, all surgical patients require the monitoring and evaluation, and sometimes benefit from optimizing their hemodynamic status. Therefore, all surgeons should have a basic understanding of the principles, indications, and therapeutic implications of hemodynamic monitoring.

Rationale for hemodynamic monitoring

The arguments to defend the use of specific types of monitoring techniques can be roughly grouped into three levels based on their level of validation [1]. At the basic level, the specific monitoring technique can be defended based on historical controls. At this level, prior experience using similar monitoring was traditionally used and presumed to be beneficial. The mechanism by which the benefit is achieved need not be understood. The second level of defense comes through an understanding of the pathophysiology of the process being treated. This physiological argument can be stated as "knowledge of how a disease process creates its effect and preventing the process from altering measured bodily functions should prevent the disease process from progressing or injuring remote physiological functions." Most of the rationale for

This work was supported by Grant federal funding HL67181 and HL0761570.
* Corresponding author.
E-mail address: pinsky@pitt.edu (M.R. Pinsky).

surgical.theclinics.com

hemodynamic monitoring resides at this level. It is not clear from recent clin-ical studies in critically ill patients that this argument is valid, primarily be-cause knowledge of the actual processes involved in the expression of disease and tissue injury is often inadequate. The third level of defense comes from documentation that the monitoring device, by altering therapy in other-wise unexpected ways, improves outcome in terms of survival and quality of life. In reality, few therapies done in medicine can claim benefit at this level. Thus, we are left with the physiological rationale as the primary defense of monitoring of critically ill patients.

The physiologic basis for hemodynamic monitoring

On a philosophical level, one may consider the monitoring of critically ill patients as serving a dual function. First, it can be used to document hemodynamic stability and the lack of need for acute interventions, and second, it can be used to monitor when measured variables vary from their defined baseline values. Accordingly, knowing the limits to which such monitoring reflects actual physiological values is an essential aspect of its utility.

On the physical side, hemodynamic monitoring can be invasive or nonin-vasive, and continuous or intermittent. Monitoring devices can measure physiologic variables directly, or derive these variables through signal pro-cessing. Signal processing does not minimize the usefulness of physiologic variable analysis; it just separates the output data from the patient by the use of the data processor. The most common signal processing physiologic variable measured clinically is the electrocardiogram.

Variables that can be measured noninvasively include body temperature, heart rate, systolic and diastolic arterial blood pressure, and respiratory frequency. Processed noninvasive variables include the electrocardiogram, transcutaneous pulse oximetry (SpO_2), expired CO_2, trans-thoracic echo-cardiography, and noninvasive respiratory plethysmography. Invasive monitoring reflects intravascular catheter insertion, transesophageal echo-cardiographic probe insertion, and blood component analysis. Invasive he-modynamic monitoring of vascular pressures is usually performed by the percutaneous insertion of a catheter into a vascular space and transducing the pressure sensed at the distal end. This allows for the continual display and monitoring of these complex pressure waveforms. Similar intrapulmo-nary vascular catheters can be used to derive thermal signals and mixed venous oxygen (O_2) saturation (SvO_2), needed to assess cardiac output and the adequacy of O_2 delivery, respectively. How useful this hemodynamic information is to diagnosis treatment and prognosis is a function of its reliability, established treatment protocols, and guidelines, and the expertise of the operator. Box 1 summarizes all the possible unitary and calculated measures derived from invasive hemodynamic monitoring.

Box 1. Physiological variables derived from invasive monitoring and their physiological relevance

Unitary measures
Arterial pressure
- Mean arterial pressure (MAP)
  Organ perfusion inflow pressure
- Arterial pulse pressure and its variation during ventilation
  Left ventricular stroke volume changes and pulsus paradoxus
  Preload-responsiveness (if assessed during intermittent positive pressure ventilation [IPPV])
- Arterial pressure waveform
  Aortic valvulopathy, input impedance, and arterial resistance
  Used to calculate stroke volume by pulse contour technique

Central venous pressure (CVP)
- Mean CVP
  If elevated, then effective circulating blood volume is not reduced
- CVP variations during ventilation
  Tricuspid insufficiency, tamponade physiology
  Preload-responsiveness (if assessed during spontaneous breathing)

Pulmonary arterial pressure (Ppa)
- Mean Ppa
  Pulmonary inflow pressure
- Systolic pulmonary artery pressure
  Right ventricular pressure load
- Diastolic pulmonary artery pressure and pulse pressure, and their variations during ventilation
  Right ventricular stroke volume, pulmonary vascular resistance
  Diastolic pressure tract changes in intrathoracic pressure during ventilation

Pulmonary artery occlusion pressure (Ppao)
- Mean Ppao
  Left atrial and left ventricular intralumenal pressure, and by inference, left ventricular preload
  Back pressure to pulmonary blood flow
- Ppao waveform and its variation during occlusion and ventilation

Mitral valvulopathy, atrial or ventricular etiology of
arrhythmia, accuracy of mean Ppao to measure intralumenal
left ventricle (LV) pressure, and pulmonary capillary pressure
(Ppc)

Calculated measures
Calculated measures using multiple measured variables
including cardiac output by thermodilution (COtd), arterial blood
gases (ABG) and mixed venous blood gases (VBG)
Vascular resistances
- Total peripheral resistance = MAP/COtd
- Systemic vascular resistance = (MAP − CVP)/COtd
- Pulmonary arterial resistance = (mean Ppa − Ppc)/COtd
- Pulmonary venous resistance = (Ppc − Ppao)/COtd
- Pulmonary vascular resistance = (mean Ppa − Ppao)/COtd

Vascular pump function
- Left ventricular stroke volume (SVlv) = COtd/HR
- Left ventricular stroke work (SWlv) = (MAP − Ppao)/SVlv
- Preload—recruitable stroke work = SWlv/Ppao

Oxygen transport and metabolism
- Global oxygen transport or delivery (DO_2) = Cao_2/COtd
- Global oxygen uptake (VO_2) = (Cao_2 − Cvo_2)/COtd
- Venous admixture
- Ratio of dead space to total tidal volume (Vd/Vt) = $Paco_2$/
  ($Paco_2$ − $Petco_2$) Right ventricular (RV) function using RV
  ejection fraction (EFrv) catheter-derived data
- Right ventricular end-diastolic volume (EDVrv) = SV/Efrv
- Right ventricular end-systolic volume (ESVrv) = EDVrv − SV

Abbreviations: HR, heart rate; Cao_2, arterial O_2 content; Cvo_2, mixed venous O_2
content; $Petco_2$, end tidal CO_2; SV, stroke volume; SV/Efrv, stroke volume/ejection
fraction of right ventricle.
   Adapted from Bellomo R, Pinsky MR. Invasive monitoring. In: Tinker J, Browne
D, Sibbald W, editors. Critical care—standards, audit and ethics. 26. London:
Arnold Publishing Co.; 1996. p. 82–104; with permission.

Arterial pressure monitoring

After pulse rate, arterial pressure is the most common hemodynamic variable monitored and recorded. Blood pressure is usually measured noninvasively using a sphygmomanometer and the auscultation technique.
Importantly, very large and obese subjects in whom the upper arm circumfer-
ence exceeds the width limitations of a normal blood pressure cuff will record

pressures that are higher than they actually are. In such patients, using the large thigh blood pressure cuff usually resolves this problem. Blood pressure can be measured automatically using computer-driven devices (eg, Dynamat) that greatly reduce nursing time. Sphygmomanometer-derived blood pressure measures display slightly higher systolic and lower diastolic pressures than simultaneously measured indwelling arterial catheters, but the mean arterial pressure is usually similar, and the actual systolic and diastolic pressure differences are often small except in the setting of increased peripheral vasomotor tone. If perfusion pressure of the finger is similar to arterial pressure, then both blood pressure and the pressure profile may be recorded noninvasively and continuously using the optical finger probe (Finapres Medical Systems BV, Amsterdam, The Netherlands). Finger perfusion is often compromised during hypovolemic shock and hypothermia, however, limiting this monitoring technique to relatively well-perfused patients.

Accurate and continuous measures of arterial pressure can be done through arterial catheterization of easily accessible arterial sites in the arm (axillary, brachial, or radial arterial) or groin (femoral arterial). Usually neither axillary nor brachial arterial sites are used because of fears of causing downstream ischemia, although there are no data supporting these fears. Arterial catheterization displaying continuous arterial pressure waveforms lends itself to arterial waveform analysis, essential in calculating pulse pressure, pulse pressure variations, and cardiac output.

Why measure arterial pressure?

Arterial pressure is the input pressure for organ perfusion. Organ perfusion is usually dependent on organ metabolic demand and perfusion pressure. With increasing tissue metabolism, organ blood flow proportionally increases by selective local vasodilation of the small resistance arterioles. If cardiac output cannot increase as well, as is the case with heart failure, then blood pressure decreases, limiting the ability of local vasomotor control to regulate organ blood flow. If local metabolic demand remains constant, however, changes in arterial pressure are usually matched by changes in arterial tone so as to maintain organ blood flow relatively constant. This local vasomotor control mechanism is referred to as autoregulation. Cerebral blood flow over the normal autoregulatory range of 65 to 120 mm Hg is remarkably constant. Although autoregulation occurs in many organs, such as the brain, liver, skeletal muscle, and skin, it is not a universal phenomenon. For example, coronary flow increases with increasing arterial pressure because the myocardial O_2 demand increases as the heart ejects into a higher arterial pressure circuit. Furthermore, renal blood flow increases in a pressure-dependent fashion over its entire pressure for similar reasons. As renal flow increases, so does renal filtrate flow into the tubules, increasing renal metabolic demand. Thus, a normal blood pressure does not mean that all organs have an adequate amount of perfusion, because increases in local vasomotor tone and mechanical vascular obstruction can still induce asymmetrical vascular ischemia.

Determinants of arterial pressure

Arterial pressure is a function of both vasomotor tone and cardiac output. The local vasomotor tone also determines blood flow distribution, which itself is usually determined by local metabolic demands. For a constant vasomotor tone, vascular resistance can be described by the relation between changes in both arterial pressure and cardiac output. The body defends organ perfusion pressure above all else in its autonomic hierarchy through alterations in α-adrenergic tone, mediated through baroreceptors located in the carotid sinus and aortic arch. This supremacy of arterial pressure in the adaptive response to circulatory shock exists because both coronary and cerebral blood flows are dependent only on perfusion pressure. The cerebral vasculature has no α-adrenergic receptors; the coronary circulation has only a few. Accordingly, hypotension always reflects cardiovascular embarrassment, but normotension does not exclude it. Hypotension decreases organ blood flow and stimulates a strong sympathetic response that induces a combined α-adrenergic (increased vasomotor tone) and β-adrenergic (increased heart rate and cardiac contractility) effect, and causes a massive adenrocorticotropic hormone (ACTH)-induced cortisol release from the adrenal glands. Thus, to understand the determinants of arterial pressure one must also know the level of vasomotor tone.

In the intensive care unit setting, arterial tone can be estimated at the bedside by calculating systemic vascular resistance. Using Ohm's Law, resistance equals the ratio of the pressure to flow, usually calculated as the ratio of the pressure gradient between aorta and central venous pressure (CVP) to cardiac output. Arterial tone can also be calculated as total peripheral resistance, which is the ratio of mean arterial pressure to cardiac output. Regrettably, neither systemic vascular resistance nor total peripheral resistance faithfully describes arterial resistance. Arterial resistance is the slope of the arterial pressure-flow relation. The calculation of systemic vascular resistance using CVP as the backpressure to flow has no physiological rationale, and the use of systemic vascular resistance for clinical decision-making should be abolished. Regrettably, both systemic vascular resistance and total peripheral resistance are still commonly used in hemodynamic monitoring because they allow for the simultaneous assessment of both pressure and flow, whereas the actual measure of arterial tone is more difficult to estimate.

The determinants of arterial pressure can simplistically be defined as systemic arterial tone and blood flow. Because blood flow distribution will vary amongst organs relative to their local vasomotor tone, and arterial pressure is similar for most organs, measurement of peripheral resistance, by any means or formula, reflects the lump parameter of all the vascular beds, and thus describes no specific vascular bed completely. If no hemodynamic instability alters normal regulatory mechanisms, then local blood flow will also be proportional to local metabolic demand. Within this construct, the only reason cardiac output becomes important is to sustain an adequate and changing blood flow to match changes in vasomotor tone, such that arterial input pressure remains constant. Because cardiac output is proportional to metabolic demand, there is no level of cardiac output that reflects normal values in the unstable and metabolically active patient; however, as blood pressures decreases below 60 mm Hg mean or cardiac indices decrease below 2.0 l/min/m^2, organ perfusion usually becomes compromised, and if sustained, will lead to organ failure and death. Presently, only one clinical trial has examined the effect of increasing mean arterial pressure on tissue blood flow [2]. When patients with circulatory shock were resuscitated with volume and vasopressors to a mean arterial pressure range of 60 to 70, 70 to 80, or 80 to 90 mm Hg, no increased organ blood flow could be identified above a mean arterial pressure of 65 mm Hg. Clearly, subjects who have prior hypertension will have their optimal perfusion pressure range increased over normotensive patients. Thus, there are no firm data supporting any one limit of arterial pressure or cardiac output values or therapeutic approaches based on these values as more beneficial than any other. Accordingly, empiricism is the rule regarding target values of both mean arterial pressure and cardiac output. At present, the literature suggests that maintaining a previously nonhypertensive patient's mean arterial pressure greater than 65 mm Hg by the use of fluid resuscitation and subsequent vasopressor therapy is an acceptable target. Previously hypertensive subjects will need a higher mean arterial pressure to insure the same degree of blood flow [2]. There is no proven value in forcing either arterial tone or cardiac output to higher levels to achieve a mean arterial pressure above this threshold. In fact, data suggest that further resuscitative efforts using vasoactive agents markedly increase mortality [3], and the relatively new concept of "delayed" and "hypotensive resuscitation" for traumatic hemorrhagic shock has shown improved outcome in some clinical and experimental studies [4–6]. Those studies, however, were in trauma patients who had penetrating wounds and no immediate access to surgical repair. Once a patient is in the hospital and the sites of active bleeding addressed, then aggressive fluid and pressor resuscitation is indicated.

Arterial pressure variations during ventilation

The majority of the critically ill surgical patients treated in the ICU are usually on mechanical ventilation. Ventilation-induced arterial pressure variations have been described since antiquity as pulsus paradoxus. Inspiratory decreases in arterial pressure were used to monitor both the severity of bronchospasm in asthmatics and their inspiratory efforts [7].

Recently renewed interest in the hemodynamic significance of heart-lung interactions has emerged. The commonly observed variations in arterial pressure and aortic flow seen during positive- pressure ventilation have been analyzed as a measure of preload responsiveness [8]. The rationale for this approach is that positive-pressure ventilation–induced changes in either systolic arterial pressure (used to describe pulsus paradoxus), arterial pulse pressure, or stroke volume can predict in which subjects cardiac output will increase in response to fluid resuscitation. Ventilation-induced changes in systolic arterial pressure (pulsus paradoxus) and arterial pulse pressure are easy to measure from arterial pressure recordings. The greater the degree of systolic arterial pressure or pulse pressure variation over the respiratory cycle, the greater the increase in cardiac output in response to a defined fluid challenge. Recently, measuring the mean change in aortic blood flow during passive leg raising in spontaneous breathing patients has also proven accurate in predicting preload responsiveness [9].

Although arterial pressure variations are a measure of preload-responsiveness [10], the "traditional" preload measures, such as right atrial pressure (Pra), Ppao, RV end-diastolic volume, and intrathoracic blood volume, poorly reflect preload-responsiveness [11]. In essence, preload is not preload-responsiveness.

Indications for arterial catheterization

The arterial catheter is frequently inserted as a "routine" at the admission of patients to the ICU for continuous monitoring of blood pressure and repetitive measurements of blood gases. There is no evidence to support this exaggerated clinical practice. Although probably the only proven indication for arterial catheterization is to synchronize the intra-aortic balloon of counterpulsation, there are some others indications whereby the information obtained is valuable in the assessment and treatment of the patient, such as cardiovascular instability or the use of vasopressors or vasodilators during resuscitation. The probable indications for arterial catheterization are summarized in Box 2. Although arterial catheterization is an invasive procedure that is not free of complications, a recent systematic review of a large number of cases [12] showed that most of the complications were minor, including temporary vascular occlusion (19.7%) and hematoma (14.4%). Permanent ischemic damage, sepsis, and pseudoaneurysm formation occurred in fewer than 1% of cases [12].

Central venous pressure monitoring

Methods of measuring central venous pressure

CVP is the pressure in the large central veins proximal to the right atrium relative to atmosphere. In the ICUs, the CVP is usually measured using a fluid-filled catheter (central venous line or Swan-Ganz catheter) with the distal tip located in the superior vena cava connected to a manometer, or more often to

---

Box 2. Arterial catheterization

Indications for arterial catheterization
- As a guide to synchronization of intra-aortic balloon counter pulsation

Probable indications for arterial catheterization
- Guide to management of potent vasodilator drug infusions to prevent systemic hypotension
- Guide to management of potent vasopressor drug infusions to maintain a target MAP
- As a port for the rapid and repetitive sampling of arterial blood inpatients in whom multiple arterial blood samples are indicated
- As a monitor of cardiovascular deterioration in patients at risk for cardiovascular instability

Useful applications of arterial pressure monitoring in the diagnosis of cardiovascular insufficiency
- Differentiating cardiac tamponade (pulsus paradoxus) from respiration-induced swings in systolic arterial pressure— tamponade reduces the pulse pressure but keeps diastolic pressure constant. Respiration reduces systolic and diastolic pressure equally, such that pulse pressure is constant.
- Differentiating hypovolemia from cardiac dysfunction as the cause of hemodynamic instability. Systolic arterial pressure decreases more following a positive pressure breath as compared to an apneic baseline during hypovolemia. Systolic arterial pressure increases more during positive pressure inspiration when LV contractility is reduced.

Adapted from Bellomo R, Pinsky MR. Invasive monitoring. In: Tinker J, Browne D, Sibbald W, editors. Critical Care—Standards, Audit and Ethics. 26. London: Arnold Publishing Co., 1996. p. 82–104; with permission.

---

a pressure transducer of a monitor, displaying the waveform in a continuous fashion. CVP can also be measured noninvasively as jugular venous pressure, the height of the column of blood distending the internal and external jugular veins when the subject is sitting in a semireclined position; small elevations in CVP will be reflected by persistent jugular venous distention.

Determinants of central venous pressure

Starling demonstrated the relationship between cardiac output, venous return, and CVP, showing that increasing the venous return (and preload) increases the stroke volume (and cardiac output [CO]) until a plateau is reached. Although the CVP is clearly influenced by the volume of blood in the central compartment and its venous compliance; there are several physiological and anatomical factors that can influence its measurement and waveform, such as the vascular tone, right ventricular function, intra-thoracic pressure changes, tricuspid valve disease, arrhythmias, and both myocardial and pericardial disease. These are summarized in Box 3.

Box 3. Factors affecting the measured CVP

Central venous blood volume
- Venous return/cardiac output
- Total blood volume
- Regional vascular tone

Compliance of central compartment
- Vascular tone
- RV compliance
- Myocardial disease
- Pericardial disease
- Tamponade

Tricuspid valve disease
- Stenosis
- Regurgitation

Cardiac rhythm
- Junctional rhythm
- Atrial fibrillation (AF)
- Atrio ventricular (A-V) dissociation

Reference level of transducer
- Positioning of patient

Intrathoracic pressure
- Respiration
- IPPV
- Positive end-expiratory pressure (PEEP)
- Tension pneumothorax

From Smith T, Grounds RM, Rhodes A. Central venous pressure: uses and limitations. In: Pinsky MR, Payen D. Functional hemodynamic monitoring. Berlin, Heidelberg (Germany): Springer-Verlag; 2006. p. 101; with kind permission of Springer Science and Business Media.

Monitoring central venous pressure

CVP has been used as a monitor of central venous blood volume and an estimate of the right atrial pressure for many years, being wrongly used as a parameter and sometimes goal for replacement of intravascular volume in shock patients. The validity of this measure as an index of RV preload is nonexistent across numerous studies. It has been shown that CVP has a poor correlation with cardiac index, stroke volume, left ventricular end-diastolic volume, and right ventricular end-diastolic volume [13–15].

Although a very high CVP demands a certain level of total circulating blood volume, one may have a CVP of 20 mm Hg and still have an under-filled left ventricle that is fluid responsive. For example, in the setting of acute RV infarction, CVP can be markedly elevated, whereas cardiac output often increases further with volume loading. In reported series, some patients who had low CVP failed to respond to fluids and some patients who had high CVP responded to challenge of fluids [16]. Based on this and the poor correlations described above, it is impossible to define ideal values of CVP; however, there is some evidence that volume loading in patients who have CVP greater than 12 mmHg is very unlikely to increase cardiac output [17]. Thus, the only usefulness of CVP is to define relative hypervolemia, because an elevated CVP only occurs in disease. Two clinical studies [18,19] showed a potential benefit in specific groups of surgical patients (hip replacement and renal transplant patients) in whom CVP was used to guide therapy; however, there is no clinical evidence that CVP monitoring improves outcome in critically ill patients, and attempts to normalize CVP in early goal directed therapy during resuscitation do not display any benefit [20].

Pulmonary artery catheterization and its associated monitored variables

Pulmonary arterial catheterization allows the measurement of many clinically relevant hemodynamic variables (see Box 1). One can measure the intrapulmonary vascular pressures including CVP, Ppa, and by intermittent balloon occlusion of the pulmonary artery, Ppao and pulmonary capillary pressure (Ppc). Furthermore, by using the thermodilution technique and the Stewart-Hamilton equation, one can estimate cardiac output and EFrv, global cardiac volume, and intrathoracic blood volume. Finally, one can measure mixed SvO_2 either intermittently by direct sampling of blood from the distal pulmonary arterial port or continuously via fiber optic reflectometry. Assuming one knows the hemoglobin concentration and can tract arterial O_2 saturation (SaO_2), easily estimated by noninvasively by pulse oximetry as SpO_2, one can calculate numerous derived variables that describe well the global cardiovascular state of the patient. These derived variables include DO_2, VO_2, venous admixture (as an estimate of intrapulmonary shunt), pulmonary and systemic vascular resistance, EDVrv and ESVrv, and both RV and LV stroke work index.

Pulmonary artery pressure

The determinants of Ppa are the volume of blood ejected into the pulmonary artery during systole, the resistance of the pulmonary vascular bed, and the downstream left atrial (LA) pressure. The pulmonary vascular bed is a low-resistance circuit with a large reserve that allows increases of cardiac output with minor changes in the Ppa. On the other hand, increases in the downstream venous pressure (eg, left ventricular failure) or in the flow resistance (eg, lung diseases) raise the Ppa. Although increases in cardiac output alone do not cause pulmonary hypertension, having an increased vascular resistance can lead to elevations in Ppa, with changes in cardiac output. Based on these considerations, the Ppa should not be used as a reliable parameter of ventricular filling under several lung diseases that cause changes in the vascular tone and cardiac output. The normal range of values for Ppa are: systolic 15 to 30 mm Hg, diastolic 4 to 12 mm Hg, and mean 9 to 18 mm Hg [21].

Pulmonary artery occlusion pressure

Methods of measuring pulmonary artery occlusion pressure

Numerous studies by physicians have demonstrated that the ability to accurately measure Ppao from a strip chart recording or a freeze-frame snapshot of the monitor screen is poor. Many initiatives have been put into place to educate physicians and nurses, but the reality is that because the pressure measured also reports changes in intrathoracic pressure, a value which is always changing, the accuracy of Ppao measures is likely to remain poor.

The Ppao value is thought to reflect the LV filling because of the unique characteristic of the pulmonary circulation. Balloon inflation of the pulmonary artery catheter (PAC) forces the tip to migrate distally into smaller vessels until the tip occludes a medium-sized (1.2 cm diameter) pulmonary artery. This occlusion stops all blood flow in that vascular tree distal to the occlusion site, until such time as other venous branches reconnect downstream to this venous draining bed. The point where such parallel pulmonary vascular beds anastomose is about 1.5 cm from the left atrium. Thus, if a continuous column of blood is present from the catheter tip to the left heart, then Ppao measures pulmonary venous pressure at this first junction, or J-1 point, of the pulmonary veins [22]. As downstream pulmonary blood flow ceases, distal pulmonary arterial pressure falls in a double exponential fashion to a minimal value, reflecting the pressure downstream in the pulmonary vasculature from the point of occlusion. The Ppa value where the first exponential pressure decay is overtaken by the second longer exponential pressure decay reflects Ppc measures, useful in calculating pulmonary arterial and venous resistances. Importantly, the column of water at the end of the catheter is now extended to include the pulmonary vascular circuit up to this J-1 point of blood flow. Because the vasculature is compliant relative to the catheter, vascular pressure signals dampen relative to the nonoccluded Ppa signal. Thus, the two primary aspects of Ppao measures that are used to identify an occluded pressure are the decrease in diastolic pressure values to less than diastolic Ppa and the damping of the pressure signal (Fig. 1). If one needed further validation that the catheter is actually in an occluded vascular bed, then one could measure the pH, pCO_2, and pO_2 of blood sampled from the occluded distal tip of the catheter. Because the sampled blood will be from the stagnant pool of blood, its removal will make it be pulled back into the PAC from the pulmonary veins. Because the blood sampled will have crossed the alveolar capillaries twice, its pCO_2 will be lower than arterial pCO_2, and its pO_2 higher, as a result of the law of mass action.

Pleural pressure and Ppao

Although one may measure Ppao accurately relative to atmosphere, the heart and large vessel pulmonary vasculature live in an intrathoracic compartment and sense pleural pressure (Ppl) as their surrounding pressure. Ventilation causes significant swings in Ppl. Pulmonary vascular pressures, when measured relative to atmospheric pressure, will reflect these respiratory changes in Ppl. To minimize this "respiratory artifact" on intrathoracic vascular pressure recordings, measures are usually made at end-expiration. During quiet spontaneous breathing, end-expiration occurs at the highest vascular pressure values, whereas during passive positive-pressure breathing, end-expiration occurs at the lowest vascular pressure values. With assisted ventilation or with forced spontaneous ventilation, it is often difficult to define end-expiration [23]. These limitations are the primary reasons for inaccuracies in estimating Ppao at the bedside.

Even if measures of Ppao are made at end-expiration and Ppao values reflect a continuous column of fluid from the catheter tip to the J-1 point, these Ppao measures may still overestimate Ppao if Ppl is elevated at end-expiration. Hyperinflation caused by air trapping, dynamic hyperinflation, or the use of extrinsic PEEP will all increase end-expiratory Ppl to a varying degree as a function of airway resistance and lung and chest wall

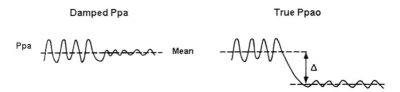

Fig. 1. This figure represents the differential characteristics of a damped Ppa and a true wedge or Ppao during the balloon inflation. Notice the flattening of the waveform on the damped Ppa tracing (*left*) without a decrease of the mean pressure, whereas in the true Ppao (*right*) there is a substantial decrease in the mean pressure.

compliance. It is not possible to predict with accuracy the degree to which increases in PEEP will increase Ppl. Because differences in lung and chest wall compliance exist among patients and within the same patient other over time, one cannot assume a fixed relation between increases in airway pressure (Paw) and Ppl [24].

Why measure pulmonary artery occlusion pressure?

Ppao is used most often in the bedside assessment of: (1) pulmonary edema, (2) pulmonary vasomotor tone, (3) intravascular volume status and LV preload, and (4) LV performance. These points were summarized recently and are restated below [25].

Pulmonary edema

Pulmonary edema can be caused by either elevations of pulmonary capillary pressure, referred to as hydrostatic or secondary pulmonary edema, or increased alveolar capillary or epithelial permeability, referred to as primary pulmonary edema. Usually hydrostatic pulmonary edema requires a pulmonary capillary increase to greater than 18 mm Hg; however, if capillary or alveolar cell injury is present, alveolar flooding can occur at much lower pulmonary capillary pressures. Furthermore, in the setting of chronic pulmonary vascular congestion, increased pulmonary lymphatic flow and increased respiratory excursions promote a rapid clearance of lung interstitial fluid, minimizing edema formation. Still, measures of Ppao are commonly used to determine the cause of pulmonary edema. Ppao values less than 18 mm Hg suggest a nonhydrostatic cause, whereas values greater than 20 mm Hg suggest a hydrostatic cause of pulmonary edema [22]; however, many exceptions to this rule exist. As mentioned above, if increased lung permeability is present, then fluid-resuscitation–induced pulmonary edema may occur at Ppao values much below 18 mm Hg, and treatment strategies aimed at reducing Ppao further will reduce pulmonary edema formation. Similarly, if pulmonary venous resistance is increased, then Ppc may be much higher than the measured Ppao, inducing hydrostatic pulmonary edema despite no increased lung permeability and a low Ppao. Similarly, Ppao may be greater than 20 mm Hg without any evidence of hydrostatic pulmonary edema, either because Ppl is also elevated or because of increased pulmonary lymphatic flow.

Pulmonary vasomotor tone

The pulmonary circulation normally has a low resistance, with pulmonary arterial diastolic pressure only slightly higher than Ppao and mean pulmonary arterial pressure a few mm Hg higher than Ppao. Pulmonary vascular resistance (PVR) can be estimated using Ohm's Law as the ratio of the pulmonary vascular pressure gradient (mean pulmonary artery pressure minus Ppao) and cardiac output (ie, PVR = (mean Ppa − Ppao)/ CO). Normal pulmonary vascular resistance is between 2 and 4 mm Hg × l/min/m^2. Usually these values are multiplied by 80 to give normal pulmonary vascular resistance range in dynes sec/cm^5 of 150 to 250. Either an increased pulmonary vascular resistance or a passive pressure buildup from the pulmonary veins can induce pulmonary hypertension. If pulmonary hypertension is associated with an increased PVR, then the causes are primarily within the lung. Diagnoses such as pulmonary embolism, pulmonary fibrosis, essential pulmonary hypertension, and pulmonary veno-occlusive disease need to be excluded. If PVR is normal, then LV dysfunction is the more likely cause of pulmonary hypertension [26]. Because the treatments for these two groups of diseases are quite different despite similar increases in pulmonary arterial pressure, the determination of PVR in the setting of pulmonary hypertension is very important. Regrettably, PVR poorly reflects true pulmonary vasomotor tone in lung disease states and during mechanical ventilation, especially with the application of PEEP. Alveolar pressure (Palv) can be the back pressure to pulmonary blood flow in certain lung regions during positive-pressure ventilation and in the presence of hyperinflation, because Palv exceeds left atrial pressure. Furthermore, because lung disease is usually nonhomogeneous, pulmonary blood flow is preferentially shifted from compressed vessels in West Zone 1 and 2 conditions (Ppao < Palv and Ppa = Palv, respectively) to those circuits with the lowest resistance (West Zone 3; ie, Ppao > Palv), thus making the lung vascular pathology appear less than it actually is.

Left ventricular preload

Ppao is often taken to reflect LV filling pressure, and by inference, LV end-diastolic volume. Patients who have cardiovascular insufficiency and a low Ppao are presumed to be hypovolemic and initially treated with fluid resuscitation, whereas patients who have similar presentations but an elevated Ppao are presumed to have impaired contractile function. Although there are no accepted high and low Ppao values for which LV underfilling is presumed to occur or not, Ppao values less than 10 mm Hg are usually used as presumed evidence of a low LV end-diastolic volume, whereas values greater than 18 mm Hg suggest a distended LV [27]. Unfortunately, there are very few data to support this approach. There are multiple documented reasons for this observed inaccuracy that relate to individual differences in LV diastolic compliance and contractile function [28]. First, the relation between Ppao and LV end-diastolic volume is curvilinear and is often very different among subjects and within subjects over time. Thus, neither absolute values of Ppao nor changes in Ppao will define a specific LV end-diastolic volume or its change [29]. Second, Ppao is not the distending pressure for LV filling. It is only the internal pressure of the pulmonary veins relative to atmospheric pressure. Assuming Ppao approximated left atrial pressure, it will poorly reflect LV end-diastolic pressure, because it poorly follows the late diastolic pressure rise induced by atrial contraction and does not measure pericardial pressure, which is the outside pressure for LV distention. With lung distention, Ppl increases increasing pericardial pressure. Although we can estimate Ppl using esophageal balloon catheters, pericardial pressure is often different. Changes in pericardial pressure will alter LV end-diastolic volume independent of Ppao. Finally, even if one knew pericardial pressure and Ppao did accurately reflect LV end-diastolic pressure, LV diastolic compliance can vary rapidly, changing the relation between LV filling pressure and LV end-diastolic volume. Myocardial ischemia, arrhythmias, and acute RV dilation can all occur over a few heartbeats. Thus, is not surprising that Ppao is a very poor predictor of preload responsiveness. Therefore, it is not recommended to use Ppao to predict response to fluid resuscitation in critically ill patients.

Left ventricular performance

The four primary determinants of LV performance are preload (LV end-diastolic volume), afterload (maximal LV wall stress), heart rate, and contractility. Ppao is often used as a substitute for LV end-diastolic volume when constructing Starling curves (ie, relationship between changing LV preload and ejection phase indices). Usually one plots Ppao versus SWlv stroke work (SVlv × developed pressure). Using this construct, patients who have heart failure can be divided into four groups, depending on their Ppao (> or <18 mm Hg) and cardiac index values (> or <2.2 l/min/m²) [27]. Those patients who have low cardiac indices and high Ppao are presumed to have primary heart failure, and a low cardiac output and low Ppao, on the other hand, reflect hypovolemia. Those who have high cardiac indices and high Ppao are presumed to be volume overloaded, and having high cardiac output and low Ppao reflects increased sympathetic tone. Although this maybe a useful construct for determining diagnosis, treatment, and prognosis of patients who have acute coronary syndrome, it poorly predicts cardiovascular status in other patient groups. As described above, however, if LV end-diastolic volume and Ppao do not trend together in response to fluid loading or inotropic drug infusion, then inferences about LV contractility based on this Ppao/SWlv relation may be incorrect. This is not a minor point. Volume loading may induce acute RV dilation, markedly reducing LV diastolic compliance, such that Ppao will increase as SWlv decreases; however, the relationship between LV end-diastolic volume and swLV need not have changed at all. Similarly, inotropic drugs such as dobutamine may reduce biventricular volumes by decreasing venous return, decreasing LV diastolic compliance, even if the heart is not responsive to inotropic therapy. Thus, the same limitations on the use of Ppao in assessing LV preload must be considered when using it to assess LV performance.

Measuring cardiac output

Cardiac output can be estimated by many techniques, including invasive hemodynamic monitoring. Pulmonary blood flow using a balloon floatation PAC equipped with a distal thermistor, and transpulmonary blood flow using an arterial thermistor, both with a central venous cold volume injection, can be used. Similarly, minimally invasive echo Doppler techniques can measure blood flow at the aortic value and descending aortic flow using esophageal Doppler monitoring. Cardiac output can be measured intermittently by bolus cold injection, or continuously by cold infusion. The advantage of the continuous cardiac output technique and the transpulmonary technique is that neither is influenced greatly by the ventilation-induced swings in pulmonary blood flow. Measurement of cardiac output by intermittent pulmonary artery flow measures using bolus cold indicator and monitoring the thermal decay curve is the most common method to measure cardiac output at the bedside; however, such intermittent measures will show profound ventilatory cycle-specific patterns [30]. By making numerous measures at random with the ventilatory cycle and then averaging all measures with proper thermal decay profiles, regardless of their values, one can derive an accurate measure of pulmonary blood flow [31].

Recently, a renewed interest in pulse contour analysis to estimate SVlv, and therefore cardiac output, from the arterial pressure profile over ejection has acquired its own set of supporters [32]. Arterial pressure and arterial pulse pressure are a function of rate of LV ejection, SVlv and the resistance, compliance, and inertance characteristics of the arterial tree and blood. If the arterial components of tone remain constant, then changes in pulse pressure most proportionally reflect changes in SVlv. Thus, it is not surprising that aortic flow variation parallels arterial pulse pressure variation [33], and pulse contour-derived estimates of stroke volume variation can be used to determine preload responsiveness [34,35]. Caution must be applied to using the pulse contour method, because it has not been validated in subjects who have rapidly changing arterial tone, as often occurs in subjects who have hemodynamic instability. Furthermore, it requires the application of abnormally large tidal volumes [34–36]. Thus, at the present time, the pulse contour-derived stroke volume variation technique represents a potentially great but still unproven clinical decision tool [37].

Currently three commercial devices that use pulse contour analysis of an arterial line waveform to obtain continuous cardiac output are approved for clinical use: PiCCO (Pulsion Medical Systems, Munich, Germany), LIDCO (Cambridge, United Kingdom), and Vigileo monitor (Edwards Lifesciences, Irvine, California) systems. Their benefit of being minimally invasive and the correlation shown with "standard" methods of measuring cardiac output in some clinical and experimental studies make them promising tools for hemodynamic monitoring [38,39].

Mixed venous oxygen saturation

Measuring venous oxygen saturation

SvO_2 reflects the pooled venous O_2 saturation, and is an important parameter in the assessment of the adequacy of DO_2 and its relation with VO_2. A decrease of SvO_2 could be explained by a decrease in DO_2 or any of the parameters that determine this, such as SaO_2, cardiac output, and hemoglobin concentration, and also by an increase in VO_2. A decrease of DO_2 will be followed by stable VO_2, with a consequent decrease of the SvO_2 until a critical value of DO_2 is reached where the tissues are no longer able to compensate having a constant VO_2, and VO_2 becomes dependent on DO_2 in an almost linear relation. At this level SvO_2, though continuing to decrease, becomes less sensitive to changes of tissue perfusion (Fig. 2).

SvO_2 measured from blood drawn from the distal tip of a PAC represents the true mixed venous value of the blood blended in the right ventricle. Care must be taken to withdraw blood slowly, so that it does not get aspirated from the downstream pulmonary capillaries. Validation of true mixed venous blood requires documentation that the measures $Pvco_2$ is greater than $Paco_2$, because blood drawn over the capillaries sees alveolar gas twice, and will have a lower Pco_2 than arterial blood. Continuous measures of SvO_2 can be made using fiber optic reflectance spectroscopy. Two techniques are commercially available. Both use one fiber optic line to send a light signal and another to receive the reflected light at a different wavelength; however, only one catheter, Abbott, uses the Shaw technique of also measuring hemoglobin reflectance, and thus remains accurate over wide changes in hemoglobin concentration. The other catheter, Edwards, requires recalibration if hemoglobin levels vary by more than 1 gm/dL. Both techniques are valuable to monitoring SvO_2 trends as cardiac output, arterial O_2 content, or metabolic demand varies.

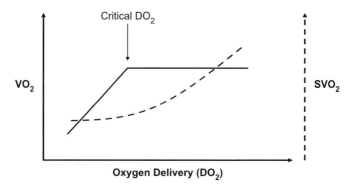

Fig. 2. This graph shows the interrelation of the determinants of SvO_2. The decrease of O_2 delivery under invariable oxygen consumption (VO_2) by the tissues will traduce a decrease of SvO_2, until a critical point where the consumption becomes dependent on the delivery almost in a linear relation; thus the SvO_2 in this case remains stable.

Superior vena caval oxygen saturation

Recent interest in superior vena caval O_2 saturation ($ScvO_2$) has evolved over the past years with the positive results of the Rivers and colleagues study [40], which demonstrated that in patients who had septic shock or severe sepsis admitted in the emergency department, an early and aggressive resuscitation guided by $ScvO_2$, CVP, and MAP reduced 28-day mortality from 46.5% to 30.5%. Measures of SvO_2, however, remain the gold standard to reflect minimal O_2 delivery. This is because although $SvcO_2$ and SvO_2 co-vary and seem to follow a parallel tracking, their differences can exceed 5%. Furthermore, during dynamic changes in cardiac output, such as occur in shock states, $ScvO_2$ may exceed SvO_2 by 5% or more, or be less than SvO_2 by 5% or more [41]. Thus, using a defined threshold value for $ScvO_2$ to identify when to start or stop resuscitation in a critically ill patient is fundamentally flawed. Still, a low $ScvO_2$ ($<65\%$) is invariably associated with a low SvO_2 ($<72\%$), making it less sensitive but still clinically useful at lower threshold values.

The meaning of cardiac output and venous oxygen saturation as end points of resuscitation

Although one may potentially measure cardiac output accurately at the bedside, there is no such thing as a normal cardiac output. Cardiac output is either adequate for the needs of the body or it is not. For example, the same cardiac output and DO_2 that is adequate at rest may be grossly inadequate and not associated with life during periods of increased metabolic demand. Because the primary goal of the cardiorespiratory system is to continuously maintain adequate amounts of O_2 (DO_2) to meet the metabolic demands of the tissues (VO_2), neither cardiac output nor mean arterial pressure are sensitive or specific measures of adequacy of cardiovascular function. Clearly, the best measures of adequacy of blood flow are the continued maintenance of normal end-organ function without evidence of excessive anaerobic metabolism. Normal urine output, gut activity, mentation, normal blood lactate levels, and spontaneous voluntary muscular activities reflect the most easily validated measures of body health [42]. Regrettably, many patients present with coexistent organ-system dysfunction, either pre-existent or caused by the insult. Furthermore, organ function cannot be monitored quickly enough to allow for titration of care. Thus, one cannot rely on these absolute markers to direct therapy [43]. Perhaps a more functional marker of adequacy of DO_2 to the tissues is SvO_2 [44]. Although values of SvO_2 greater than 70% do not ensure that all vascular beds are adequately perfused, SvO_2 values less than 60% are associated with oxidative impairment of tissues with a high metabolic rate, and values less than 50% are uniformly associated with evidence of anaerobic metabolism in some vascular beds [45]. Thus, as a negative predictive marker, preventing SvO_2 from decreasing below 50% and keeping it above

70% by fluid resuscitation, sedation, and ancillary support (eg, mechanical ventilation to reduce the work cost of breathing) all may improve O_2 delivery to metabolically active tissues.

If metabolic demand changes, cardiac output should co-vary with it [46]. Because this puts an added variable on the analysis of hemodynamic stability, a common approach in the cardiovascular management of the critically ill patient is to minimize the extraneous metabolic demands of the patient during intervals in which therapeutic interventions and diagnostic processes are being performed, so as to maintain stable baseline O_2 consumption for comparison. Thus, minimizing the work cost of breathing by using mechanical ventilation and reducing sympathetic responses by infusion of sedative agents reflect stabilizing processes that allow for accurate hemodynamic assessment. This is often more difficult to achieve than imagined [31]. Even a sedated and mechanically ventilated subject can be expending much effort assisting or resisting the ventilator-derived breaths. Muscular activities, such as moving in bed or being turned, "fighting the ventilator," and breathing spontaneously can easily double resting VO_2 [47]. O_2 supply and demand must co-vary as a normal and expected aspect of homeostasis under almost all conditions. In cardiovascular insufficiency states, such as cardiogenic shock or hypovolemic shock, total cardiac output is often limited and cannot increase enough in response to increasing metabolic demand to match the demand. Under these severe conditions VO_2 tends to remain constant by varying the extraction of O_2 in the tissues rather than by varying total blood flow. Thus, measures of SvO_2 can be used to identify patients in circulatory shock. Furthermore, resuscitation efforts that increase SvO_2 to greater than 70% should be associated with improved end-organ function.

The controversy of the pulmonary artery catheter

One would think that the clinical use of the PAC in the management of the hemodynamically unstable patient would be invaluable; however, that utility has not been documented. Although currently there are no proven indications for the insertion of a PAC, there are potential indications (not yet proven) for its use based on the need to assess cardiac function, global DO_2, intravascular volume status, and pulmonary pressures, among others summarized in Box 4.

The controversy over the use of the PAC in the management of critically ill patients continues to rage. Proponents of its use cite a physiologic rationale to diagnosis and titration of complex treatments that may otherwise be detrimental. Opponents of its use cite the almost total lack of data showing that its use in the management of critically ill patients improves outcome. Still, one truth remains: no catheter will improve outcome unless coupled to a treatment that itself improves outcome.

Despite some exciting initial uncontrolled reports of markedly improved outcome in high-risk surgery patients [48,49], further well-controlled studies in both high-risk surgical patients [50] and trauma patients [51,52] failed to

---

Box 4. Probable indications for pulmonary arterial catheterization

Data necessary for diagnosis
Distinguishing primary (noncardiogenic) from secondary (cardiogenic) pulmonary edema
Diagnosis of acute ventricular septal defect
Diagnosis of acute cardiac tamponade

Data necessary for management
Vasoactive drug therapy for cardiogenic shock with or without acute mitral regurgitation
Cardiac dysfunction with ischemia requiring intra-aortic balloon counter-pulsation
Balancing fluid and vasoactive therapy in acute lung injury states (acute respiratory distress syndrome [ARDS])
Assessing pulmonary pathology and response to ventilator therapy in acute lung injury states
To assess global cardiac output and systemic oxygen delivery
To direct vasodilator therapy in the management of pulmonary hypertension associated with acute cor pulmonale
To continuously monitor mixed venous oxygen saturation as an estimate of the adequacy of oxygen delivery to oxygen requirements in hemodynamically unstable patients

---

Adapted from Bellomo R, Pinsky MR. Invasive monitoring. In: Tinker J, Browne D, Sibbald W, editors. Critical care: Standards, Audit and Ethics. London: Hodder-Arnold, 1996; with permission.

---

document any improved survival when patients were treated based on pulmonary arterial catheter-derived data. In fact, the patients resuscitated aggressively to increase O_2 delivery into these survivor levels suffered a much higher mortality rate than did the control group treated conservatively [3]. Interestingly, as mentioned above, using only arterial pressure and $ScvO_2$, but with a defined physiology-based treatment algorithm, Rivers and coworkers [40] demonstrated a markedly improved survival in septic shock patients without the need of a PAC. On the other hand, a recent statistical analysis of the National Trauma Data Bank that included over 50,000 patients [53] showed for the first time a decrease in mortality in a selective group of trauma patients (severely injured, elderly, who arrived in shock) with the use of PAC.

Because of this unclear benefit on the use of PAC, the fact that it is an invasive monitoring procedure with potential serious complications acquires a major relevance when deciding about the risk-benefit of its use. Two recent

---

Box 5. Complications of the pulmonary artery catheter

Arrhythmia
Complete heart block
Catheter malpositioning
Extracardiac
Catheter knotting
Catheter fragmentation and meteorism
Pulmonary infarction
Pulmonary artery rupture
Thrombosis
Vascular infection

---

large prospective multicenter studies showed incidence of 5% and 10% of complications [54,55]. The most frequent complications described in these series were hematomas, arterial puncture, arrhythmias, and PAC-related infections, although a long list of complications has been described, as listed in Box 5. No deaths attributable to PAC were found on this series, but other authors had previously reported mortality generally due to right heart and pulmonary artery perforation [56,57].

Beyond the controversial use of the PAC, two recent randomized clinical trials using active protocols of hemodynamic monitoring and algorithms of goal-directed therapy guided by esophageal Doppler flowmetry [58] and pulse contour analysis for cardiac output [59] in postoperative surgical patients showed a decreased duration of hospital stay and morbidity. Thus the literature suggests that the generalized use of hemodynamic monitoring and aggressive goal-directed therapy could improve outcome, but that one does not need to use a PAC to achieve these goals. These arguments, however, miss the point that the utility of hemodynamic monitoring is relative— no monitoring device, no matter how accurate, safe and simple to use, will improve outcome unless coupled to a treatment that itself improves outcome. Thus, the question should not be, "Does the PAC improve outcome?" but rather, "Do treatment protocols that require information only attainable from pulmonary arterial catheterization improve outcome?" Furthermore, the treatment protocol itself should also be shown to improve outcome, because otherwise if the trial shows no difference in outcome with or without a PAC, the results may well reflect the fact that there was no benefit for the protocol in either arm of the study.

Summary

All surgical patients require monitoring to assess cardiovascular stability, and sometimes may benefit from optimization of their hemodynamic status. Therefore, all surgeons require a basic understanding of physiological underpinnings of hemodynamic monitoring. The physiological rationale is still the primary level of defense for monitoring critically ill patients.

Arterial catheterization to monitor arterial pressure is a safe procedure with a low complication rate; however, it should be used only when clear indications exist. There is no evidence that achieving pressures over 65 mm Hg increases organ perfusion or favors outcome. The analysis of pulse pressure variation is a useful method to assess preload responsiveness and a potential tool for resuscitation.

CVP has been wrongly used as a parameter of goal for replacement of intravascular volume in shock patients. Volume loading in patients who have CVP greater than 12 mmHg is unlikely to increase cardiac output, and attempts to normalize CVP in early goal-directed therapy during resuscitation have no proven benefit.

The use of PAC provides direct access to several physiological parameters, both as raw data and derived measurements (CO, SvO_2, DO_2). At present, targeting specific levels of DO_2 has proven effective only in high-risk surgery patients in the perioperative time. Ppao is often used as a bedside assessment of pulmonary edema, pulmonary vasomotor tone, intravascular volume status, and LV preload and performance. Several publications have explored the potential indications and benefits of the PAC to direct goal therapies. Beyond this controversy, there is a trend toward less invasive methods of hemodynamic monitoring, and current data support protocols of monitoring and goal-directed therapy that could improve outcome in selected group of surgical patients.

References

[1] Bellomo R, Pinsky MR. Invasive monitoring. In: Tinker J, Browne D, Sibbald W, editors. Critical care—standards, audit and ethics. London: Arnold Publishing Co., 2006. p. 82–104.

[2] Ledoux D, Astiz ME, Carpati CM, et al. Effects of perfusion pressure on tissue perfusion in septic shock. Crit Care Med 2000;28(8):2729–32.

[3] Hayes MA, Timmins AC, Yau EH, et al. Elevation of systemic oxygen delivery in the treatment of critically ill patients. N Engl J Med 1994;330(24):1717–22.

[4] Bickell WH, Wall MJ Jr, Pepe PE, et al. Immediate versus delayed fluid resuscitation for hypotensive patients with penetrating torso injuries. N Engl J Med 1994;331(17):1105–9.

[5] Capone AC, Safar P, Stezoski W, et al. Improved outcome with fluid restriction in treatment of uncontrolled hemorrhagic shock. J Am Coll Surg 1995;180(1):49–56.

[6] Kowalenko T, Stern S, Dronen S, et al. Improved outcome with hypotensive resuscitation of uncontrolled hemorrhagic shock in a swine model. J Trauma 1992;33(3):349–53.

[7] Rebuck AS, Read J. Assessment and management of severe asthma. Am J Med 1971;51(6): 788–98.

[8] Michard F, Boussat S, Chemla D, et al. Relation between respiratory changes in arterial pulse pressure and fluid responsiveness in septic patients with acute circulatory failure. Am J Respir Crit Care Med 2000;162(1):134–8.

[9] Monnet X, Rienzo M, Osman D, et al. Passive leg raising predicts fluid responsiveness in the critically ill. Crit Care Med 2006;34(5):1402–7.

[10] Gunn SR, Pinsky MR. Implications of arterial pressure variation in patients in the intensive care unit. Curr Opin Crit Care 2001;7(3):212–7.

[11] Michard F, Teboul JL. Predicting fluid responsiveness in ICU patients: a critical analysis of the evidence. Chest 2002;121(6):2000–8.

[12] Scheer B, Perel A, Pfeiffer UJ. Clinical review: complications and risk factors of peripheral arterial catheters used for haemodynamic monitoring in anaesthesia and intensive care medicine. Crit Care 2002;6(3):199–204.

[13] Michard F, Alaya S, Zarka V, et al. Global end-diastolic volume as an indicator of cardiac preload in patients with septic shock. Chest 2003;124(5):1900–8.

[14] Godje O, Peyerl M, Seebauer T, et al. Central venous pressure, pulmonary capillary wedge pressure and intrathoracic blood volumes as preload indicators in cardiac surgery patients. Eur J Cardiothorac Surg 1998;13(5):533–9.

[15] Buhre W, Weyland A, Schorn B, et al. Changes in central venous pressure and pulmonary capillary wedge pressure do not indicate changes in right and left heart volume in patients undergoing coronary artery bypass surgery. Eur J Anaesthesiol 1999;16(1):11–7.

[16] Magder S, Georgiadis G, Tuck C. Respiratory variations in right atrial pressure predict-response to fluid challenge. J Crit Care 2004;7:76–85.

[17] Magder S. How to use central venous pressure measurements. Curr Opin Crit Care 2005; 11(3):264–70.

[18] Venn R, Steele A, Richardson P, et al. Randomized controlled trial to investigate influence of the fluid challenge on duration of hospital stay and perioperative morbidity in patients with hip fractures. Br J Anaesth 2002;88(1):65–71.

[19] Thomsen HS, Lokkegaard H, Munck O. Influence of normal central venous pressure on onset of function in renal allografts. Scand J Urol Nephrol 1987;21(2):143–5.

[20] Shoemaker WC, Kram HB, Appel PL, et al. The efficacy of central venous and pulmonary artery catheters and therapy based upon them in reducing mortality and morbidity. Arch Surg 1990;125(10):1332–7.

[21] Sharkey SW. Beyond the wedge: clinical physiology and the Swan-Ganz catheter. Am J Med 1987;83(1):111–22.

[22] Swan HJ, Ganz W, Forrester J, et al. Catheterization of the heart in man with use of a flow-directed balloon-tipped catheter. N Engl J Med 1970;283(9):447–51.

[23] Hoyt JD, Leatherman JW. Interpretation of the pulmonary artery occlusion pressure in mechanically ventilated patients with large respiratory excursions in intrathoracic pressure. Intensive Care Med 1997;23(11):1125–31.

[24] Pinsky M, Vincent JL, De Smet JM. Estimating left ventricular filling pressure during positive end-expiratory pressure in humans. Am Rev Respir Dis 1991;143(1):25–31.

[25] Pinsky MR. Clinical significance of pulmonary artery occlusion pressure. Intensive Care Med 2003;29(2):175–8.

[26] Abraham AS, Cole RB, Green ID, et al. Factors contributing to the reversible pulmonary hypertension of patients with acute respiratory failure studies by serial observations during recovery. Circ Res 1969;24(1):51–60.

[27] Forrester JS, Diamond G, Chatterjee K, et al. Medical therapy of acute myocardial infarction by application of hemodynamic subsets (first of two parts). N Engl J Med 1976;295(24): 1356–62.

[28] Raper R, Sibbald WJ. Misled by the wedge? The Swan-Ganz catheter and left ventricular preload. Chest 1986;89(3):427–34.

[29] Kumar A, Anel R, Bunnell E, et al. Pulmonary artery occlusion pressure and central venous pressure fail to predict ventricular filling volume, cardiac performance, or the response to volume infusion in normal subjects. Crit Care Med 2004;32(3):691–9.

[30] Jansen JR, Bogaard JM, Versprille A. Extrapolation of thermodilution curves obtained during a pause in artificial ventilation. J Appl Physiol 1987;63(4):1551–7.

[31] Synder JV, Powner DJ. Effects of mechanical ventilation on the measurement of cardiac output by thermodilution. Crit Care Med 1982;10(10):677–82.

[32] Wesseling K, Wit BD, Weber J, et al. A simple device for the continuous measurement of cardiac output. Adv Cardiovasc Physiol 1983;(5):16–52.

[33] Feissel M, Michard F, Mangin I, et al. Respiratory changes in aortic blood velocity as an indicator of fluid responsiveness in ventilated patients with septic shock. Chest 2001;119(3): 867–73.

[34] Reuter DA, Felbinger TW, Schmidt C, et al. Stroke volume variations for assessment of cardiac responsiveness to volume loading in mechanically ventilated patients after cardiac surgery. Intensive Care Med 2002;28(4):392–8.

[35] Reuter DA, Felbinger TW, Kilger E, et al. Optimizing fluid therapy in mechanically ventilated patients after cardiac surgery by on-line monitoring of left ventricular stroke volume variations. Comparison with aortic systolic pressure variations. Br J Anaesth 2002;88(1): 124–6.

[36] Berkenstadt H, Margalit N, Hadani M, et al. Stroke volume variation as a predictor of fluid responsiveness in patients undergoing brain surgery. Anesth Analg 2001;92(4):984–9.

[37] Pinsky MR, Payen D. Functional hemodynamic monitoring. Crit Care 2005;9(6):566–72.

[38] Linton R, Band D, O'Brien T, et al. Lithium dilution cardiac output measurement: a comparison with thermodilution. Crit Care Med 1997;25(11):1796–800.

[39] Kurita T, Morita K, Kato S, et al. Comparison of the accuracy of the lithium dilution technique with the thermodilution technique for measurement of cardiac output. Br J Anaesth 1997;79(6):770–5.

[40] Rivers E, Nguyen B, Havstad S, et al. Early goal-directed therapy in the treatment of severe sepsis and septic shock. N Engl J Med 2001;345(19):1368–77.

[41] Reinhart K, Kuhn HJ, Hartog C, et al. Continuous central venous and pulmonary artery oxygen saturation monitoring in the critically ill. Intensive Care Med 2004;30(8): 1572–8.

[42] Marik PE. Gastric intramucosal pH. A better predictor of multiorgan dysfunction syndrome and death than oxygen-derived variables in patients with sepsis. Chest 1993;104(1):225–9.

[43] Pinsky MR. Beyond global oxygen supply-demand relations: in search of measures of dysoxia. Intensive Care Med 1994;20(1):1–3.

[44] Kandel G, Aberman A. Mixed venous oxygen saturation. Its role in the assessment of the critically ill patient. Arch Intern Med 1983;143(7):1400–2.

[45] Miller MJ, Cook W, Mithoefer J. Limitations of the use of mixed venous pO_2 as an indicator of tissue hypoxia. Clin Res 1979;(27):401A.

[46] Pinsky MR. The meaning of cardiac output. Intensive Care Med 1990;16(7):415–7.

[47] Weissman C, Kemper M, Damask MC, et al. Effect of routine intensive care interactions on metabolic rate. Chest 1984;86(6):815–8.

[48] Tuchschmidt J, Fried J, Astiz M, et al. Elevation of cardiac output and oxygen delivery improves outcome in septic shock. Chest 1992;102(1):216–20.

[49] Boyd O, Grounds RM, Bennett ED. A randomized clinical trial of the effect of deliberate perioperative increase of oxygen delivery on mortality in high-risk surgical patients. JAMA 1993;270(22):2699–707.

[50] Sandham JD, Hull RD, Brant RF, et al. A randomized, controlled trial of the use of pulmonary-artery catheters in high-risk surgical patients. N Engl J Med 2003;348(1):5–14.

[51] McKinley BA, Kozar RA, Cocanour CS, et al. Normal versus supranormal oxygen delivery goals in shock resuscitation: the response is the same. J Trauma 2002;53(5): 825–32.

[52] Velmahos GC, Demetriades D, Shoemaker WC, et al. Endpoints of resuscitation of critically injured patients: normal or supranormal? A prospective randomized trial. Ann Surg 2000; 232(3):409–18.

[53] Friese RS, Shafi S, Gentilello LM. Pulmonary artery catheter use is associated with reduced mortality in severely injured patients: a National Trauma Data Bank analysis of 53,312 patients. Crit Care Med 2006;34:1597–1601.

[54] Binanay C, Califf RM, Hasselblad V, et al. Evaluation study of congestive heart failure and pulmonary artery catheterization effectiveness: the ESCAPE trial. JAMA 2005;294(13): 1625–33.

[55] Harvey S, Harrison DA, Singer M, et al. Assessment of the clinical effectiveness of pulmonary artery catheters in management of patients in intensive care (PAC-Man): a randomised controlled trial. Lancet 2005;366(9484):472–7.

[56] Ducatman BS, McMichan JC, Edwards WD. Catheter-induced lesions of the right side of the heart. A one-year prospective study of 141 autopsies. JAMA 1985;253(6):791–5.

[57] Kearney TJ, Shabot MM. Pulmonary artery rupture associated with the Swan-Ganz catheter. Chest 1995;108(5):1349–52.

[58] McKendry M, McGloin H, Saberi D, et al. Randomised controlled trial assessing the impact of a nurse delivered, flow monitored protocol for optimisation of circulatory status after cardiac surgery. BMJ 2004;329(7460):258.

[59] Pearse R, Dawson D, Fawcett J, et al. Early goal-directed therapy after major surgery reduces complications and duration of hospital stay. A randomised, controlled trial [ISRCTN38797445]. Crit Care 2005;9(6):R687–93.

ELSEVIER
SAUNDERS

SURGICAL
CLINICS OF
NORTH AMERICA

Surg Clin N Am 86 (2006) 1457–1481

Management of Severe Sepsis in the Surgical Patient

Kristen C. Sihler, MD, MS[a],
Avery B. Nathens, MD, PhD, MPH[b,c],*

[a]Section of General Surgery, TC-2924D, University of Michigan Health System,
1500 E. Medical Center Drive, Ann Arbor, MI 48109-0331, USA
[b]Department of Surgery, Harborview Medical Center, 325 9th Avenue, Seattle,
WA 98104-2499, USA
[c]Department of Surgery, University of Washington, 325 9th Avenue, Seattle,
WA 98104-2499, USA

Sepsis and septic shock are not uncommon conditions in the surgical intensive care unit (ICU). There are many aspects to the term sepsis; thus before focusing on therapy, the terminology needs to be clarified. Sepsis is a generalized activation of the immune system in the presence of clinically suspected or culture-proven infection. Severe sepsis is sepsis with organ system dysfunction. Septic shock is sepsis with hypotension (systolic blood pressure <90 mm Hg) without other causes [1].

Epidemiology

In the year 2000 the incidence of sepsis in the United States was 240 per 100,000 population, based on the National Hospital Discharge Survey, and was increasing at 9% per year [2]. The incidence of severe sepsis is estimated at three cases per 100,000 population, based on hospital discharge data from seven states. The curve of the incidence across ages is J-shaped, with a high rate in infants, low rates in children and young adults, and steadily increasing rates thereafter (Fig. 1). More than half of the cases of sepsis are in patients 65 years of age or older. The overall incidence of severe sepsis is similar in men and women, but the age-adjusted incidence in women is lower. Overall mortality from severe sepsis is 28.6%, with the lowest mortality (10.0%) in children and the highest (38.4%) in adults 85 years of age or

* Corresponding author. Department of Surgery, Box 359796, Harborview Medical Center, 325 Ninth Avenue, Seattle, WA 98104-2499.
E-mail address: anathens@u.washington.edu (A.B. Nathens).

0039-6109/06/$ - see front matter © 2006 Elsevier Inc. All rights reserved.
doi:10.1016/j.suc.2006.09.005
surgical.theclinics.com

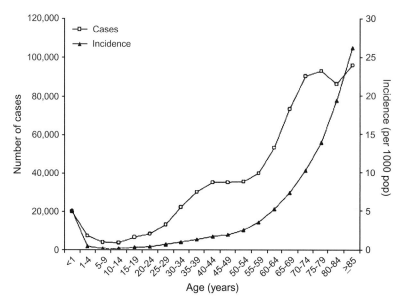

Fig. 1. National age-specific number and incidence of cases of severe sepsis. (*From* Angus DC, Linde-Zwirble WT, Lidicker J, et al. Epidemiology of severe sepsis in the United States: analysis of incidence, outcome, and associated costs of care. Crit Care Med 2001;29:1306; with permission.)

older. For adults who have comorbidities, however, mortality is higher and does not vary much with age. Overall mortality is higher for males than females, but when adjusted for age, comorbidities, and site of infection, the morality rates are the same for both genders.

The burden of disease associated with severe sepsis is staggering. Total hospital cost for the care of severe sepsis in the United States in 1995 was estimated at $16.7 billion [3]. In addition to the high in-hospital mortality, patients who have severe sepsis are still at a higher risk of dying once they are discharged from the hospital. In a study by Weycker and colleagues [4], in-hospital morality for adult patients who had severe sepsis was 21.2%, and at 1 year after diagnosis it had risen to 51.4%.

Surgical patients compose 28.6% of all severe sepsis patients and have similar mortality to medical patients [3]. In a study of 1125 patients who were hospitalized for more than 48 hours after surgery, 6.5% developed severe sepsis [5]. Among patients having major oncologic surgery, 20.4% developed severe sepsis, and 36.8% of these patients died. The most common source of sepsis was the lungs. Preoperative risk factors for severe sepsis included male gender and a higher burden of coexisting disease. Intra- and postoperative factors that put patients at increased risk for severe sepsis included presence of a pronounced systemic inflammatory response and a greater degree of early postoperative organ dysfunction, evident as early as postoperative day 2 [6]. In patients who had intra-abdominal infection and who required surgery, 11%

developed severe sepsis. Organ dysfunction was most commonly limited to the respiratory and cardiovascular system. The mortality was 34% in patients who had severe sepsis, compared with 6% overall. As in the prior study, pre-existing comorbidities, specifically cardiovascular, pulmonary, hepatic, renal, or neurologic disease, increased the risk of severe sepsis. Severe sepsis was more likely to complicate peritonitis if there was a nonappendiceal source or there was evidence of recurrent infection [7].

The Surviving Sepsis Campaign

Given the availability of clinical strategies and pharmacologic agents for the treatment of severe sepsis, there has been an increased emphasis on the identification and evidence-based management of severe sepsis. The Surviving Sepsis Campaign is the result of an international effort to develop guidelines for the treatment of severe sepsis [8]. The recommendations were developed by a modified Delphi technique, with recommendations graded based on the strength of the evidence behind them. In this article, the authors focus on the Severe Sepsis guidelines and modify the recommendations where necessary, such that they might better meet the needs of the surgical patient.

Initial resuscitation

It is generally believed that earlier and aggressive resuscitation to restore tissue perfusion reduces the risk of organ dysfunction and mortality in patients who have severe sepsis. Early attempts at resuscitation initially focused on providing supraphysiologic levels of tissue oxygen delivery, a concept referred to as supranormal oxygen delivery; however, two randomized controlled trials based on interpretation of data from pulmonary artery catheters and in which the intervention arm made liberal use of inotropic support failed to show benefit, and suggested the potential for harm [9,10]. In both of these studies, this goal-directed therapy was started when patients arrived in the ICU.

Providing resuscitation at an earlier phase of care in the emergency department and limiting the resuscitation goals to relatively conservative end points might offer greater benefits. This concept of early goal-directed therapy is derived from a trial in which 263 patients presenting to the emergency department with signs of severe sepsis or septic shock were randomized to receive either standard care or goal-directed therapy for the first 6 hours of resuscitation [11]. The experimental group received central venous catheters capable of measuring superior vena caval oxygen saturation as a surrogate for mixed venous oxygen saturation (SvO_2) and arterial catheters for measuring blood pressure. Central venous pressure (CVP) was maintained at 8 to 12 mm Hg with boluses of 500 mL of crystalloid intravenous fluid. Mean arterial pressure (MAP) was kept at 65 mm Hg or higher with intravenous fluid (Fig. 2). Patients were placed on mechanical ventilation if necessary and sedated as needed. Using this relatively simple approach, in-hospital mortality was reduced from 47% to 31%. Because these interventions (fluid, transfusions, SvO_2 monitoring) were evaluated together, it is difficult to ascertain how much each intervention contributed to the reduction in mortality. As a result, many institutions have simply emulated this protocol with the hope of reproducing these results at their institutions. Trzeciak and coworkers [12] studied their implementation of early goal-directed therapy and concluded that it could be implemented effectively without changes to the emergency department physical plant or staffing.

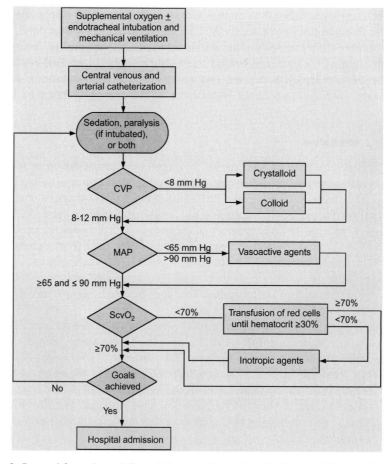

Fig. 2. Protocol for early goal-directed therapy. (*From* Rivers E, Nguyen B, Havstad S, et al. Early goal-directed therapy in the treatment of severe sepsis and septic shock. N Engl J Med 2001;345(19):1371; with permission.)

Fluid resuscitation

Septic shock is a form of distributive shock, and large volumes of fluid may be required to compensate for the profound vasodilation. Hypotensive patients should receive fluid boluses of 500 to 1000 mL of crystalloid, rather than simply increasing the rate of their maintenance fluids, to more rapidly assess their fluid responsiveness. Increasing the maintainance IV fluid rate from 100 mL/hr to 200 mL/hr will take 10 hours to infuse an extra liter of fluid, compared with 1 hour or less to infuse the same amount as a bolus. These patients can require massive amounts of fluid, and the input/output ratio is not useful for monitoring fluid needs during resuscitation. Patients should be monitored for fluid tolerance by watching for signs of pulmonary edema and congestive heart failure. Peripheral edema is to be expected because of the profound capillary leak that accompanies the systematic inflammatory response, and should not be taken as a sign of fluid intolerance.

Because of this capillary leak, there has been an interest in using albumin for resuscitation, with the thought that it would remain within the intravascular space. Results of two meta-analyses comparing albumin and crystalloid suggested that mortality was higher in patients receiving albumin [13,14]. The authors also found that trials with higher methodologic quality showed a trend toward reduced mortality with albumin [14]. A subsequent randomized controlled trial of almost 7000 critically ill, hypovolemic patients, of whom 18% had sepsis, demonstrated a trend toward reduced survival in septic patients receiving albumin (31% mortality versus 35%, $P = 0.09$) [15]. In light of the lack of clear benefit of albumin coupled with its increased cost, crystalloid remains the resuscitation fluid of choice at this time. Lactated Ringer's solution should be used to prevent the hyperchloremic metabolic acidosis seen with the administration of large volumes of saline. Because lactated ringer's contains potassium, repeat assessments of serum potassium levels should be considered, particularly in patients who have oliguria or renal dysfunction.

A CVP monitor should be placed to better guide fluid management in patients who have severe sepsis, with a target CVP of 8 to 12 cm H_2O. Fluid status can also be assessed by monitoring the respiratory variation of the arterial line tracing. When the systolic pressure varies by more than 5 to 10 mmHg with respiration, the patient remains hypovolemic [16]. This measurement is only useful in patients receiving positive pressure ventilation. A slightly more complex measurement is assessment of the pulse pressure (systolic minus diastolic blood pressure). The maximal pulse pressure (Pp_{max}) is measured during inspiration and the minimal pulse pressure (Pp_{min}) is measured during expiration. The percentage difference is then calculated by the formula $\Delta Pp(\%) = 100 \times (Pp_{max} - Pp_{min})/[(Pp_{max} + Pp_{min})/2]$. A ΔPp of 13% or more is indicative of a patient who will be volume responsive. This was a more reliable indicator of fluid responsiveness than systolic pressure variation in a study of 40 patients who had septic shock [17]. Although this is more difficult to calculate, it is one of the calculations performed automatically by the lithium indicator dilution cardiac output monitor device, which provides real-time cardiac output data from the arterial line tracing [18].

In septic patients who develop acute lung injury, a more conservative approach to intravascular volume may be useful. A trial of 1000 patients who had acute lung injury, of whom about 25% had sepsis [19], showed that limited fluid administration once patients were no longer hypotensive and liberal use of diuretics shortened time on the ventilator by 1.5 days, and reduced ICU length of stay by 2.3 days. There was no difference in mortality. Of note, in this same trial, subjects were also randomized to a central venous catheter or pulmonary artery catheter (PAC). Patients randomized to a PAC had no better outcome and a higher risk of catheter-related complications [20]. The extent to which these data from either trial can be generalized to the surgical patient is unclear. Only 44% of subjects randomized were in a surgical ICU, and care was highly protocolized. Nevertheless, there is no reason to believe that patients undergoing operation for sepsis would have a significantly different risk/benefit ratio using these approaches than critically ill medical patients.

Management of metabolic acidosis

Metabolic acidosis, particularly lactic acidosis, commonly complicates sepsis and septic shock. Lactic acidosis is sometimes divided into type A (caused by tissue hypoxia) and type B (no clinical evidence of tissue hypoxia), but in sepsis both mechanisms may be involved. Clinicians commonly correct a low pH with bicarbonate, usually citing the negative effects of acidemia on myocardial dysfunction; however, studies of myocardial function in acidemia have found conflicting results. Moreover, as experience grows with permissive hypercapnia in acute respiratory distress syndrome (ARDS) and asthma, it has become clear that patients can often tolerate a pH as low as 7.20. There is even some evidence that acidemia is protective in critical illness, with delayed onset of cell death in acidotic hepatocytes undergoing anoxia, and acidosis during reperfusion has been shown to limit the size of infarcted myocardium [21].

The other issue is the direct effect of bicarbonate. Bicarbonate has been shown to raise PCO_2 (CO_2 being a weak acid) when given to mechanically ventilated patients who have lactic acidosis [22]. Bicarbonate has also been shown to increase lactic acid production [23]. A variety of mechanisms have been proposed for this effect, including a shift in the oxyhemoglobin saturation relationship, increased anaerobic glycolysis (mediated by pH-sensitive phosphofructokinase, the rate-limiting step), and changes in hepatic blood flow or lactate clearance. Because bicarbonate raises CO_2 levels, and CO_2 is more diffusible than bicarbonate, pH in intracellular spaces and cerebrospinal fluid may actually drop. This mechanism might explain the increase in intracranial pressure sometimes seen with bicarbonate boluses. Animal studies have not shown a hemodynamic benefit to bicarbonate infusion over saline. Two human studies showed no changes in hemodynamics or catecholamine responsiveness, despite an increase in pH and serum bicarbonate concentrations. Both studies compared bicarbonate to saline and suggested that the commonly observed hemodynamic improvement seen with bicarbonate may in fact be due to increased preload from the volume of the infusion [22,24].

Therefore bicarbonate administration is not recommended for pH greater than 7.15 [25], and may not be necessary at even a lower pH. It is, however, still recommended for bicarbonate-losing acidoses, such as renal tubular acidosis.

Antimicrobial therapy

Empiric selection of antimicrobials

In patients who have suspected sepsis, it is critical to initiate early empiric antimicrobial therapy, because several cohort studies have demonstrated an increased incidence of adverse outcomes in patients who had bacteremia or pneumonia and who experienced a delay in receiving the appropriate antimicrobials [26,27]. Similar data exist for patients who have intra-abdominal infection, with inappropriate empiric choices associated with a twofold greater risk of death [28]. Agents should be broad-spectrum and should cover likely causative organisms, based on patient presentation and susceptibility patterns in the hospital and community. Empiric treatment of patients who have complicated skin and soft tissue infections should take into account the prevalence of community-acquired, methicillin-resistant *Staphylococcus aureus*, which might necessitate empiric therapy with vancomycin or linezolid [29]. The goal should be to initiate empiric antimicrobial therapy within 1 hour of arrival in the ICU or emergency department, after drawing blood cultures. Once the causative organism has been identified, the spectrum of antimicrobial therapy may be narrowed. This de-escalation of antimicrobial therapy offers the best balance between appropriate early coverage and prevention of the later emergence of resistant organisms [30].

Surgical patients are at significant risk for fungal infections, and their diagnosis is frequently not suspected ante mortem, a phenomenon related to the limited predictive utility of culture-based (eg, blood cultures) means of making the diagnosis [31]. Even in those patients in whom the diagnosis is suspected, delays in instituting therapy have a significant impact on outcome [32]. Given these data, early presumptive therapy in specific subgroups of surgical patients may be warranted. For example, the addition of fluconazole to an empiric antimicrobial regimen in patients who have severe sepsis and peritonitis lowers the risk of fungal infections [33]. The risk factors for yeast in the peritoneal cavity have been well studied, and include female gender, prior antimicrobials, shock, and upper gastrointestinal (GI) perforation [34]. Patients who have severe sepsis caused by intra-abdominal infection and any of these risk factors should be treated with an antifungal agent.

The agent of choice will vary with the risk of non-albicans species and the patterns of institutional antifungal resistance [35].

Duration of antimicrobial therapy

Duration of therapy is guided by the patient's response to therapy. There is some evidence from a randomized trial of patients who had ventilator-associated pneumonia [36] that 8 days of therapy is as efficacious as 15 days, with the possible exception of non-lactose–fermenting, gram-negative rod infections, which had a higher pulmonary reinfection rate, but no increased mortality. For other infections, antibiotics should be stopped after 7 to 10 days, assuming the patient has improved clinically [37]. Failure to respond should mandate a careful search for either other sources of infection, superinfection, antimicrobial resistance, or inadequacy of source control.

Source control

Source control addresses the root cause of the sepsis by reducing or eliminating the focus of infection. There are three principles to source control: (1) drainage of infected fluid collections, (2) removal of infected or dead tissue and infected foreign bodies, and (3) correction of the abnormality that set the stage for the development of infection. Although all of these things need to be done, the patient must be resuscitated first. Investigations to determine the source of the infection can be done simultaneously if they can be done at the bedside (eg, portable ultrasound). Control should then be obtained with the least physiologic insult possible (eg, percutaneous catheter drainage of abscesses) until the patient is able to withstand a more definitive procedure if necessary. Necrotizing soft tissue infections and necrotic bowel are two surgical emergencies that necessitate rapid resuscitation and operation without delay once the patient is able to tolerate induction of general anesthesia [38].

Central lines should be removed if identified as a source of infection or if no other source can be found [39]. In the patient who has difficult or limited central venous access, the line can be exchanged over a guide wire, but this is associated with an increased risk of catheter exit site infection and failure of resolution of bacteremia. The risk of mechanical complications, however, is reduced with guide wire exchange [40]. Absence of inflammation at the site of catheter insertion should not be used to judge the presence of a catheter infection [41]. Ideally, a patient who has suspected catheter-related sepsis would have a 24 hour period without any central lines to help clear the infection and avoid seeding the new line, but this is frequently not possible in a critically ill patient. A new site of insertion should be used whenever possible.

Vasopressors

When adequate blood volume has been restored as evidenced by a central venous pressure (CVP) of 8 to 12 cmH$_2$O, persistent hypotension should be treated with vasopressors. If the patient is severely hypotensive, vasopressors may need to be started before fluid resuscitation can be completed. Target MAP is generally 60 to 65 mm Hg, but there is limited evidence for this goal. Ideally, the appropriate MAP for a given patient is determined by evaluating organ perfusion as vasopressors are titrated. Organ perfusion can be monitored by SvO$_2$, urine output, and lactate levels.

First-line agents for blood pressure support are norepinephrine and dopamine, with dobutamine added as needed for support of cardiac output. Dopamine is a precursor to norepinephrine and epinephrine. At low doses of dopamine the stimulation of DA1 receptors in the renal, coronary, and mesenteric beds predominates. At higher doses β-adrenergic effects start to dominate, increasing cardiac contractility and heart rate. At even higher doses α-adrenergic effects become dominant, with arterial vasoconstriction and increased blood pressure occurring. Norepinephrine is an α-adrenergic agonist with some β-adrenergic effects. Therefore it has a predominately vasoconstrictive effect, and may require the addition of dobutamine to augment cardiac output in patients who have sepsis-induced myocardial depression or pre-existing heart disease. Dobutamine is a β$_1$- and β$_2$-adrenergic agonist. It increases stroke volume and heart rate, and therefore cardiac output. Cardiac output can either be measured with a pulmonary artery catheter or other means of assessment (arterial wave form analysis, transesophageal echocardiography). Adequacy of cardiac output may also be inferred from central venous oxygen values. Because of the increase in afterload from norepinephrine, goal MAP should be as low as possible to maintain end-organ perfusion so as not to compromise cardiac output.

No large-scale clinical trials have been completed to provide recommendations as to which agents are associated with improved outcomes. A Cochrane review concluded that there was insufficient evidence to recommend one pressor strategy over another [42]; however, a large-scale observational trial conducted across multiple ICUs in Europe evaluated 1058 patients [43]. Of the patients in septic shock, 80% received norepinephrine and 35% received dopamine. Most patients received multiple agents. In a multivariate analysis, patients in shock who received any dopamine had higher 30-day mortality when compared with patients who did not receive any dopamine. Because this was an observational study, it is not sufficient to change practice, but it is an intriguing finding that warrants further study. Until a randomized controlled trial can be performed, practitioners should base choice of pressor agent on familiarity with the agent and individual patient response.

Vasopressin at 0.04 units/min without titration can be added to either dopamine or norepinephrine if high doses of the initial pressor are required to maintain MAP. Normally vasopressin has minimal effect on blood pressure with an intact tonic inhibitory baroreceptor input; however, this input is attenuated in septic shock, making the system much more sensitive to the vasoconstrictive effects of vasopressin [44]. In septic shock there is also a relative deficiency of vasopressin because of depletion of neurohypophyseal stores, inhibition of release by norepinephrine, and inhibition of production by nitric oxide [45]. The addition of vasopressin has been shown to reduce the dose of norepinephrine needed [46]. Higher doses of vasopressin (>0.1 –units/min) are associated with complications such as significant depression in cardiac output, myocardial ischemia, and cardiac arrest, and should not be used. Phenylephrine and epinephrine should not be used as first-line agents [47]. Phenylephrine can decrease stroke volume. Epinephrine may impair splanchnic circulation and exacerbate tachycardia.

Corticosteroids

Because the manifestations of sepsis are the result of a profound systemic inflammatory response, attempts to modify this response using corticosteroids have been evaluated for almost 50 years. Early studies evaluated very high, supraphysiologic doses for short durations (<72 hours). Taken together, these studies demonstrated no benefit to this approach and a significant potential for harm [48]. There are several potential reasons for the adverse effects of corticosteroids administered in this fashion. First, these higher doses typically have immunosuppressive effects and might limit the ability to clear an infection. These doses are also associated with significant hyperglycemia, which has been shown to adversely effect prognosis [49]. Lastly, this short duration is insufficient to adequately counter the more prolonged inflammatory response (Fig. 3).

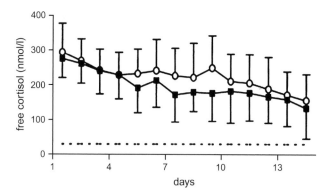

Fig. 3. The time course of cortisol concentrations in patients with septic shock (*open circles*) and multitrauma (*closed squares*). The upper limit of normal values is displayed as a dashed line. (*From* Beishuizen A, Thijs LG, Veres I. Patterns of corticosteroid-binding globulin and the free cortisol index during septic shock and multitrauma. Intensive Care Med 2001; 27:1584–91; with kind permission of Springer Science and Business Media.)

More recent reassessment of the role of corticosteroids has focused on providing lower doses for longer durations and identifying patients who have relative adrenal insufficiency. This approach is derived from a large prospective cohort study in which dynamic testing of the hypothalamic-pituitary-adrenal axis was used to predict outcome in patients who had septic shock [50]. Patients who had less than a 9 µg/dL increase in serum cortisol levels after a 250 µg corticotropin challenge were identified as at high risk of death, leading to the belief that these patients suffered relative adrenal insufficiency. In this context, there is insufficient adrenal reserve to respond in the face of the significant physiologic stressor represented by critical illness. Although high baseline cortisol levels were also an adverse prognostic marker, it was recognized that this cannot be affected by intervention (Fig. 4). Thus the goal changed from providing pharmacologic doses of corticosteroid to physiologic doses in the range of 300 to 400 mg of hydrocortisol equivalents daily. A subsequent randomized controlled trial [51] of 50 mg hydrocortisone every 6 hours for 7 days (and fludrocortisone) following the onset of septic shock demonstrated a significant mortality reduction and a faster rate of shock reversal in patients randomized to receive corticosteroid. In this study, 77% of all patients were nonresponders (<9 ug/dL increase in cortisol after a stimulation test), and there was no evidence of harm in administering this dose of corticosteroid to the responders.

As a result of these and other compelling data, patients who require vasopressors should undergo a cortisol stimulation test and be started on physiologic cortisol replacement until the results are available. Patients who have an adequate response to a cosyntropin stimulation test may have their corticosteroid replacement stopped, whereas those with an inadequate response should continue to receive corticosteroids for a total of 7 days. There is no need to taper the dose at the end of the course.

Activated protein C

The inflammatory response to sepsis is intimately associated with the coagulation cascade. Several inflammatory cytokines activate coagulation and inhibit fibrinolysis. Endogenous activated protein C promotes fibrinolysis and inhibits thrombosis and inflammation. Recombinant activated protein C (also known as drotrecogin alpha) is recommended for patients who have severe sepsis and an APACHE II score greater than 25 without significant risk of bleeding [52]. In this group it reduced mortality from 30.8% to 24.7%. Activated protein C has not been shown to be beneficial in patients who has single organ system failure or APACHE II lower than 25 [53]. A more extensive discussion of the role of APC in surgical patients is in an article elsewhere in this issue.

Transfusion

Transfusions are common in the ICU, with 37% to 40% of ICU patients receiving at least one unit of blood [54,55]. Patients who have sepsis may

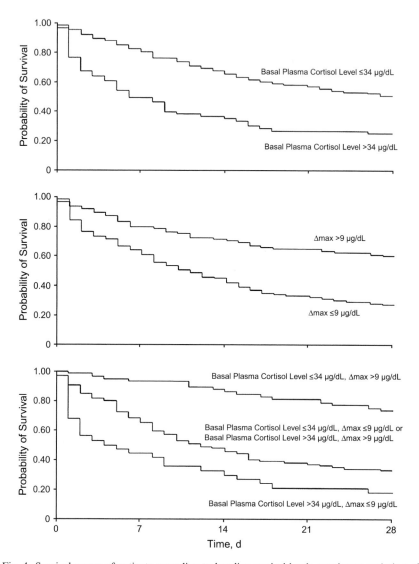

Fig. 4. Survival curves of patients according to baseline cortisol levels, maximum variation of cortisol levels after stimulation, and the combination of baseline levels and maximum variation. (*From* Annane D, Sebile V, Troche G, et al. A 3-level prognostic classification in septic shock based on cortisol levels and cortisol response to corticotropin. JAMA 2000;283:1038–45; with permission.)

become anemic through multiple mechanisms. They may have preexisting anemia, either from medical causes or from recent surgery. Anemia may be acquired through phlebotomy for laboratory testing, with blood loss from this source averaging about 40 mL per day [56]. Additionally, normal mechanisms of red cell replacement are suppressed in critical illness. There is a blunted increase in erythropoietin for a given hemoglobin concentration, a phenomenon attributed to the inhibitory effects of proinflammatory cytokines such as interleukin-1β and tumor necrosis factor-α, and by IL-1 and bacterial endotoxin. Acute renal failure, when present, is another contributor. Proliferation and differentiation of erythroid precursors are also inhibited. These effects are compounded by the alteration in iron metabolism, resulting in low concentrations of circulating iron [57].

Blood transfusion, however, is a double-edged sword. On one edge are the benefits of increased oxygen-carrying capacity and increased oncotic pressure from a colloid infusion that stays within the intravascular space. On the other edge are the numerous problems with transfusion: disease transmission, transfusion reactions, immunosuppression, inflammation, use of a limited resource, and cost. Traditional transfusion thresholds have been challenged by recent studies, most notably by the Transfusion Requirements in Critical Care trial [58], which demonstrated no harm from a transfusion threshold of 7 to 9 g/dL compared with a more traditional 10 to 12 g/dL and possible benefit in patients older than 55 and those who had an APACHE II of 25 or lower. Only 6% of patients in the restrictive group and only 4% in the traditional transfusion group were admitted to the ICU with a diagnosis of sepsis, however. In a post-hoc subgroup analysis there was no difference in mortality in patients who had cardiovascular disease using a restrictive transfusion threshold [59]. These results need to be viewed with caution because a significant number of patients screened for the original trial were not enrolled and the population was limited to euvolemic patients.

At this time, in light of evidence that restrictive transfusion thresholds are not harmful and may reduce mortality, transfusions should be limited to patients who have a hemoglobin of less than 7.0 g/dL. Some patients may tolerate an even lower hemoglobin level, whereas others, particularly those who have ongoing myocardial ischemia, will benefit from a higher hemoglobin level [60]. Transfusion for low SvO$_2$ was performed as part of the study on early goal directed therapy by Rivers and colleagues [11], but this has not been well-studied as an independent intervention. In a small study of 29 patients, transfusion did not result in a statistically significant increase in SvO$_2$ [61].

One often proposed solution to reduce transfusion needs is recombinant human erythropoietin. It has been widely used in patients who have chronic renal failure, but no studies exist of exogenous erythropoietin use in sepsis. A large trial of erythropoietin in critically ill patients [62], however, of whom 9% had sepsis or systemic inflammatory response syndrome (SIRS), showed a reduction in the likelihood of receiving a transfusion, with an odds ratio of 0.65 for the erythropoietin group. Of those who received blood, the erythropoietin group received a median of one unit, versus two units for the placebo group [62]. Because the effect required at least a week of treatment to be evident, erythropoietin should be reserved for those patients who are not only anemic, but also have an anticipated ICU length of stay of more than 7 days. Practitioners who choose to use erythropoietin should be aware that a trial of erythropoietin in patients who had metastatic breast cancer was terminated prematurely after 28.5% of patients in the erythropoietin arm developed thrombotic events, compared with no patients in the control arm [63]; however, patients who have metastatic breast cancer have a different thrombotic risk profile than septic patients, so it is unclear how this finding applies to these patients.

Mechanical ventilation

The most common site of organ failure in severe sepsis is the respiratory system. Respiratory failure, defined as the need for mechanical ventilation, occurs in 46% of cases of severe sepsis [3]. Mechanical ventilation should be instituted as needed. One of the most common manifestations of organ failure in patients who have sepsis is acute lung injury (ALI). Specific ventilatory strategies have been advocated in the management of ALI and are covered in greater detail in an article elsewhere in this issue.

Sedation and analgesia

Patients who have sepsis frequently require analgesia and sedatives, particularly if they are intubated. There are few randomized, controlled trials that provide evidence of superiority of one agent over another. The profiles and side effects of various drugs in concert with the patient's particular illness, and comorbidities will guide the selection.

Sedation is most often achieved with either propofol or benzodiazepines. Propofol has the benefit of a short duration of action, and is thus a good choice for patients who require short-term sedation or frequent neurological examinations; however, propofol can cause or worsen hypotension because of its myocardial depressant and vasodilatory properties. Among the benzodiazepines, midazolam and lorazepam have shorter half-lives than diazepam, and lorazepam does not have active metabolites. In a randomized, double-blind trial of 64 patients, Swart and coworkers [64] found no difference in the duration of sedation, but cost was lower and patients were sedated at the appropriate level for a higher percentage of time in the lorazepam group compared with the midazolam group. The authors also noted a large interpatient variability in the half-life of midazolam. They postulated this might be caused by variable hepatic function in critically ill patients and part of the mechanism behind the more appropriate sedation levels with lorazepam [64]. Another alternative for sedation is dexmedetomidine, a selective α_2 agonist approved for short-term sedation in adults. It generally does not cause hypotension, but no studies have been published on its use in septic patients.

Analgesia is generally provided by opioids. Fentanyl has a rapid onset and short half-life, although prolonged use may lead to a longer duration of action because of accumulation of the parent compound. It is useful for short-term use such as painful procedures. Morphine is longer-acting, but may cause hypotension because of histamine release and venodilation. Its metabolites can accumulate in renal failure. Despite these limitations, it is commonly used as a first-line agent and generally works well. Hydromorphone does not have the same hemodynamic effects as morphine, nor does it have active metabolites; therefore it may be beneficial in patients who cannot tolerate morphine. Merperidine has active metabolites that can lead to seizure if they accumulate, and is therefore generally avoided in critically ill patients needing analgesia. Side effects of opioids include depressed levels of consciousness and respiration, and inhibition of gastric and intestinal motility. Acetaminophen has an opioid-sparing effect [65] in addition to its antipyretic effect, and may be given as long as there is no hepatic insufficiency.

Sedation and analgesia should not be given continuously, but rather as boluses, unless large doses are required. In a prospective cohort trial, Kollef and colleagues [66] demonstrated that patients who received bolus sedation or analgesia had significantly shorter duration of mechanical ventilation and ICU and hospital lengths of stay compared with those who received continuous infusions. Patients should have a daily "sedation vacation"; that is, withdrawal of sedative and opiate infusions until the patient is awake or agitated enough to require resumption of the infusions. At this point patient sedation needs should be reassessed, commonly by starting the infusions back at half their previous rate. Kress and coworkers [67] performed a randomized controlled trial of 128 intubated patients, and showed that daily sedation vacations resulted in a decrease in ventilator days from 7.3 to 4.9 and a reduction in ICU length of stay from 9.9 to 6.4 days. In a retrospective blinded chart review of the same study population, Schweickert and colleagues [68] found that overall complications were reduced from 6.2 to 2.8%, likely directly related to the reduction in ventilator and ICU days.

Neuromuscular blockade is occasionally needed in critically ill patients, although indications for its use are not well-defined. It is often used with profound patient-ventilator dyssynchrony or when the patient is unable to oxygenate satisfactorily; however, multiple studies have shown an association between neuromuscular blockade and long-term neuromuscular dysfunction, referred to as critical illness polyneuropathy [69]. Therefore neuromuscular blockade should only be used when there are no other alternatives and maximal use of sedation has been unsuccessful. Sedation and analgesia should be continued and train-of-four monitoring should be used to monitor the degree of blockade. Patients should be maintained with one or two twitches, and patients whose twitches disappear entirely should have the paralytics stopped until twitches return.

Glycemic control

Hyperglycemia, defined as a blood sugar more than 110 mg/dL, is seen in over 95% of mechanically ventilated patients in the surgical ICU [49]. This rise in glucose has been attributed to increased amounts of circulating stress hormones, peripheral insulin resistance, drugs, including steroids, and exogenous dextrose administration. Elevated glucose levels have a number of detrimental effects, including increased leukocyte adhesion to vascular endothelium, and impaired neutrophil chemotaxis and phagocytosis. Hyperglycemia also enhances the procoagulant state of critically ill patients [70].

Tight glycemic control has become an integral part of critical care. It has been shown to improve mortality in a randomized, controlled trial of 1548 surgical patients, the majority of whom were patients admitted following cardiac surgery [49]. ICU mortality was significantly lower (4.3% versus 8.0%) in patients randomized to tight glycemic control (80–110 mg/dL) compared with those who only received insulin after their blood glucose rose above 200 mg/dL. The beneficial effect appeared to be caused by a reduction in the risk of deaths caused by sepsis-induced multiple organ failure. In addition to the mortality benefit, patients randomized to tight glycemic control also had a shorter ICU length of stay (LOS), decreased rate of mechanical ventilatory support lasting longer than 14 days, an attenuated inflammatory response, less antibiotic use, and decreased incidence and duration of critical illness polyneuropathy. Benefits from intensive insulin therapy appear to be related to control of glucose levels and not to the dose of insulin used [71]. In a later study [72], the same investigators found that the effects of tight glycemic control in a medical ICU population were not as profound. This may relate to the higher attributable mortality of sepsis in surgical patients.

Renal failure

Acute renal failure (ARF) occurs in 19% to 50% of patients who have sepsis, and is associated with a mortality of almost 70% [73]. Conversely, almost half of all cases of ARF (defined as urine output less than 200 mL in 12 hours or blood urea nitrogen greater than 84 mg/dL) are associated with septic shock, making it the leading etiology of ARF in the ICU [74]. Estimates of the true incidence are complicated by the lack of a standard definition. In a large epidemiologic study of severe sepsis [75], renal failure was the acute organ system failure most strongly associated with death, with an odds ratio of 3.1.

The etiology of renal failure in sepsis is multifactorial. Tumor necrosis factor appears to cause direct injury [76], but hypovolemia, nephrotoxic drugs, and iodinated contrast for radiographic studies also play roles. Adequate hydration and avoidance of hypotension are the mainstays of prevention of ARF. Low-dose dopamine was long thought to be beneficial to preserving renal function; however, a randomized, double-blind study of 328 patients who had SIRS and early renal dysfunction [77] found no difference in peak serum creatinine, need for renal replacement therapy, or mortality. Although not truly a preventative trial because patients were already showing signs of renal dysfunction, it does strongly suggest that low-dose dopamine is not beneficial. Norepinephrine and vasopressin have both been shown in small-scale studies to improve urine output and glomerular filtration rate [78].

It is critical to avoid nephrotoxic agents, such as aminoglycosides and intravenous iodinated contrast media. Most nephrotoxic medications have satisfactory alternatives, but there is often no satisfactory alternative for iodinated contrast in septic patients, who often need studies for source identification or evaluation for pulmonary embolism. Iodinated contrast is thought to induce renal failure through direct tubular toxicity, generation of oxygen free radicals, and a reduction of renal blood flow. Patients who have pre-existing renal impairment and those who have diabetes are at highest risk. Hydration is the first line of defense against contrast-induced nephropathy (CIN). Trevedi and colleagues [79] showed that patients randomized to IV normal saline at 1 mg/kg/hr beginning 12 hours before contrast administration for angiography and continuing for 24 hours had a lower rate of CIN than patients randomized to unrestricted oral fluids. The relative risk for the saline group was 0.11. Mueller and coworkers [80] demonstrated that patients randomized to normal saline hydration had lower rates of CIN than those who were hydrated with half normal saline with 5% dextrose (0.9% versus 2%), with an odds ratio of 0.3.

N-acetylcysteine (NAC) has been proposed as a pharmacologic means of preventing CIN because of its free radical scavenging properties, yet trials of NAC in this context have yielded conflicting results. Further, most of the trials enroll patients receiving radiocontrast for angiography (cardiac catheterization). There is a paucity of data addressing the prevention of ARF in patients who have sepsis. In a meta-analysis of 9 trials [81], the relative risk for CIN was 0.51 (95% CI, 0.35 to 0.74) with NAC. NAC is inexpensive, nontoxic, and possibly beneficial; however, the study authors note that renal failure requiring dialysis was rare (0.2%) and that emergent studies requiring IV contrast should not be delayed for administration of NAC [81].

Because free radical formation is enhanced in an acidic environment, bicarbonate infusion has been proposed as protection from CIN. A study of 137 patients who had chronic renal insufficiency [82] randomized to hydration with sodium chloride or sodium bicarbonate before receiving iodinated intravenous contrast demonstrated significant benefit with this approach. Glomerular filtration increased by 8.5% in the bicarbonate group, yet declined by 0.1% in the sodium chloride group. Absolute risk reduction of CIN (defined as >25% increase in creatinine) was 11.9%, yielding a need to treat 8.4 patients to prevent one case of CIN. The study had several methodologic limitations, however, and was not adequately blinded [82].

A full discussion of the advantages and disadvantages of various renal replacement therapies is beyond the scope of this article. Intermittent hemodialysis (IHD) is thought to induce hemodynamic instability because of the large amount of fluid removed in a short time period. Therefore continuous renal replacement therapy (CRRT), which removes fluid and toxins at a slower rate, is traditionally used in unstable, critically ill patients. A small trial of 27 patients did not show a difference in blood pressure changes or vasopressor requirements for patients on IHD compared to those on CRRT [83], however. Studies comparing outcomes of CRRT and IHD have been limited by methodologic issues and have yielded conflicting results [78]. At this time there is no evidence to suggest that there is a difference in outcomes among the various methods of extracorporeal renal replacement; however, there is a report suggesting that daily hemodialysis results in earlier recovery of renal function in ICU patients when compared with every-other-day hemodialysis [84].

Stress ulcer prophylaxis

Clinically significant gastrointestinal bleeding occurs in about 2% of critically ill patients. Risk factors include mechanical ventilation for more than 48 hours and coagulopathy [85], both of which can complicate sepsis. The relative effectiveness of various classes of pharmacologic prophylaxis (H_2 receptor antagonists, proton pump inhibitors, and sucralfate) is controversial. The clinical trials designed to address efficacy have been hampered by varying definitions of end points (any bleeding; clinically significant bleeding) and the use of a placebo or active treatment groups. The largest trial (1200 patients) by Cook and colleagues [86] compared ranitidine and sucralfate in a double-blinded fashion and examined clinically significant GI bleeding as the end point. The risk of bleeding was significantly lower in the ranitidine group (1.7%) versus the sucralfate group (3.8%). The number of critically ill, mechanically ventilated patients who would need to receive ranitidine instead of sucralfate to prevent one gastrointestinal bleed was 48 [86]. A meta-analysis published 2 years later [87] looked at the effectiveness of ranitidine and sucralfate in placebo-controlled trials. Ranitidine was statistically indistinguishable from placebo for the prevention of GI bleeding. There was only one study looking at sucralfate versus placebo for GI bleeding and it did not show a difference [87]. Recently two small trials, one comparing ranitidine to sucralfate to placebo [88], and one comparing famotidine to omeprazole to sucralfate to placebo, found no difference in the rates of gastrointestinal hemorrhage [89]. Also, a historical observational study of over 1400 patients [90] found no difference in clinically significant gastrointestinal hemorrhage before and after the institution of stress ulcer prophylaxis, largely using sucralfate. These studies suggest that the issue of overall efficacy of stress ulcer prophylaxis is not completely resolved, and that a large, placebo-controlled trial with multiple intervention groups is needed. The incidence of clinically significant stress ulcer bleeding is so low, however, that a study to definitively settle the issue is no longer practical.

H_2 receptor antagonists and proton pump inhibitors raise the gastric pH, thus defeating one of the natural mechanisms against bacteria colonization in the upper GI tract. There is concern that using these agents might result in a greater risk of ventilator-associated pneumonia as a result of microaspiration of heavily colonized gastric secretions. The study by Cook and colleagues [86] was adequately powered to detect a 25% reduction in ventilator-associated pneumonia in the sucralfate group, yet no significant difference was identified. The meta-analysis mentioned above [87] examined the risk of pneumonia with ranitidine versus placebo, sucralfate versus placebo, and ranitidine versus sucralfate. In the placebo-controlled studies, neither raniditine nor sucralfate had an effect on ventilator-associated pneumonia rates, but in head-to-head studies, ranitidine had a higher risk of ventilator-associated pneumonia [87].

Given the available evidence, H_2 receptor antagonist therapy is recommended over sulcalfate in patients meeting high risk criteria for stress ulcer bleeding. If neither is available or can be used, a proton pump inhibitor should be considered. Stress ulcer prophylaxis should be discontinued once patients are receiving enteral feeds, unless they are also receiving steroids.

Long-term outcomes after severe sepsis

There are very few studies of long-term outcomes after sepsis. One study by Granja and colleagues [91] compared 104 patients admitted to the ICU with severe sepsis to 133 ICU patients who did not have sepsis. The study authors looked at health-related quality of life 6 months after ICU discharge. The patients' health-related quality of life was similar, with the exception of anxiety and depression, which were less prevalent in the patients who had sepsis; however, about half of both groups of patients reported that they had trouble with or were unable to perform their usual activities, suggesting that illness resulting in an ICU stay results in prolonged decline in health status [91].

Other evaluations of long-term outcome following critical illness suggest that older age and increased severity of illness are associated with decreased general health perception and poorer physical functioning [92]. Post-traumatic stress disorder might occur after an episode of critical care, and might be related to the depth of sedation. Specifically, less sedation may be protective because it mitigates the need to fill in a memory void with delusional thoughts [93]. Physical weakness is also a problem. A study by Herridge and coworkers [94] of survivors from ARDS found that patients had proximal muscle weakness and poor physical status at 3 months after discharge. This weakness improved over the first year after discharge but did not return to baseline. Most of the decline in physical status was nonpulmonary. Factors associated with poor physical function were illness acquired during the ICU stay, any corticosteroid treatment during the ICU stay, rate of resolution of the lung injury, and multiorgan dysfunction [94].

As we learn more about how to keep critically ill patients alive, we also need to learn how to maintain the quality of that life in the months and years after they leave our ICUs. Despite the poorer prognosis of elderly patients, many of them are able to return to functional lives, and age should not be used as a reason to withhold treatment [93].

Summary

The incidence of sepsis is increasing, but the case fatality rate is decreasing. Several aspects of care likely contribute to these better outcomes, including:

- Early care
- Provide large amounts of crystalloid intravenous fluids.
- Culture and then start broad-spectrum antibiotics quickly.
- Use pressors as needed to maintain blood pressure. This should be either dopamine or norepinephrine with vasopressin at a fixed dose of 0.04 units/min if high doses are needed. Dobutamine can be added for inotropic support.
- Monitor CVP and administer fluids to maintain a pressure of 8–12 cm H_2O. Monitor superior vena caval oxygen content and transfuse as needed to keep it at 70%.
- Treatment with bicarbonate is not necessary for pH >7.15.
- Determine the source of infection and obtain source control with the least physiologic stress possible. If no source can be found, assume central lines are the source and remove or replace them at new sites.
- Begin antimicrobial therapy with broad-spectrum antibiotics and narrow coverage once the organisms and sensitivities are determined. Duration of therapy should be 8 days for VAP and 7–10 days for other conditions, with the exact duration determined by the patient's clinical response. Antifungal therapy should be added if the patient fails to respond or there is clinical suspicion of fungal infection.
- Patients who have hypotension should receive a cosyntropin stimulation test, and if the rise is ≤ 9 µg/dL, then physiologic stress doses of hydrocortisone should be administered for 7 days.
- Activated protein C should be considered in appropriate patients.
- Red cell transfusions can be withheld until the hemoglobin concentration drops to 7 g/dL, unless the patient has an SvO_2 $<70\%$ (during acute resuscitation) or is experiencing an acute coronary syndrome.
- Sedation and analgesia should be provided through boluses if possible, and a daily sedation vacation should be performed. Neuromuscular blockage should be avoided unless absolutely necessary.
- Maintain blood sugars in the range of 80–110 mg/dL.
- Reduce the risk of renal failure through aggressive hydration and minimization of hypotension. Hydrate patients when they receive iodinated contrast and consider NAC and bicarbonate.

- Stress ulcer prophylaxis should be provided to high-risk patients using H_2-receptor blocking medications or proton pump inhibitors, and should be discontinued once enteral feeds are started.

References

[1] Levy MM, Fink MP, Marshall JC, et al. 2001 SCCM/ESICM/ACCP/ATS/SIS International Sepsis Definitions Conference. Crit Care Med 2003;31:1250–6.

[2] Martin GS, Mannino DM, Eaton S, et al. The epidemiology of sepsis in the United States from 1979 through 2000. N Engl J Med 2003;348:1546–54.

[3] Angus DC, Linde-Zwirble WT, Lidicker J, et al. Epidemiology of severe sepsis in the United States: analysis of incidence, outcome, and associated costs of care. Crit Care Med 2001;29: 1303–10.

[4] Weycker D, Akhras KS, Edelsberg J, et al. Long-term mortality and medical care charges in patients with severe sepsis. Crit Care Med 2003;31:2316–23.

[5] Bellomo R, Goldsmith D, Russell S, et al. Postoperative serious adverse events in a teaching hospital: a prospective study. Med J Aust 2002;176:216–8.

[6] Mokart D, Leone M, Sannini A, et al. Predictive perioperative factors for developing severe sepsis after major surgery. Br J Anaesth 2005;95:776–81.

[7] Anaya DA, Nathens AB. Risk factors for severe sepsis in secondary peritonitis. Surg Infect (Larchmt) 2003;4:355–62.

[8] Dellinger RP, Carlet JM, Masur H, et al. Surviving Sepsis Campaign guidelines for management of severe sepsis and shock. Crit Care Med 2004;32:858–73.

[9] Hayes MA, Timmins AC, Yau E, et al. Elevation of systemic oxygen delivery in the treatment of critically ill patients. N Engl J Med 1994;330:1717–22.

[10] Gattinoni L, Brazzi L, Pelosi R, et al. A trial of goal-oriented hemodynamic therapy in critically ill patients. SvO2 Collaborative Group. N Engl J Med 1995;333:1025–32.

[11] Rivers E, Nguyen B, Havstad S, et al. Early goal-directed therapy in the treatment of severe sepsis and septic shock. N Engl J Med 2001;35:1368–77.

[12] Trzeciak S, Dellinger RP, Abate NL, et al. Translating research to clinical practice: a 1-year experience with implementing early goal-directed therapy for septic shock in the emergency department. Chest 2006;129:225–32.

[13] Cochrane Injuries Group Albumen Reviewers. Human albumin administration in critically ill patients: systematic review of randomised controlled trials. BMJ 1998;317:235–40.

[14] Wilkes MM, Navickis RJ. Patient survival after human albumin administration: a meta-analysis of randomized, controlled trials. Ann Intern Med 2001;135:149–64.

[15] The SAFE Study Investigators. A comparison of albumin and saline for fluid resuscitation in the intensive care unit. N Engl J Med 2004;350:2247–56.

[16] Rooke GA, Schwid HA, Shapira Y. The effect of graded hemorrhage and intravascular volume replacement on systolic pressure variation in humans during mechanical and spontaneous ventilation. Anesth Analg 1995;80:925–32.

[17] Michard F, Boussat S, Chemla D, et al. Relation between respiratory changes in arterial pulse pressure and fluid responsiveness in septic patients with acute circulatory failure. Am J Respir Crit Care Med 2000;162:134–8.

[18] Pearse RM, Ikram K, Barry J. Equipment review: an appraisal of the LiDCO plus method of measuring cardiac output. Crit Care 2004;8:190–5.

[19] The National Heart. Lung, and Blood Institute Acute Respiratory Distress Syndrome (ARDS) Clinical Trials Network. Comparison of two fluid management strategies in acute lung injury: the Fluid and Catheter Treatment Trial. N Engl J Med 2006;354:2564–75.

[20] The National Heart, Lung, and Blood Institute Acute Respiratory Distress Syndrome (ARDS) Clinical Trials Network. Pulmonary-artery versus central venous catheter to guide treatment of acute lung injury. N Engl J Med 2006;354:2213–24.

[21] Forsythe SM, Schmidt GA. Sodium bicarbonate for the treatment of lactic acidosis. Chest 2000;117:260–7.

[22] Cooper DJ, Walley KR, Wiggs BR, et al. Bicarbonate does not improve hemodynamics in critically ill patients who have lactic acidosis. A prospective, controlled clinical study. Ann Intern Med 1990;112:492–8.

[23] Graf H, Leach W, Arieff AI. Evidence for a detrimental effect of bicarbonate therapy in hypoxic lactic acidosis. Science 1985;227:754–6.

[24] Mathieu D, Neviere R, Billard V, et al. Effects of bicarbonate therapy on hemodynamics and tissue oxygenation in patients with lactic acidosis: a prospective, controlled clinical study. Crit Care Med 1991;19:1352–6.

[25] Cariou A, Vinsonneau C, Dhainaut J-F. Adjunctive therapies in sepsis: an evidence-based review. Crit Care Med 2004;32(Suppl):S562–70.

[26] Ibrahim EH, Sherman G, Ward S, et al. The influence of inadequate antimicrobial treatment of bloodstream infections on patient outcomes in the ICU setting. Chest 2000;118:146–55.

[27] Iregui M, Ward S, Sherman G, et al. Clinical importance of delays in the initiation of appropriate antibiotic treatment for ventilator-associated pneumonia. Chest 2002;122:262–8.

[28] Montravers P, Gauzit R, Marmuse JP, et al. Emergence of antibiotic-resistant bacteria in cases of peritonitis after intraabdominal surgery affects the efficacy of empirical antimicrobial therapy. Clin Infect Dis 1996;23:486–94.

[29] Kollef MH, Micek ST. Methicillin-resistant Staphylococcus aureus: a new community-acquired pathogen? Curr Opin Infect Dis 2006;19:161–8.

[30] Rello J, Vidaur L, Sandiumenge A, et al. De-escalation therapy in ventilator-associated pneumonia. Crit Care Med 2004;32:2183–90.

[31] Mort TC, Yeston NS. The relationship of pre mortem diagnoses and post mortem findings in a surgical intensive care unit. Crit Care Med 1999;27:299–303.

[32] Morrell M, Fraser VJ, Kollef MH. Delaying the empiric treatment of Candida bloodstream infection until positive blood culture results are obtained: a potential risk factor for hospital mortality. Antimicrob Agents Chemother 2005;49:3640–5.

[33] Eggimann P, Francioli P, Bille J, et al. Fluconazole prophylaxis prevents intra-abdominal candidiasis in high-risk surgical patients. Crit Care Med 1999;27:1066–72.

[34] Dupont H, Bourichon A, Paugam-Burtz C, et al. Can yeast isolation in peritoneal fluid be predicted in intensive care unit patients with peritonitis? Crit Care Med 2003;31:752–7.

[35] Golan Y, Wolf MP, Pauker SG, et al. Empirical anti-Candida therapy among selected patients in the intensive care unit: a cost-effectiveness analysis. Ann Intern Med 2005;143:857–69.

[36] Chastre J, Wolff M, Fagon J-Y, et al. Comparison of 8 vs 15 days of antibiotic therapy for ventilator-associated pneumonia in adults: A randomized trial. JAMA 2003;290:2588–98.

[37] Bochud P-Y, Bonten M, Marchetti O, et al. Antimicrobial therapy for patients with severe sepsis and septic shock: an evidence-based review. Crit Care Med 1997;25:1417–24.

[38] Marshall JC, Maier RV, Jemenez M, et al. Source control in the management of severe sepsis and septic shock: an evidence-based review. Crit Care Med 2004;32(Suppl):S513–26.

[39] O'Grady NP, Barie P, Bartlett J, et al. Practice parameters for evaluating new fever in critically ill adult patients. Crit Care Med 1998;26:392–408.

[40] Cook D, Randolph A, Kernerman P, et al. Central venous catheter replacement strategies: a systematic review of the literature. Crit Care Med 1997;25:1417–24.

[41] Safdar N, Maki DG. Inflammation at the insertion site is not predictive of catheter-related bloodstream infection with short-term, noncuffed central venous catheters. Crit Care Med 2002;30:2632–5.

[42] Mullner M, Urbanek B, Havel C, et al. Vasopressors for shock. Cochrane Database Syst Rev 2004;(3):CD003709.

[43] Sakr Y, Reinhart K, Vincent J-L, et al. Does dopamine administration in shock influence outcome? Results of the Sepsis Occurrence in Acute Ill Patients (SOAP) study. Crit Care Med 2006;34:589–97.

[44] den Ouden DT, Meinders AE. Vasopressin: physiology and clinical use in patients with vaso-dilatory shock. Neth J Med 2005;63:4–13.

[45] Homes CL, Patel BM, Russell JA, et al. Physiology of vasopressin relevant to management of septic shock. Chest 2001;120:989–1002.

[46] Dunser MW, Mayr AJ, Umer H, et al. Arginine vasopressin in advanced vasodilatory shock. A prospective, randomized, controlled study. Circulation 2003;107:2313–9.

[47] Beale RJ, Hollenberg SM, Vincent J-L, et al. Vasopressor and inotropic support in septic shock: an evidence-based review. Crit Care Med 2004;32(Suppl):S455–65.

[48] Annane D, Bellissant E, Bollaert PE, et al. Corticosteroids for severe sepsis and septic shock: a systematic review and meta-analysis. BMJ 2004;329:480–8.

[49] Van den Berghe G, Wouters P, Weekers F, et al. Intensive insulin therapy in critically ill patients. N Engl J Med 2001;345:1359–67.

[50] Annane D, Sébille V, Troché G, et al. A 3-level prognostic classification in septic shock based on cortisol levels and cortisol response to corticotrophin. JAMA 2000;283:1038–45.

[51] Annane D, Sebille V, Charpentier G, et al. Effect of treatment with low doses of hydro-cortisone and fluoricortisone on mortality in patients with septic shock. JAMA 2002;288: 862–7.

[52] Bernard GR, Vincent JL, Laterre PF, et al. Efficacy and safety of recombinant human acti-vated protein C for severe sepsis. N Engl J Med 2001;344:699–709.

[53] Abraham E, Laterre PF, Garg R, et al. Drotrecogin alfa (activated) for adults with severe sepsis and a low risk of death. N Engl J Med 2005;353:1332–41.

[54] Chohan SS, McArdle F, McClelland DBL, et al. Red cell transfusion practice following the Transfusion Requirements in Critical Care (TRICC) study: prospective observational cohort study in a large UK intensive care unit. Vox Sang 2003;84:211–8.

[55] Walsh TS, Garrioch M, Maciver C, et al. Red cell requirements for intensive care units ad-hering to evidence-based transfusion guidelines. Transfusion 2004;44:1405–11.

[56] Vincent J-L, Baron J-F, Reinhart K, et al. Anemia and blood transfusion in critically ill patients. JAMA 2002;288:1499–507.

[57] Scharte M, Fink MP. Red blood cell physiology in critical illness. Crit Care Med 2003; 31(Suppl):S651–7.

[58] Hébert PC, Wells G, Blajchman MA, et al. A multicenter, randomized, controlled clinical trial of transfusion requirements in critical care. N Engl J Med 1999;340:409–17.

[59] Hébert PC, Yetisir E, Martin C, et al. Is a low transfusion threshold safe in critically ill patients with cardiovascular diseases? Crit Care Med 2001;29:227–34.

[60] Wu W-C, Rathore SS, Wang Y, et al. Blood transfusion in elderly patients with acute myo-cardial infarction. N Engl J Med 2001;345:1230–6.

[61] Mazza BF, Machado FR, Mazza DD, et al. Evaluation of blood transfusion effects on mixed venous oxygen saturation and lactate levels in patients with SIRS/sepsis. Clinics 2005;60: 311–6.

[62] Corwin HL, Gettinger A, Pearl RG, et al. Efficacy of recombinant human erythropoietin in critically ill patients. A randomized controlled trial. JAMA 2002;288:2827–35.

[63] Rosenzweig MQ, Bender CM, Lucke JP, et al. The decision to prematurely terminate a trial of R-HuEPO due to thrombotic events. J Pain Symptom Manage 2004;27:185–90.

[64] Swart EL, van Schijndel RJ, van Loenen AC, et al. Continuous infusion of lorazepam versus midazolam in patients in the intensive care unit: sedation with lorazepam is easier to manage and is more cost-effective. Crit Care Med 1999;27:1461–5.

[65] Peduta VA, Ballabio M, Sefanini S. Efficacy of propacetamol in the treatment of postoper-ative pain: morphine sparing effect in orthopedic surgery. Acta Anaesthesiol Scand 1998; 42:293–8.

[66] Kollef MH, Levy NT, Ahrens TS, et al. The use of continuous i.v. sedation is associated with prolongation of mechanical ventilation. Chest 1998;114:541–8.

[67] Kress JP, Pohlman AS, O'Conner MF, et al. Daily interruption of sedative infusions in crit-ically ill patients undergoing mechanical ventilation. N Engl J Med 2000;324:1471–7.

[68] Schweickert WD, Gehlbach BK, Pohlman AS, et al. Daily interruption of sedative infusions and complications of critical illness in mechanically ventilated patients. Crit Care Med 2004; 32:1272–6.

[69] Vender JS, Szokol JW, Murphy GS, et al. Sedation, analgesia, and neuromuscular blockade in sepsis: an evidence-based review. Crit Care Med 2004;34(Suppl):S554–61.

[70] Turina M, Fry DE, Polk HC. Acute hyperglycemia and the innate immune system: clinical, cellular, and molecular aspects. Crit Care Med 2005;33:1624–33.

[71] Van den Berghe G, Wouters PJ, Weekers F, et al. Outcome benefit of intensive insulin therapy in the critically ill: insulin dose versus glycemic control. Crit Care Med 2003;31:359–66.

[72] Van den Berghe G, Wilmer A, Hermans G, et al. Intensive insulin therapy in the medical ICU. N Engl J Med 2006;354:449–61.

[73] Schrier RW, Wang W. Acute renal failure and sepsis. N Engl J Med 2004;351:159–69.

[74] Uchino S, Kellum JA, Bellomo R, et al. Acute renal failure in critically ill patients. A multinational, multicenter study. JAMA 2005;294:813–8.

[75] The EPISEPSIS Group. EPISEPSIS: a reappraisal of the epidemiology and outcome of severe sepsis in French intensive care units. Intensive Care Med 2004;30:580–8.

[76] Wan L, Bellomo R, Giantomasso DD, et al. The pathogenesis of septic acute renal failure. Curr Opin Crit Care 2003;9:496–502.

[77] Bellomo R, Chapman M, Finfer S, et al. Low-dose dopamine in patients with early renal dysfunction: a placebo-controlled randomised trial. Australia and New Zealand Intensive Care Society Clinical Trials Group. Lancet 2000;356:2139–43.

[78] De Vriese AS. Prevention and treatmesnt of acute renal failure in sepsis. J Am Soc Nephrol 2003;14:792–805.

[79] Trivedi HS, Moore H, Nasr S, et al. A randomized prospective trial to assess the role of saline hydration on the development of contrast nephrotoxicity. Nephron Clin Pract 2003;93: C29–34.

[80] Mueller C, Buerkle G, Buettner HJ, et al. Prevention of contrast media-associated nephropathy: randomized comparison of 2 hydration regimens in 1620 patients undergoing coronary angioplasty. Arch Intern Med 2002;162:329–36.

[81] Liu R, Nair D, Ix J, et al. N-acetylcysteine for the prevention of contrast-induced nephropathy: a systematic review and meta-analysis. J Gen Intern Med 2005;20:193–200.

[82] Merten GJ, Burgess WP, Gray LV, et al. Prevention of contrast-induced nephropathy with sodium bicarbonate: a randomized controlled trial. JAMA 2004;291:2328–34.

[83] Misset B, Timsit JF, Chevret S, et al. A randomized cross-over comparison of the hemodynamic response to intermittent hemodialysis and continuous hemofiltration in ICU patients with acute renal failure. Intensive Care Med 1996;22:742–6.

[84] Schiffl H, Lang SM, Fischer R. Daily hemodialysis and the outcome of acute renal failure. N Engl J Med 2002;346:305–10.

[85] Cook DJ, Fuller HD, Guyantt GH, et al. Risk factors for gastrointestinal bleeding in critically ill patients. N Engl J Med 1994;330:377–81.

[86] Cook D, Guyatt G, Marshall J, et al. A comparison of sucralfate and ranitidine for the prevention of upper gastrointestinal bleeding in patients requiring mechanical ventilation. N Engl J Med 1998;338:791–7.

[87] Messori A, Trippoli S, Vaiani M, et al. Bleeding and pneumonia in intensive care patients given ranitidine and sucralfate for prevention of stress ulcer: meta-analysis of randomized controlled trials. BMJ 2000;321:1–7.

[88] Misra UK, Kalita J, Pandey S, et al. A randomized placebo controlled trial of ranitidine versus sucralfate in patients with spontaneous intracerebral hemorrhage for prevention of gastric hemorrhage. J Neurol Sci 2005;239:5–10.

[89] Kantrova I, Svoboda P, Scheer P. Stress ulcer prophylaxis in critically ill patients: a randomized controlled trial. Hepatogastroenterology 2004;51:757–61.

[90] Faisy C, Guerot E, Diehl JL, et al. Clinically significant gastrointestinal bleeding in critically ill patients with and without stress-ulcer prophylaxis. Intensive Care Med 2003;29:1306–13.

[91] Granja C, Dias C, Costa-Pereira A, et al. Quality of life of survivors from severe sepsis and septic shock may be similar to that of others who survive critical illness. Crit Care 2004;8: R91–8.

[92] Dowdy DW, Eid MP, Sedrakyan A, et al. Quality of life in adult survivors of critical illness: a systematic review of the literature. Intensive Care Med 2005;31:611–20.

[93] Wood KA, Ely EW. What does it mean to be critically ill and elderly? Curr Opin Crit Care 2003;9:316–20.

[94] Herridge MS, Cheung AM, Tansey CM, et al. One-year outcomes in survivors of the acute respiratory distress syndrome. N Engl J Med 2003;348:683–93.

SURGICAL
CLINICS OF
NORTH AMERICA

Surg Clin N Am 86 (2006) 1483–1493

Advances in Surgical Nutrition

Juan B. Ochoa, MD[a,b,*], David Caba, MD, MS[a]

[a]*Department of Surgery, University of Pittsburgh Medical Center Presbyterian,
200 Lothrop Street, Pittsburgh, PA 15213, USA*
[b]*Department of Critical Care, University of Pittsburgh Medical Center Presbyterian,
200 Lothrop Street, Pittsburgh, PA 15213, USA*

Dr. Stanley Dudrick, a surgery resident working under Dr. Jonathan Rhoads, invented total parenteral nutrition (TPN) in 1968, providing a desperately needed therapy to those patients who could not eat [1]. Before this, patients who had a nonfunctional gastrointestinal tract were condemned to die of malnutrition. TPN has since saved thousands of patients worldwide. It is not surprising, therefore, that medicine embraced TPN with fervor, despite the absence of adequate evaluation of its benefits and limitations.

Work on TPN had the unforeseen effect of bringing the discipline of nutrition into the spotlight of mainstream medicine. Suddenly, it was important for clinicians in virtually every discipline to embrace nutrition. It was expected of interns and residents to be able to calculate calories and protein in TPN bags, and to demonstrate that nutrition intervention (NI) were being done. It became fashionable for clinicians to order high amounts of calories and protein in what was called "hyperalimentation." This was done in a naïve attempt to curtail the progression toward malnutrition caused by the hypermetabolism of injury [2].

Appropriate trials comparing TPN and enteral nutrition (EN) were eventually done, with humbling results. These studies, and the meta-analyses performed on them, demonstrated that under virtually any circumstance EN produces better outcomes than TPN whenever the patient's gastrointestinal tract can be used [3]. These results are observed even though TPN consistently delivers 30% to 50% more calories and protein than conventional enteral nutrition. Thus we have learned that the benefits of nutrition far surpass the mere provision of nutrients.

NI has gained significantly in complexity, with an increasing array of possible but not always intuitive decisions. NI, like any other form of medical

---

* Corresponding author.
E-mail address: ochoajb@upmc.edu (J.B. Ochoa).

0039-6109/06/$ - see front matter © 2006 Elsevier Inc. All rights reserved.
doi:10.1016/j.suc.2006.09.002
                                  surgical.theclinics.com

or surgical therapy, has to demonstrate a beneficial effect on clinical outcomes. In addition, and more than with other therapies, NI is also expected to demonstrate adequate cost-effectiveness [4]. The purpose of this article, therefore, is to review what we know of the different forms of NI, and to evaluate their practical roles at the bedside. This article analyzes five forms of NI that virtually cover any decision-making process in surgical/trauma patients. These are: (1) controlled starvation (CS), (2) TPN, (3) EN, (4) oral nutritional supplements (ONS), and (5) nutrients with pharmacological properties.

Forms of nutrition intervention

Controlled starvation and early enteral nutrition

Short periods of CS have traditionally been allowed in most surgical patient populations, including patients undergoing elective surgery and the critically ill. Arguments suggesting that oral intake can only be resumed until bowel function returns still abound on surgical floors [5]. Most surgical patients, however, will tolerate oral/enteral intake. The benefits of early oral/enteral intake cannot be minimized, and a concerted effort toward changing clinical practices at individual institutions is important.

In 2001, Lewis and colleagues [6] published a meta-analysis on 11 different studies in patients undergoing elective gastrointestinal surgery (Fig. 1). Six of these studies used early oral/enteral nutrition (EEN), whereas 5 used a nasoenteral device or a jejunostomy. In general, oral/enteral intake

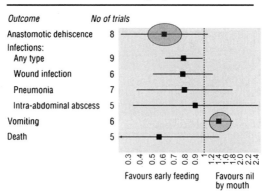

Fig. 1. Early enteral nutrition outcome. (*Adapted from* Lewis SJ, Egger M, Sylvester PA, et al. Early enteral feeding versus "nil by mouth" after gastrointestinal surgery: systematic review and meta-analysis of controlled trials. BMJ 2001;323:775; with permission.)

was started within 24 hours after surgery. The results of this study demonstrate several important issues:

Early use of oral or enteral intake is associated with a statistically significant decrease in infection rates (relative risk 0.72, 95% confidence interval, 0.54 to 0.98, $P = 0.036$). The mean length of stay in hospital was also reduced ($P = 0.001$). This observation is also confirmed in critically ill trauma patients [7]. The decrease in infections is probably caused by a systemic effect, because decreased infections are observed at different sites, including the lung, wounds, and the urinary tract.

There is no evidence of increased breakdown of gastrointestinal anastomoses. In fact, EEN is associated with a clear trend toward decreased anastomotic breakdown (relative risk 0.53, 95% confidence interval, 0.26 to 1.08, $P = 0.080$). Studies performed in rodents demonstrate that oral intake is associated with a significant increase in collagen deposition at the anastomosis and wound strength [8]. Thus, there is no validity to the widespread idea that nutrients in the lumen will disrupt anastomoses.

There is a trend toward decreased mortality when patients are fed early, although this did not reach statistical significance.

There is a small (approximately 10%) statistically significant increase in rates of vomiting. Vomiting, however, does not appear to be associated with negative physiologic consequences. A recent meta-analysis encourages the use of selective rather than routine nasogastric tube decompression, demonstrating that its use delays the return of bowel function and may actually increase pulmonary complications [9].

Lewis and coworkers [6] did not report as to whether caloric goals had been met in the group of patients receiving early oral intake. Thus, so far we do not know whether the benefits of early oral intake are independent of the amounts of calories given.

EEN is also clearly indicated in the critically ill surgical/trauma patient. A systematic review of EEN has been done by Heyland and colleagues, from the Canadian Critical Care Nutrition Taskforce (CCCNT) [10]. Eight Level II studies demonstrate a significant decrease in infection rates without affecting mortality.

In conclusion, there is now clear evidence supporting the idea that controlled short periods of starvation are not indicated in most surgical patients. In addition, the accumulating data demonstrate that the gastrointestinal tract can be used successfully in most surgical/critically ill patients.

Permissive underfeeding

An interesting observation of virtually all studies on EEN is the realization that in most, there is a failure to meet intake of planned caloric goals. In general, most patients on EEN meet between 50% and 70% of caloric goals [11]. Yet, there appears to be a benefit from lower caloric intake, which has raised considerable interest in the concept of "permissive underfeeding." This observation raises several interesting possibilities.

The first is that caloric intake has been set at inappropriately high levels. Historically, caloric goals (CGs) were decided on in an attempt to curtail the catabolic response and loss of muscle and visceral mass that invariably occurs after surgery/trauma and critical illness. In the absence of stress, provision of small amounts of carbohydrate (400 calories/d) leads to sparing of muscle breakdown—the so called "protein-sparing" effect of glucose. In the presence of traumatic or septic stress, however, the provision of carbohydrates, even at caloric goals, fails to protect muscle mass, thus making CG unnecessary.

Guidelines to determine CGs have been written by several organizations. In 1997 the American College of Chest Physicians (ACCP) published guidelines based on expert opinion [12]. Similar, though more modest guidelines have been published by the American Society of Parenteral and Enteral Nutrition (ASPEN) [13]. Finally, the Canadian Critical Care Task force has determined that there are insufficient data to suggest what number of calories should be given to critically ill patients [10]. Thus, all the hospital nutrition authoritative organizations agree that CGs in surgical/trauma critically ill patients have never been successfully determined.

The second possibility is that EEN produces benefits through mechanisms that are independent of CGs. Starvation is associated with significant abnormalities in gastrointestinal function, including mucosal atrophy and loss of gastrointestinal associated lymphoid tissue (GALT). EEN maintains normal gastrointestinal function even when CGs are not met. Thus, it is suggested that a small amount of nutrients, which "bathe" the gut mucosa, is all that is necessary or desirable. It appears to be important to provide at least some protein, though again how much should be provided initially is still undetermined.

Another possibility is that meeting CGs is associated with complications, including overfeeding. Provision of EN is associated with an increased number of side effects as the dietary volume delivered is increased in an attempt to meet caloric goals. In addition, calorically dense formulas with high concentrations of fat can overwhelm the digestive and absorptive capacity of the gastrointestinal tract. Thus, investigators have noticed increased gastric residuals, bloating, and diarrhea when high volumes are delivered or when high fat formulas are provided to critically ill surgical/trauma patients. Furthermore, overfeeding is associated with a large number of complications, and may indeed increase mortality. Overfeeding negatively affects function of every organ (Fig. 2) [14]. Overfeeding causes encephalopathy, increases cardiac and respiratory demands, prolongs ventilator dependency, and causes immune dysfunction. Thus, the dangers of overfeeding cannot be overemphasized.

It would be simple to avoid overfeeding if clinicians used a reliable of way of determining the caloric needs of a given patient. Most clinicians

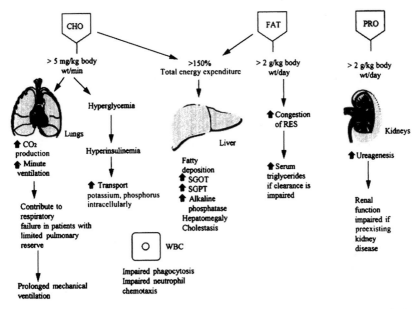

Fig. 2. Negative Effects of overfeeding. (*From* Klein CJ, Stanek GS, Wiles III CE. Overfeeding macronutrients to critically ill adults: metabolic complications. J Am Diet Assoc 1998;98:796; with permission.)

(including nutritionists) rely on population-based calculated formulas such as the Harris-Benedict formulas. These formulas were generated far before the availability of intensive care units, and thus it is unclear as to whether they are applicable to that setting. Unfortunately, the use of these formulas may lead to overfeeding in up to 30% of patients, and thus may cause harm. The use of indirect calorimetry may provide a more reliable mechanism of determining the appropriate calories needed by a given patient [15]. Unfortunately, indirect calorimetry is labor intensive and difficult to do, and is not available in many institutions. Furthermore, there is no significant evidence that performing indirect calorimetry is cost-effective.

Early enteral nutrition

Enteral nutrition has shown its greatest effectiveness when started early. Even though there is significant heterogeneity between the different studies, EEN is defined as that nutrition started within 24 to 48 hours of admission to the ICU. Across all critically ill patient populations, patients receiving EEN exhibit a clear trend toward a decrease in mortality ($P = 0.08$) and infection rates [10,16]. In practical terms, EEN is started as soon as the patient's hemodynamic status is stabilized. Ideally, a small-bore feeding tube is placed and diet is started at low volumes. Low volumes are associated with decreased complications such as abdominal distention, increased gastric residuals, and vomiting. The authors routinely supplement these patients with additional protein to meet goals of 1.5 to 2 g/kg/d. Consideration to providing additional early micronutrients should also be given.

In conclusion, CS is not necessary or desirable in most patients. Oral or enteral nutrition can be achieved in most surgical/trauma and in critically ill patients. Enteral nutrition should be started as early as possible, ideally within the first 24 hours of arrival. Meeting caloric goals is not necessary or desirable, though the degree of underfeeding that is beneficial remains undetermined.

Total parenteral nutrition

Compared with EN, TPN appears to offer distinct advantages. Establishing delivery access is far simpler and more reliable for TPN. In addition, TPN delivery does not have to be stopped for surgical procedures or trips outside of the ICU. Not surprisingly, patients on TPN consistently meet caloric goals more often than those given EN. These observations led clinicians to advocate the use of TPN, implying that its use would be of benefit. This, however, is not the case.

Multiple studies have demonstrated that in surgical patients, trauma victims, and critically ill patients, TPN is inferior to EN. In the ICU, for example, 13 different studies have demonstrated that EN is associated with decreased rates of infections when compared with TPN, though there is no evidence of an effect on mortality [10,16]. In critically ill trauma patients also, the use of TPN is associated with increased morbidity, including infections, a longer length of stay in the ICU, and prolonged ventilator dependency [17].

In 1993, a carefully performed prospective randomized study compared the use of postoperative TPN with simple starvation [18]. Three hundred patients divided equally into two groups scheduled to undergo elective gastrointestinal or urologic surgery received TPN or D10W plus electrolytes starting on the first postoperative day. This regimen was maintained until the patient started eating, or for up to 2 weeks if the patient failed to take adequate oral intake. Although most patients in both groups were able to initiate oral intake, a small number of patients (24/150 in the TPN group, 28/150 in the D10W controls) failed to eat. One would have predicted that those patients that received D10W for 2 weeks would have had a significantly poorer outcome when compared with those receiving TPN, because of the previous knowledge of a protective role of TPN from the progression toward malnutrition. Contrary to the predicted outcome, however, those patients placed on TPN exhibited increased morbidity and mortality (Fig. 3) [18]. Thus this well-performed study demonstrated that there is no role for prophylactic TPN in surgical patients. Similarly, TPN used only as a means of achieving caloric goals has failed to demonstrate clear benefits in other patient populations such as trauma and surgical critically ill. The

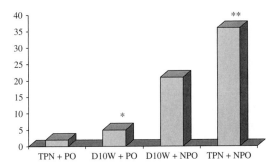

Fig. 3. Mortality in the use of TPN. (*Data from* Sandstrom R, Drott C, Hyltander A, et al. The effect of postoperative intravenous feeding (TPN) on outcome following major surgery evaluated in a randomized study. Ann Surg 1993;217:192–5.)

role of TPN has therefore been progressively reduced. Nevertheless it remains invaluable in several situations:

Nonstressed patient who has severe protein-calorie malnutrition, who is scheduled to undergo surgery. A perfect example is the patient scheduled to undergo esophageal surgery because of obstruction. In the malnourished patient, TPN given 7 days before surgery is associated with a significant decrease in infection rates [19].

The patient who has short gut. Indefinite survival of patients who have short gut is now possible thanks to the use of TPN. TPN can be used for long-term management or as a bridge to intestinal transplant.

Patients who fail oral/enteral nutrition. A frequent consult to any nutrition intervention team is that of failure to achieve adequate enteral nutrition support in a given patient. This is often used as an excuse to start TPN. More often, however, adequate evaluation of the patient and implementation of simple measures lead to successfully achieving adequate EN. It is only after an adequate attempt at enteral nutrition that TPN should be implemented. There are currently no clear guidelines as to what constitutes a failed attempt at EN. It is clear though, that it is not necessary, at least early on, to meet caloric goals through the enteral route to see its benefits. There is no role for the use of combined TPN and EN [10].

Oral nutritional supplements

ONS are a frequent addition to the therapy of many patients in the hospital. ONS are often concentrates of high amounts of calories with proteins and micronutrients, including vitamins, and are heavily commercially advertised. There is little evidence, however, that ONS indiscriminately administered to hospitalized patients will benefit outcome.

In a prospective randomized trial [20] conducted in patients undergoing elective gastrointestinal surgery, for example, ONS demonstrated no difference in outcome when compared with controls. There was also no demonstrable effect on prevention of weight loss. Similarly, ONS failed to show any benefit at all in stroke patients admitted to a prospective randomized multi-center trial [21]. Several studies have been performed in patients undergoing hip replacements [22,23]. In this patient population, high protein supplementation may be associated with a modest improvement in survival, though the quality of the studies does not permit a definitive demonstration of benefit.

Thus one cannot advocate the routine use of ONS.

Nutrients with pharmacologic properties

Surgery and trauma are associated with depression of adaptive T-cell function, including decreased T-cell numbers, abnormally low circulating CD4 counts, decreased T-cell proliferation, involution of the thymus, and depressed delayed type hypersensitivity (DTH) [24,25]. In the late 1970s Barbul and colleagues [26,27] demonstrated that arginine supplementation in a rodent model of surgical trauma prevented thymic involution. These changes in T-cell function have been considered pathologic and thought to increase the susceptibility to infections that accompany any major surgery or severe trauma. This hypothesis, though logical, has never been thoroughly tested or proven. Nevertheless, therapy to "normalize" T-cell function was deemed necessary and desirable. Arginine supplementation was thus a potentially effective therapy for surgery/trauma-induced T-cell suppression.

Independent of the arginine work, other investigators demonstrated that a host of nutrients, including omega-3 fatty acids (ω-FA), nucleic acids, and glutamine, also affected immune function. These nutrients, along with arginine, were eventually incorporated and commercialized as "immune enhancing diets" (IEDs) [28]. At least seven of these different diets exist in the market, each one with its own proprietary mix of nutrients. Blending was done despite incomplete knowledge of their mechanisms of action, possible side effects, and unknown interactions between the different substances. Nevertheless, multiple trials in different patient populations have tested the use of IEDs and attempted to prove (or disprove) a beneficial effect on outcome.

It is therefore not surprising that the results of these multiple studies are conflicting, difficult to interpret, and even more difficult to incorporate into practical clinical practices. Nevertheless, and acknowledging the multiple shortcomings of this area of research, the "dust has begun to settle," allowing us to suggest some practical guidelines.

Arginine deficiency develops in several disease processes, including surgery and trauma, hemorrhagic shock, ischemia reperfusion of the liver, in hemoytic diseases, and in certain forms of cancer. Arginine deficiency in these diseases is the result of the abnormal expression of arginase, an enzyme that metabolizes arginine to ornithine and urea.

Arginine deficiency affects key biological functions, including the generation of nitric oxide and T lymphocyte function. T lymphocyte changes caused by arginine deficiency are characteristic, and include a decrease in T-cell proliferation and the loss of the ζ chain, an essential component of the T-cell receptor complex. Arginine supplementation at supraphysiologic doses designed to overcome arginine deficiency restores nitric oxide production and T-cell function.

In the immune system, arginase expression is upregulated by surgery/trauma, and in cancer in a group of specialized myeloid cells, now called myeloid suppressor cells (MSC) [29]. Granulocytes appear to play a role as MSC in humans. MSC deplete arginine necessary for normal T0-cell function, including that of T-cell receptor expression. It is hypothesized, but only partially tested, that arginine supplementation may overcome the effects of MSC.

A combination of arginine, ω-3 FA, and nucleotides, given as a dietary supplement perioperatively, decreases infection rates around 40% in patients undergoing high-risk surgery. The benefits of this dietary combination are well-demonstrated in all meta-analyses, and currently considered Level I evidence of benefit [30]. Thus the use of an IED should be standard of care in all major surgical interventions, including cardiac and gastrointestinal surgery.

The use of arginine-containing IEDs is highly controversial in septic, critically ill patients, with contradictory studies showing either increased or decreased mortality. Glutamine, a neutral amino acid, which is also a precursor of arginine, may benefit patients who have sepsis.

Diets containing ω-3 FA may be of benefit in patients who have respiratory failure.

Summary

Nutrition interventions in surgical/trauma and critically ill patients have evolved dramatically during the last 20 years, evolving from a supportive therapy to a clear therapeutic role. Like any other form of therapy, NI will benefit patients when adequately indicated and prescribed. NI, however, may cause significant side effects and harm when poorly ordered.

References

[1] Dudrick SJ, Wilmore DW, Vars HM, et al. Long-term total parenteral nutrition with growth, development, and positive nitrogen balance. Surgery 1968;64:134–42.
[2] Dudrick SJ, Copeland EM. Parenteral hyperalimentation. Surg Annu 1973;5:69–95.
[3] Heyland DK, Cook DJ, Guyatt GH. Enteral nutrition in the critically ill patient: a critical review of the evidence. Intensive Care Med 1993;19:435–42.

[4] Koretz RL. Death, morbidity and economics are the only end points for trials. Proc Nutr Soc 2005;64:277–84.

[5] Correia MI, da Silva RG. The impact of early nutrition on metabolic response and postoperative ileus. Curr Opin Clin Nutr Metab Care 2004;7:577–83.

[6] Lewis SJ, Egger M, Sylvester PA, et al. Early enteral feeding versus "nil by mouth" after gastrointestinal surgery: systematic review and meta-analysis of controlled trials. BMJ 2001; 323:773–6.

[7] Moore EE, Moore FA. Immediate enteral nutrition following multisystem trauma: a decade perspective. J Am Coll Nutr 1991;10:633–48.

[8] Kiyama T, Onda M, Tokunaga A, et al. Effect of early postoperative feeding on the healing of colonic anastomoses in the presence of intra-abdominal sepsis in rats. Dis Colon Rectum 2000;43:S54–8.

[9] Nelson R, Tse B, Edwards S. Systematic review of prophylactic nasogastric decompression after abdominal operations. Br J Surg 2005;92:673–80.

[10] Heyland DK, Dhaliwal R, Drover JW, et al. Canadian clinical practice guidelines for nutrition support in mechanically ventilated, critically ill adult patients. JPEN J Parenter Enteral Nutr 2003;27:355–73.

[11] Jeejeebhoy KN. Permissive underfeeding of the critically ill patient. Nutr Clin Pract 2004;19: 477–80.

[12] Cerra FB, Benitez MR, Blackburn GL, et al. Applied nutrition in ICU patients. A consensus statement of the American College of Chest Physicians. Chest 1997;111:769–78.

[13] Guidelines for the use of parenteral and enteral nutrition in adult and pediatric patients. JPEN J Parenter Enteral Nutr 2002;26(1 Suppl):1SA–138SA.

[14] Klein CJ, Stanek GS, Wiles CE III. Overfeeding macronutrients to critically ill adults: metabolic complications. J Am Diet Assoc 1998;98:795–806.

[15] Brandi LS, Santini L, Bertolini R, et al. Energy expenditure and severity of injury and illness indices in multiple trauma patients. Crit Care Med 1999;27:2684–9.

[16] Heyland DK, Dhaliwal R, Day A, et al. Validation of the Canadian clinical practice guidelines for nutrition support in mechanically ventilated, critically ill adult patients: results of a prospective observational study. Crit Care Med 2004;32:2260–6.

[17] Moore FA, Feliciano DV, Andrassy RJ, et al. Early enteral feeding, compared with parenteral, reduces postoperative septic complications. Annals of Surgery 1992;216:172–83.

[18] Sandstrom R, Drott C, Hyltander A, et al. The effect of postoperative intravenous feeding (TPN) on outcome following major surgery evaluated in a randomized study. Ann Surg 1993;217:185–95.

[19] Perioperative total parenteral nutrition in surgical patients. The Veterans Affairs Total Parenteral Nutrition Cooperative Study Group. N Engl J Med 1991;325:525–32.

[20] MacFie J, Woodcock NP, Palmer MD, et al. Oral dietary supplements in pre- and postoperative surgical patients: a prospective and randomized clinical trial. Nutrition 2000;16:723–8.

[21] Dennis MS, Lewis SC, Warlow C. Routine oral nutritional supplementation for stroke patients in hospital (FOOD): a multicentre randomised controlled trial. Lancet 2005;365: 755–63.

[22] Avenell A, Handoll HH. Nutritional supplementation for hip fracture aftercare in the elderly. Cochrane Database Syst Rev 2005;2:CD001880.

[23] Avenell A, Handoll HH. A systematic review of protein and energy supplementation for hip fracture aftercare in older people. Eur J Clin Nutr 2003;57:895–903.

[24] Mannick JA, Rodrick ML, Lederer JA. The immunologic response to injury. J Am Coll Surg 2001;193:237–44.

[25] Miller-Graziano CL, Szabo G, Griffey K, et al. Role of elevated monocyte transforming growth factor beta (TGF beta) production in posttrauma immunosuppression. J Clin Immunol 1991;11:95–102.

[26] Barbul A, Sisto DA, Wasserkrug HL, et al. Metabolic and immune effects of arginine in postinjury hyperalimentation. J Trauma 1981;21:970–4.

[27] Barbul A, Sisto D, Rettura G, et al. Thymic inhibition of wound healing: abrogation by adult thymectomy. J Surg Res 1982;32:338–42.

[28] Bansal V, Ochoa JB. Arginine availability, arginase, and the immune response. Curr Opin Clin Nutr Metab Care 2003;6:223–8.

[29] Makarenkova VP, Bansal V, Matta BM, et al. CD11b + /Gr-1 + myeloid suppressor cells cause T cell dysfunction after traumatic stress. J Immunol 2006;176:2085–94.

[30] Consensus recommendations from the US summitt on immune-enhancing enteral therapy. JPEN J Parenter Enteral Nutr 2001;25:S61–3.

ELSEVIER
SAUNDERS

SURGICAL
CLINICS OF
NORTH AMERICA

Surg Clin N Am 86 (2006) 1495–1502

Jaundice in the Intensive Care Unit

Vishal Bansal, MD[a], Vaishali Dixit Schuchert, MD[b],*

[a]Department of Surgery, University of California at San Diego, San Diego, CA, USA
[b]Department of Critical Care, University of Pittsburgh Medical Center Presbyterian,
200 Lothrop Street, Pittsburgh, PA 15212, USA

Hyperbilirubinemia, or jaundice, is commonly encountered in the ICU, with an incidence as high as 40% among critically ill patients. Unfortunately, jaundice in the critically ill is poorly understood, and its presence all too often presents a diagnostic dilemma to the intensive care physician. Causes of jaundice in the ICU are multiple; the etiology in any given patient multifactorial. Acute jaundice can be a harbinger or marker of sepsis, multisystem organ failure (MSOF), or a reflection of transient hypotension (shock liver), right-sided heart failure, the metabolic breakdown of red blood cells, or pharmacologic toxicity. The persistence of jaundice is associated with a significant increase in patient morbidity and mortality [1].

Acute ICU jaundice is best divided into two categories: obstructive and non-obstructive, as detailed in Box 1. Stratifying jaundice into one of these categories directs subsequent management and therapeutic decisions.

Obstructive jaundice

Mechanical or functional obstruction of the bile ducts increases intraluminal ductal pressure proximal to the obstruction and prevents hepatocellular excretion of bile into the ductal system, leading to ductal dilatation seen on ultrasound imaging. Subsequent hepatocellular overflow eventually causes a rise in serum direct bilirubin and high levels of serum alkaline phosphatase and gamma-glutamyl transpeptidase (GGTP). A past medical history of cholelithiasis or prior hepatobiliary surgery may help narrow the differential. Causes of obstructive jaundice are outlined above in Box 1.

Choledocholithiasis is a frequent presentation of previously unrecognized cholelithiasis. Gallstones migrate via the cystic duct to the common bile duct

---

* Corresponding author.
E-mail address: schuchertv@upmc.edu (V.D. Schuchert).

surgical.theclinics.com

Box 1. Etiologies of jaundice in the ICU

Obstructive jaundice
Choledocholithiasis
Cholangitis
Cholangiocarcinoma
Pancreatic duct stricture
Pancreatic head mass

Nonobstructive jaundice
Hemolysis
Massive transfusion
Hypotension/"shock liver"
Disseminated intravascular coagulation
Soft tissue trauma and hematoma resorption
Sepsis
Liver trauma/biloma
Liver failure/MSOF
Medications/hepatotoxins
Viral hepatitis

---

and may lodge at the ampulla of Vater, causing pancreatitis and or cholangitis. Even though most patients can be managed without intensive monitoring, some develop cholangitis with severe sepsis. Recognition of the classic triad of right upper quadrant tenderness, fever, and acute jaundice, as described by Charcot, may be hampered by an obtunded or sedated patient. Patients can often present with a mixed picture of acute cholecystitis and choledocholithiasis. In elderly patients, nearly 20% of acute cholecystis occurs with choledocholithiasis. The incidence of de novo acute choledocholithiasis in an ICU setting is unknown, but should be considered in patients with acute jaundice and a history of cholelithiasis.

Biliary stricture most commonly presents from iatrogenic injury to the bile ducts following a cholecystectomy. Fortunately, this remains a rare cause of biliary stricture, with the incidence of bile duct injury following open cholecystectomy being 0.2% to 0.3%, and incidence in laparoscopic cholecystectomy being 0.4% to 0.5% [2]. Early jaundice, within days of the operation, may indicate a retained gallstone, ligation or transection of the common bile duct, a leaking cystic duct stump, or injury and leakage of either the common and or hepatic bile ducts, all of which can lead to perihepatic bilomas. Late jaundice, within 1 year after a cholecystectomy, may indicate an unrecognized partial injury to the ducts, with subsequent scarring and obstruction. Patients who have surgical histories involving the porta hepatis (ie, pancreaticoduodenectomy or hepaticojejunosotmy) may develop anastamotic stricture and subsequent obstruction.

Patients who have a cholangiocarcinoma or a pancreatic head mass most often present with painless jaundice, although the primary presentation may include acute cholangitis requiring ICU resuscitation.

Nonobstructive jaundice

Hyperbilirubinemia in the ICU is usually nonobstructive and multifactorial in etiology. Patient characteristics are as diverse as the causes of hypotension, involving the entire spectrum of critically ill patients, including cardiac failure, sepsis, trauma, and hemodynamic instability during the perioperative period. Hepatocyte damage and the rise in serum hepatic enzymes and bilirubin temporally lag behind the acute hypotensive episode. Patients often have a recent history of profound hypotension, with mean arterial pressures maintained by inotropic or vasoactive pressor agents. Common therapeutic interventions in the ICU that are associated with an increase in hepatic injury include mechanical ventilation, the administration of catecholamines, and total parenteral nutrition (TPN) [3]. Mechanical ventilatory support with positive end-expiratory pressure (PEEP) is associated with decreased portal venous blood flow and increased hepatic venous resistance, and has thus been implicated in ICU-related liver dysfunction [4].

Jaundice secondary to heart failure is associated with two distinct forms of liver dysfunction: passive hepatic vascular congestion and acute hepatocellular necrosis [5]. Passive hepatic congestion is a consequence of right-sided or global cardiac dysfunction. Ischemic hepatitis, or shock liver, results from impaired blood flow and inadequate oxygen perfusion. The end results are similar, marked by a significant elevation of serum aminotransaminases, lactate dehyrogenase, and hyperbilirubinemia. Patients who have liver dysfunction secondary to heart failure almost universally have dyspnea, if not frank respiratory failure, with abnormal electrocardiograms (EKGs) and echocardiograms [6]. Just as in other acute hepatic dysfunction states such as viral hepatitis, cirrhosis, or chemical-induced hepatitis, shock liver can strain hepatic synthetic capabilities, including the production of clotting factors, gluconeogensesis, and the ability to metabolize toxins and medications through the cytochrome P-450 pathway. Ischemic hepatitis is generally self-limited, though progressive liver failure may occur in patients who have pre-existing liver disease or congestive heart failure.

Jaundice is present in up to 40% of patients suffering from multiple trauma. There are several causative factors of jaundice in trauma patients. Shock liver is common following severe hemorrhage and hypotension. Direct hepatic parenchymal injury from blunt trauma usually presents as acute bleeding and is frequently managed nonoperatively [7]. Missed hepatic duct injuries and bilomas following nonoperative management occur infrequently (3%). Most of these injuries remain minor, and the developing bilomas usually resolve spontaneously. If the biloma persists or secondarily becomes infected, percutaneous drainage provides rapid therapy. Late stricture rates following hepatic injury are low, though long-term outcomes are still unknown [7]. The major causes of jaundice in trauma patients are likely to be bilirubin overload from the breakdown of transfused and extravasated blood and hepatic dysfunction secondary to hypotension and sepsis [8]. Massive packed red blood cell transfusion can cause peripheral hemolysis, leading to elevated bilirubin and clinical jaundice. On average, 10% of crossmatched, transfused, packed red blood cells undergo hemolysis yielding 200 to 250 mg of bilirubin. A healthy liver excretes approximately 300 mg of bilirubin daily, with production of bilirubin estimated to be 200 to 300 mg daily [9,10]. Large hematomas, either from solid organs, retroperitoneal, or soft tissue injury, undergo breakdown and reabsorption with a release of unconjugated bilirubin and transient conjugated bilirubin, leading to jaundice [11]. These patients are often in stages of healing and recovery, are tolerating a regular diet, and voice concern over why they "look so yellow." Because of the affinity of bilirubin for albumin, and because of the long half-life of albumin (about 14 days), clinical jaundice may persist beyond the normalization of the patient's physiology and serum laboratory tests [10].

Persistent or progressive jaundice has prognostic implications in critically ill trauma patients. Progressive jaundice beyond the twelfth day post-trauma has been shown to be associated with poor survival, with deaths occurring in the setting of multisystem organ failure and sepsis [12]. Animal studies suggest that chronic ethanol consumption, often a comorbidity in hospitalized trauma patients, exacerbates microvascular failure after shock and resuscitation [13].

Jaundice is present in 30% to 50% of patients who have an extrahepatic source of sepsis, with "pneumonia biliosa" recognized as early as 1836 by Garvin [14]. Extrahepatic infections cause intrahepatic cholestasis, with a resulting conjugated hyperbilirubinemia. In addition to cholestasis, bile canalicular dilatation and loss of microvilli have been demonstrated to occur 2 to 3 days following gram-negative bacteremia. Although endotoxin has been shown to play an important part in the pathophysiologic changes that occur in gram-negative sepsis, it is clearly not the exclusive offending agent [14]. Studies using animal models of gram-negative intraperitoneal sepsis suggest that jaundice is primarily the result of impaired bilirubin transport in the liver while cytosolic and synthetic function remains preserved [15,16]. Several investigators have proposed a link between obstructive jaundice upregulating Toll-like receptor 4 and increasing sensitivity to lipopolysaccharide (LPS)-induced sepsis [17,18]. LPS directly activates Kupffer cells, the macrophages of the liver, to produce TNF-α and other inflammatory cytokines, causing liver injury [19]. The exact link between jaundice and sepsis is unknown; however, the inflammatory response and cytokine cascade in acute sepsis and the physiologic effects of hypotension and hepatic ischemia all contribute to hepatic dysfunction and clinical jaundice.

Another commonly encountered etiology for jaundice in the ICU is the administration of TPN. The pathophysiology remains unclear, but, as in sepsis, is associated with hepatic cholestasis [20]. TPN-related hepatic dysfunction likely represents a combination of excessive calories with deficiency in micronutrients, hormonal imbalances, and possibly bacterial overgrowth and translocation from the gut [21]. Increases in serum alkaline phosphatase and GGTP are detected as early as 24 hours following the start of TPN administration, and should serve as indicators for hepatocellular injury [22]. Various trials of altering TPN nutritional components have not been shown to significantly decrease the incidence of cholestasis [23]. Cyclic TPN, as opposed to continuous TPN, may prevent further deterioration of liver function in patients who are jaundiced and require ongoing TPN [24]. For these and other reasons, TPN should only be used sparingly in an ICU patient, with emphasis on enteral feeding being foremost.

Diagnosis and treatment

The history of the patient directs subsequent diagnostic and therapeutic initiatives. A jaundiced patient should undergo a battery of serum laboratory tests, including comprehensive liver function assays with total bilirubin as well as fractionated bilirubin levels, a complete blood cell count, coagulation profile, and serum electrolytes. Jaundice generally does not appear until a patient's serum total bilirubin exceeds 2.5 mg/dL. Indirect bilirubin is circulating unconjugated bilirubin, and generally accounts for over 90% of the total measured bilirubin. Direct bilirubin is conjugated bilirubin plus delta bilirubin (conjugated bilirubin that has refluxed into the circulation and has combined with albumin) [10]. Haptoglobin, reticulocyte count, lactate dehydrogenase (LDH), and Coomb's test should be considered in patients who have unconjugated hyperbilirubinemia [11].

Though hyperbilirubinemia in critically ill patients is more commonly nonobstructive, or nonsurgical, in nature, obstruction within the biliary tree is generally readily diagnosed by ultrasonography. This should be an early step in the evaluation of the jaundiced patient. Abdominal ultrasonography may detect biliary or pancreatic ductal dilation, the presence of gallstones, or a possible subhepatic biloma. Ultrasonography has the additional benefits that it does not require administration of nephrotoxic contrast dye, and it can be performed at the bedside in even the most unstable patient. This initial radiographic step is imperative in stratifying a patient into obstructive or nonobstructive jaundice, and therefore in guiding therapy.

If, based on ultrasonographic findings, there is high suspicion of obstruction, endoscopic retrograde cholangiopancreatography (ERCP) is recommended for ductal decompression and restoration of biliary flow. If ERCP cannot be accomplished, percutaneous transhepatic cholangiography (PTC) should be considered. CT imaging may be helpful, especially in trauma patients, to determine the degree, if any, of hepatic injury or ductal disruption. Bilomas are readily drained through percutaneous ultrasound or CT-guided techniques, and the majority of bile leaks resolve and seal spontaneously.

Supportive therapy is the mainstay of management of nonobstructive jaundice. Nonsurgical causes of cholestasis such as sepsis or TPN lead to a conjugated hyperbilirubinemia. Medications may cause an unconjugated or a conjugated hyperbilirubinemia. Hemolysis as seen with massive blood transfusion, resorbing hematoma, or in hemolytic disorders, is associated with an unconjugated hyperbilirubinemia. A concerted effort to maintain hemodynamic stability with adequate intravenous fluid, appropriate antibiotics, and cessation of offending agents is paramount. In cases of shock liver secondary to impaired cardiac function, pharmacological support of cardiac output with an inotrope such as dobutamine may be beneficial for hepatic blood flow and may lead to improved outcome [25].

Future directions in therapy

Presently there is no treatment for progressive liver failure other than liver transplantation. Ongoing laboratory efforts continue to shed insight into the pathophysiology of liver failure, and experimental designs that target these changes at a cellular level are providing exciting new directions for future therapy of liver failure. Agents that modulate tumor necrosis factor-alpha (TNF-α) or the pathways leading to apoptosis (programmed cell death) show promise in future investigations and therapies. Fibronectin was shown to be protective in a murine model of hepatotoxin and LPS-induced liver failure by a mechanism that involves inhibition of NFκB activation by downregulation of TNF-α, but upregulation of Bcl-xL, with resulting inhibition of hepatocyte apoptosis [19]. Phosphodiesterase inhibitors were shown to decrease systemic release of TNF-α and protect from T-cell-mediated liver failure in another mouse model [26]. Nitric oxide (NO) and heme oxygenase-1 (HO-1) have been shown to be cytoprotective in animal models of liver failure [27,28]. It has more recently been shown that exogenous carbon monoxide protects against liver failure in a mouse model through NO-induced HO-1. In turn, the protective effect of carbon monoxide appears to be NFκB-mediated [29].

Research is also ongoing in hepatocyte transplantation. Although clinical results have thus far been disappointing, laboratory results using hepatocytes with stem cells have shown promise, and may ultimately provide an alternative to liver transplantation [30].

References

[1] Hawker F. Liver dysfunction in critical illness. Anaesth Intensive Care 1991;19(2):165–81.
[2] Lillemoe KD. Benign biliary stricture. In: Cameron JL, editor. Current surgical therapy. 7th edition. Philadelphia (PA): Mosby; 2001. p. 454–61.
[3] Strassburg CP. Gastrointestinal disorders of the critically ill. Shock liver. Best Pract Res Clin Gastroenterol 2003;17(3):369–81.

[4] Brienza N, Revelly JP, Ayuse T, et al. Effects of PEEP on liver arterial and venous blood flows. Am J Respir Crit Care Med 1995;152(2):504–10.

[5] Giallourakis CC, Rosenberg PM, Friedman LS. The liver in heart failure. Clin Liver Dis 2002;6(4):947–67.

[6] van Lingen R, Warshow U, Dalton HR, et al. Jaundice as a presentation of heart failure. J R Soc Med 2005;98(8):357–9.

[7] Croce MA, Fabian TC, Menke PG, et al. Nonoperative management of blunt hepatic trauma is the treatment of choice for hemodynamically stable patients. Results of a prospective trial. Ann Surg 1995;221(6):744–53.

[8] Labori KJ, Raeder MG. Diagnostic approach to the patient with jaundice following trauma. Scand J Surg 2004;93(3):176–83.

[9] Fink MP. Hyperbilirubinemia. In: Fink MP, Abraham E, Vincent J-L, et al, editors. Textbook of critical care. 5th edition. Philadelphia: Elsevier Saunders; 2005. p. 99–100.

[10] Hass P. Differentiation and diagnosis of jaundice. AACN Clinical Issues: Advanced Practice in Acute Critical Care 1999;10(4):433–41.

[11] Faust TW, Reddy KR. Postoperative jaundice. Clin Liver Dis 2004;8(1):151–66.

[12] Labori KJ, Bjornbeth BA, Raeder MG. Aetiology and prognostic implication of severe jaundice in surgical trauma patients. Scand J Gastroenterol 2003;38(1):102–8.

[13] Bauer I, Bauer M, Pannen BH, et al. Chronic ethanol consumption exacerbates liver injury following hemorrhagic shock: role of sinusoidal perfusion failure. Shock 1995; 4(5):324–31.

[14] Gimson AE. Hepatic dysfunction during bacterial sepsis. Intensive Care Med 1987;13(30): 162–6.

[15] Pirovino M, Meister F, Rubli E, et al. Preserved cytosolic and synthetic liver function in jaundice of severe extrahepatic infection. Gastroenterology 1989;96:1589–95.

[16] Roelofsen H, van der Veere CN, Ottenhoff R, et al. Decreased bilirubin transport in the perfused liver of endotoxemic rats. Gastroenterology 1994;107:1075–84.

[17] Miyaso H, Morimoto Y, Ozaki M, et al. Obstructive jaundice increases sensitivity to lipopolysaccharide via TLR4 upregulation: possible involvement in gut-derived hepatocyte growth factor-protection of hepatocytes. J Gastroenterol Hepatol 2005;20(12):1859–66.

[18] Ito Y, Machen NW, Urbaschek R, et al. Biliary obstruction exacerbates the hepatic microvascular inflammatory response to endotoxin. Shock 2000;14(6):599–604.

[19] Qiu Z, Kwon A, Tsuji K, et al. Fibronectin prevents D-galactosamine/lipopolysaccharide-induced lethal hepatic failure in mice. Shock 2006;25(1):80–7.

[20] Forbes A. Parenteral nutrition: new advances and observations. Curr Opin Gastroenterol 2004;20(2):114–8.

[21] Chung C, Buchman AL. Postoperative jaundice and total parenteral nutrition-associated hepatic dysfunction. Clin Liver Dis 2002;6(4):1067–84.

[22] Nanji AA, Anderson FH. Sensitivity and specificity of liver function tests in the detection of parenteral nutrition-associated cholestasis. JPEN J Parenter Enteral Nutr 1985;9(3): 307–8.

[23] Colomb V, Jobert-Giraud A, Lacaille F, et al. Role of lipid emulsions in cholestasis associated with long-term parenteral nutrition in children. JPEN J Parenter Enteral Nutr 2000; 24(6):345–50.

[24] Hwang TL, Lue MC, Chen LL. Early use of cyclic TPN prevents further deterioration of liver functions for the TPN patients with impaired liver function. Hepatogastroenterology 2000;47(35):1347–50.

[25] Kram HB, Evans T, Bundage B, et al. Use of dobutamine for treatment of shock liver syndrome. Crit Care Med 1988;16(6):644–5.

[26] Gantner F, Kusters S, Wendel A, et al. Protection from T cell-mediated murine liver failure by phosphodiesterase inhibitors. J Pharmacol Exp Ther 1997;280(1):53–60.

[27] Saavedra JE, Billiar TR, Williams DL, et al. Targeting nitric oxide (NO) delivery in vivo. Design of a liver-selective NO donor prodrug that blocks tumor necrosis factor-alpha-induced apoptosis and toxicity in the liver. J Med Chem 1997;40:1947–54.

[28] Amersi F, Buelow R, Kato H, et al. Upregulation of heme oxygenase-1 protects genetically fat Zucker rat livers from ischemia/reperfusion injury. J Clin Invest 1999;104:1631–9.

[29] Zuckerbraun BS, Billiar TR, Otterbein SL, et al. Carbon monoxide protects against liver failure through nitric oxide-induced heme oxygenase 1. J Exp Med 2003;198(11):1707–16.

[30] Mizuguchi T, Mitaka T, Katsuramaki T, et al. Hepatocyte transplantation for total liver repopulation. J Hepatobiliary Pancreat Surg 2005;12(5):378–85.

SURGICAL
CLINICS OF
NORTH AMERICA

ELSEVIER
SAUNDERS

Surg Clin N Am 86 (2006) 1503–1521

Pharmacologic Support of the Failing Heart

Jason A. London, MD, MPH*, Matthew J. Sena, MD

*Department of Surgery, Division of Trauma and Emergency Surgery, University of California,
Davis Medical Center, 2315 Stockton Boulevard, Suite 4209, Sacramento, CA 95817, USA*

Cardiovascular failure is a frequent event in critically ill patients. It can be defined as hypotension despite adequate fluid resuscitation or the need for vasopressors to maintain a normotensive state. Although a useful tool in categorizing organ failure, this definition fails to capture the physiologic state as it relates to organ perfusion and oxygen delivery at the tissue level. When viewed from this perspective, it is important to understand that cardiovascular failure is related to the shock state in so far as the latter is an inevitable consequence of the former without prompt and aggressive intervention.

A second important concept in understanding the failing heart is that the heart and blood vessels function as a single unit. Therapy directed at one component of the system invariably affects the other. This becomes critical when the intervention has significant untoward effects, such as the consequences of increasing blood pressure using a vasoconstricting agent and the associated increase in myocardial oxygen demand. For this reason, therapeutic measures should be directed at reversing the state of physiologic failure to achieve clinically significant end points. These are restoration of adequate oxygen delivery with the reversal of the clinical signs of cardiovascular failure (use of vasoactive-cardiotonic agents or aortic counterpulsation for acute ischemic pump failure); and treatment of the underlying cause (antibiotics for sepsis, revascularization of the ischemic myocardium).

Cardiovascular physiology

Physiology

The heart's function is modulated by both internal and external stimuli. Internal stimuli result from changes in myocardial fiber length, tension, and

* Corresponding author.
  E-mail address: jason.london@ucdmc.ucdavis.edu (J.A. London).

0039-6109/06/$ - see front matter © 2006 Elsevier Inc. All rights reserved.
doi:10.1016/j.suc.2006.08.003   *surgical.theclinics.com*

alterations in the electrical conduction system. External stimuli may be mechanical (intrathoracic, intrapericardial, or intra-abdominal pressures) or neurohumoral. Neurohumoral factors may affect the myocardium directly or indirectly depending on the hormonal distribution, neural innervation, and the receptor location and density. It is often difficult to predict the net effect of an intervention on cardiovascular physiology; it is critical to establish well-defined therapeutic end points that result in improved patient outcomes.

Myocardial oxygen delivery and consumption

The heart is almost exclusively an aerobic organ receiving its blood flow primarily during diastole. Under resting conditions, approximately 70% to 75% of the delivered oxygen is extracted at the capillary level. This results in an extremely low Po_2 in the blood draining from the coronary sinus that is partially reflected in the differences between mixed venous and central venous oximetry [1]. Because of this high oxygen extraction ratio, the primary mechanism for increasing oxygen delivery is coronary arteriolar dilation.

Determinants of myocardial oxygen consumption include heart rate, contractility, and wall tension. Of these, heart rate has the largest proportional effect on myocardial oxygen consumption demonstrating a near linear relationship. Increasing heart rate also reduces myocardial blood flow during diastole, potentially creating an imbalance between oxygen supply and demand. In contrast, increased wall tension has the lowest metabolic cost in terms of oxygen consumption and almost no impact on diastolic coronary perfusion [2].

Conduction system

The conducting system is composed of specialized cardiac myocytes that are responsible for synchronizing cardiac contraction. Normal electrical activity begins in the sinoatrial node and travels through the atria to the atrioventricular node, and ultimately to the ventricular myocardium. This process uses only 1% of the total myocardial oxygen demand at rest, but the location of these cells makes them susceptible to ischemia, which can result in arrhythmias and significant changes in myocardial performance.

The atrial and ventricular myocytes involved in contraction can generate spontaneous electrical signals, a property termed "automaticity." Automaticity may be altered by adrenergic stimuli, ischemia, or electrolyte abnormalities. The clinical implication is that these cells can serve as the origin for abnormal and sometimes life-threatening arrhythmias resulting from ischemia or excessive adrenergic stimulation.

Innervation of the heart and blood vessels

The myocardium is innervated by both sympathetic and parasympathetic (vagal) fibers. Sympathetic activation occurs both directly through local innervation and indirectly through systemic catecholamines secreted by the adrenal medulla. β_1 and β_2 adrenergic receptors mediate the response to catecholamines and are located on both the conducting and contractile cardiac myocytes throughout the heart. Vagal stimulation results in acetylcholine release, which acts on muscarinic receptors. In contrast to the extensive distribution of sympathetic nerves, vagal stimulation affects primarily the atria, sinoatrial node, and atrioventricular nodes.

Stimulation of the β receptors results in cardio acceleration (by increasing the automaticity of sinoatrial node discharge and the conduction through the atrioventricular node) and increased contractility leading to increased stroke volume and cardiac output. Sympathetic fibers exhibit a normal tonic discharge, which if inhibited causes a decrease in heart rate and stroke volume as much as 30% below normal. In contrast, vagal discharge causes a decrease in heart rate by decreasing the automaticity of the sinoatrial node and decreasing the excitability of the atrioventricular node. As there is minimal vagal innervation of the ventricles, vagal stimulation results in no significant change in the force of contraction [3].

The vasculature are innervated by two types of adrenergic receptors: α and β (primarily β_2). Stimulation of α_1 receptors results in arteriolar vasoconstriction, and β_2 stimulation causes arteriolar vasodilatation. In addition, α_1 receptors found in venules induce constriction, increasing venous return and preload. In contrast to the competing effect of the parasympathetic system in the heart, there is little parasympathetic input into the vascular tone of the arteries or veins. Although the effect of adrenergic stimulation in a particular organ depends on the density and proportion of α and β receptors located in that vascular bed (Table 1), the global response to sympathetic stimulation is an increase in cardiac output, systemic vascular resistance, and blood pressure. Sympathectomy, such as that which occurs with a high spinal cord injury, results in loss of vascular tone in both the arteries and veins and results in hypotension because of diminished cardiac output (decreased preload) and a decrease in systemic vascular resistance.

Review of commonly used medications

Patients with cardiovascular failure and persistent shock should be considered for pharmacologic hemodynamic support after preload has been optimized. Pharmacologic agents used in the treatment of cardiac dysfunction effect the following physiologic variables: heart rate, preload, myocardial contractility, and afterload. The most commonly used agents fall into four broad categories; cardiotonic agents, vasoconstricting agents, vasodilators, and adjuncts.

Cardiotonic and vasoconstricting agents

Agents that primarily affect the peripheral vasculature and cause vasoconstriction are vasopressors. Agents that work primarily on the heart are

Table 1
Effects of adrenergic stimulation on cardiovascular system

Effector organs	Receptor type	Adrenergic response
Heart		
SA	β1, β2	Increase automaticity
AV	β1, β2	Increase automaticity and conduction velocity
Atria	β1, β2	Increase contractility and conduction velocity
Ventricles	β1, β2	Increase automaticity, contractility, and conduction velocity
Arterioles		
Coronary	α, β2	VC+, VD++
Skin and mucosa	α	VC+++
Skeletal muscle	α, β2	VC++, VD++
Cerebral	α	VC+
Abdominal viscera	α, β2	VC+++, VD+
Pulmonary	α, β2	VC+
Renal	α, β1, β2	VC+++, VD+
Veins	α, β1, β2	VC++, VD++

Abbreviations: AV, atrioventricular node; SA, sinoatrial; VC, vasoconstriction; VD, vasodilation.

considered cardiotonic and have ionotropic (increased contractility) or chronotropic (increased heart rate) effects. Because many of these agents are structurally related or identical to endogenous catecholamines, they frequently have complex actions bridging both categories. The mechanism of action of these agents and their cardiovascular effects are summarized in Table 2.

Vasodilators

Nitrates (nitroglycerin and nitroprusside)
These agents are potent vasodilators of the peripheral vasculature. Vasodilating agents achieve their actions primarily through increasing local nitric oxide concentrations or sympathetic blockade. The primary role of these agents is in hypertensive emergencies and myocardial ischemic or infarction. At lower doses nitroglycerin is more selective for veins than nitroprusside. At higher doses, it causes a decrease in both systemic and pulmonary arterial resistance decreasing ventricular afterload. Nitroglycerin also causes coronary vasodilatation improving blood flow to the myocardium. Nitroprusside causes dilation of both arterioles and veins, reducing ventricular filling pressures, increasing aortic wall compliance, and decreasing left ventricular afterload, potentially increasing cardiac output. Nitroprusside also dilates the pulmonary vasculature and reduces right ventricular afterload.

Adjuncts

Corticosteroids
CS are required for normal homeostasis and have multiple effects on immunity, metabolism, and maintenance of vascular tone. CS exert their vascular

Table 2
Common vasoactive agents used in cardiovascular failure

Agent	Mechanism	Dose	α	β	DA	CV effects	Notes
Norepinephrine	Direct agonist	1–12 µg/min	+++	++	0	↑ SBP, DBP ↔CO VC most vascular beds	Primary vasopressor used in VD shock
Epinephrine	Direct agonist	1–200 µg/min	++	+++	0	↑ HR, SV, CO ↑ SBP, DBP, PP, PAP VC most vascular beds	↑ MVo_2 May induce tachyarrythmias
Dopamine	Direct agonist	1–2 µg/kg/h	+	+	+++	VD renal mesenteric and coronary beds	Causes NE release from nerve terminals
		2–10 µg/kg/h	++	++	+++	↑ CO, ↔ SVR	May induce tachyarrythmias and ↑ MVo_2 2nd line agent in VD shock
		10–20 µg/kg/h	+++	++	+++	↑ SVR, VC most vascular beds	
Phenylephrine	Direct agonist	20–200 µg/min	+++	0	0	↑ SVR May cause reflex bradycardia Potentially ↓ CO	Limited role in VD shock Primary agent in neurogenic shock
Dobutamine	Direct agonist	2–20 µg/kg/min	+	+++	0	↑ contractility, automaticity, CO, SV May induce hypotension by ↓ SVR	Primary inotrope in cardiogenic shock or in VD shock with myocardial depression
Milrinone	Phosphodiesterase inhibitor	50 µg/kg load 0.25–1 µg/kg/min	0	0	0	↑contractility, CO VD of systemic and pulmonary vasculature May induce hypotension	Long half-life (30–60 min) limits usefulness in acute setting

Abbreviations: CO, cardiac output; CV, cardiovascular; DA, dopamine; DBP, diastolic blood pressure; HR, heart rate; MVo_2, myocardial oxygen consumption; NE, norepinephrine; PAP, pulmonary artery pressure; PP, pulse pressure; SBP, systolic blood pressure; SV, stroke volume; SVR, systemic vascular resistance; VC, vasoconstriction; VD, vasodilation.

effects through potentiation of angiotensin II and adrenergic vasoconstriction, up-regulation of α receptors, and inhibition of nitric oxide and prostaglandin synthesis [10]. Regardless of baseline levels, the adrenal glands of critically illpatients may secrete an insufficient amount of cortisol in response to stress [11–14]. This relative deficiency of CS leads to an inability to control the inflammatory response and support the circulatory system. Administration of CS in patients with septic shock and evidence of relative adrenal insufficiency allows for tapering of vasopressor support and may improve mortality [15–19].

Vasopressin

AVP is an endogenous vasoconstrictor secreted in response to decreased atrial filling and arterial blood pressure. In addition, proinflammatory cytokines (interleukin-1 and -6, tumor necrosis factor-α), angiotensin II, catecholamines, hypoxia, and acidosis are potent secretogogues of AVP [20,21]. AVP may cause an increased responsiveness to catecholamines, an increased production of cortisol, and may improve urine output by vasoconstriction of efferent arterioles in the glomerulus [20,21]. The strongest effects of AVP are seen in the splanchnic, muscular, and cutaneous vasculature, which may lead to hypoperfusion of these organs [22,23]. In addition to its vasoconstricting properties, AVP attenuates the vasodilatation caused by endotoxin and interleukin-1 by decreasing generation of nitric oxide [20].

Patients with catecholamine-dependent vasodilatory shock may have inappropriately low AVP levels. Administration of low doses of AVP (0.04 U/min) may reverse hypotension and allow for discontinuation or reduction of vasopressor dose in many patients [24,25].

Pulmonary artery catheter

Following the introduction of the pulmonary artery catheter (PAC) in1970, invasive hemodynamic monitoring became an integral component in the care of critically ill patients with cardiopulmonary failure [4]. The rapid acceptance of this technique occurred as a result of technologic advances combined with the assumption that additional hemodynamic data necessarily improve clinical decision making. Today's PAC provides a continuous stream of data concerning right ventricular end diastolic volume, continuous cardiac output, and mixed venous oximetry, and allows constant patient assessment before and after therapeutic interventions. This provides the intensivist with a real-time trajectory of cardiovascular physiology at the bedside. For several decades, the theoretical benefits of this type of monitoring were unchallenged.

In 1987, Gore and colleagues [5] published an observational study that questioned the use of the PAC in patients with acute myocardial infarction (AMI). Since that time, several randomized trials have assessed the impact of PAC use on patient outcome in a variety of clinical scenarios [6–9]. These studies have consistently failed to demonstrate a beneficial effect and suggest that the role of the catheter in managing critically ill patients is limited. The authors believe there remains a subgroup of patients in whom the hemodynamic data provided by the PAC can be used in conjunction with clinical, radiographic, and laboratory data to improve clinical decisions in the ICU.

The following represent clinical scenarios in which a PAC should be considered:

1. Persistent shock despite adequate fluid resuscitation
2. Differentiation of acute respiratory distress syndrome from cardiogenic pulmonary edema
3. Assessing the effects of ventilatory support on cardiovascular function
4. Guiding use of vasoactive and cardiotonic medications

Invasive hemodynamic monitoring can be an essential adjunct to the care of the patient with compromised circulatory function. Determining central pressures and cardiac function are important in determining the etiology cardiovascular failure and guiding initial and subsequent therapy (Table 2). Critical information in the form of cardiac filling pressures and volumes, intrinsic cardiac function, and mixed venous oxygen saturation are easily obtained at the bedside. These data provide the potential to rapidly tailor therapy and potentially improve outcome. Ultimately, it is not the information provided, but how that information is used that determines the clinical utility of the device.

Algorithms of treatment

The following section outlines the authors' approach to patients with cardiovascular failure from primary cardiac dysfunction or secondary to sepsis (vasodilatory shock). Approaches can and should be modified according to the individual patient. Cardiovascular failure from extracardiac compressive, hypovolemic, and neurogenic etiologies are not discussed in detail. Prolonged tissue hypoperfusion from these and other causes of cardiovascular failure can lead to the production of excess inflammatory mediators responsible for systemic vasodilatation, and produce a syndrome virtually indistinguishable from primary vasodilatory shock. Vasodilatory shock is often the final common pathway resulting from prolonged cardiovascular failure from many etiologies.

Evidence-based approach to pharmacologic support of the cardiovascular system

Acute myocardial infarction and cardiogenic shock

The most common cause of acute heart failure in the surgical patient is AMI. Ischemic heart disease is a common comorbid condition in patients in the ICU with a prevalence of approximately 30%. Up to one quarter of patients admitted to the ICU develop ECG or biochemical evidence of AMI at some point during their ICU admission [26,27]. The clinical presentation and underlying pathophysiology of these events may be different from that seen in the emergency department because critically ill patients often have noncardiac conditions that induce myocardial ischemia as a secondary phenomenon. The underlying pathology in this scenario may be more related to systemic factors (fever or infection, hypoxemia, tachycardia, hypotension, and acute anemia) than to plaque instability and rupture [28].

The cardiovascular consequences of AMI are variable depending on the location and amount of ischemic myocardium. In the most severe form patients present with cardiogenic shock, the most common etiology of which is left ventricular failure. Other causes, including acute mitral regurgitation, ventricular septal defects, and right ventricular failure should be considered [29].

The goals of therapy when initially evaluating the patient with suspected myocardial ischemia are as follows:

1. Establish diagnosis and estimate severity of the infarct
2. Ensure adequate blood oxygenation
3. Ensure adequate vital organ perfusion
4. Minimize myocardial oxygen demand
5. Prevent recurrent thrombosis or propagation
6. Evaluate for myocardial revascularization or adjunct mechanical support

Establish diagnosis and initial assessment

AMI is defined by the typical rise and fall of biochemical markers plus one of the following: (1) ischemic symptoms, (2) development of Q waves, or (3) ECG evidence of ischemia. Small infarcts may cause elevations in biochemical markers without characteristic ECG changes [30]. Cardiac enzymes are biomarkers that detect evidence of myocardial damage, but do not reflect mechanism. Serial determination of cardiac enzymes greatly increases the sensitivity and specificity in comparison with a single measurement [31].

Evaluation of patients with cardiovascular failure from an AMI can be facilitated by echocardiography or a PAC. A transthoracic or transesophageal echocardiogram can visualize wall motion abnormalities in patients with suspected ischemia and nondiagnostic ECG or enzymes [30]. In the setting of AMI, echocardiogram can be used to estimate left ventricular ejection fraction, evaluate for diastolic dysfunction, estimate pulmonary pressures, detect wall motion abnormalities, and detect problems with valves or their supporting structures [32].

Ensure adequate blood oxygenation

Hypoxemia results in inadequate oxygen delivery to both the heart and periphery and can potentiate shock. In the setting of myocardial ischemia, acute left ventricular failure may exacerbate hypoxemia because of an increased left atrial pressure and pulmonary edema. The oxygen-carrying capacity of blood is determined by the formula $Cao_2 = 1.36(Hbg)(Sao_2) + 0.003(Pao_2)$, where Hbg is the hemoglobin concentration, Sao_2 is the oxygen saturation of hemoglobin, and Pao_2 is the partial pressure of oxygen in arterial blood. Hypoxemia can be treated by ensuring adequate hemoglobin concentration and saturation, or increasing the fraction of inspired oxygen. The addition of positive end-expiratory pressure in the ventilated patient may have the added benefit of decreasing preload and left ventricular wall tension, both of which decrease myocardial oxygen consumption [33].

Ensure adequate noncardiac oxygen delivery

Delivery of oxygen is a product of cardiac output and oxygen-carrying capacity of the blood ($Do_2 = CO \times Cao_2$). Transfusion of packed red blood cells, ensuring euvolemia, and pharmacologic or mechanical support of cardiac function should be considered. Secondary myocardial ischemia is common and occurs as result of alteration in supply or demand, both of which may be compromised by pharmacologic therapy. It should be emphasized that clinically important end points should be the goal of therapy. Inadequate oxygen delivery may be assessed by alterations in mixed venous oxygen saturation (SVo_2), lactate, base deficit, and clinical indicators of end organ perfusion (urine output, creatinine, mental status, liver function, and so forth). Arbitrarily increasing the blood pressure to a fixed value is not nearly as valuable as increasing renal blood flow in an oliguric patient and preventing acute renal failure. It may be necessary to augment myocardial performance at the expense of myocardial oxygen demand to prevent progressive organ failure and death. Evaluation by echocardiogram and the PAC can indicate the specific pathophysiology and how to guide therapy.

Left heart failure. An echocardiogram may show evidence of hypokinesis of the left ventricle, and the expected PAC pressures are shown in Table 3. Once euvolemia is ensured by adequate fluid resuscitation, the patient's hemodynamic status and the PAC values guide initial therapy. Although filling pressures needed to optimize CO may be higher than needed without infarction, overzealous resuscitation may lead to pulmonary edema. Normotensive patients with inadequate oxygen delivery secondary to a low cardiac output may benefit from increasing contractility with an inotrope, such as dobutamine, or afterload reduction with addition of nitrates or an angiotensin-converting enzyme inhibitor. Hypotensive patients with myocardial dysfunction usually need both inotropes and vasopressors, although occasionally only an inotrope may suffice. The authors consider dobutamine

Table 3
Hemodynamic parameters in shock

Type of shock	CO	PCWP	CVP	SVR	PAP	SVo$_2$
Cardiogenic						
LV failure	↓↓	↑↑	↑↑	↑	↑	↓
RV failure	↓↓	↔or↑	↑↑	↑	↔or↑	↓
Hypovolemic	↓↓	↓↓	↓↓	↑	↓	↓
Vasodilatory (septic)						
Early	↑↑	↓	↓	↓or↓↓	↓	↑or↑↑
Late	↔or↓	↓ or ↔	↓ or ↔	↓or↓↓	↓	↑or↑↑
Extracardiac Compressive	↓or↓↓	↔or ↓	↑↑	↑	↑↑	↓
Neurogenic	↑or↔ or↓	↓	↓	↓	↓	↓

Abbreviations: CO, cardiac output; CVP, central venous pressure; LV, left ventricle; PAP, pulmonary artery pressure; PCWP, pulmonary capillary wedge pressure; RV, right ventricle; SVo$_2$, mixed venous oxygen saturation; SVR, systemic vascular resistance.
↓-decrease, ↑-increase, ↔-equal.

with or without norepinephrine (NE) as first-line agents. Dopamine and epinephrine are considered second- and third-line agents because of their propensity to increase automaticity, myocardial oxygen consumption, and splanchnic vasoconstriction [34–36]. The long half-life of phosphodiesterase inhibitors limits their usefulness in the acute setting. Use of a pure α agonist, such as phenylephrine, without a β agonist increases afterload without improving contractility, potentially inducing reflex bradycardia and reducing cardiac output.

Right heart failure. Echocardiogram findings in isolated right heart failure may show hypokinesis of the right ventricle, and PAC values are listed in Table 3. Elevation of right ventricular systolic and pulmonary artery diastolic pressures may be seen. Patients with right heart failure may present with hypotension, distended neck veins, and clear lung fields. These patients generally have a better prognosis than those with left-sided failure [37]. Right heart failure is treated differently than other forms of cardiogenic shock, because it requires more fluid administration and inotropes rather than vasopressors. The most important aspect of management is to maintain right ventricular preload with adequate volume resuscitation. Overzealous fluid resuscitation can cause overdilation of right ventricle and septal shift decreasing left ventricular filling and cardiac output. The agent that best improves cardiac contractility while decreasing right ventricular afterload (pulmonary artery pressures) is dobutamine.

Valvular defects. Ischemic papillary muscle rupture causing acute mitral regurgitation usually occurs 3 to 7 days after an infarction in the left anterior descending distribution. It may present insidiously with a new-onset murmur or catastrophically with pulmonary edema, hypotension, and cardiogenic shock. Suspicion is confirmed by echocardiogram. Management is aimed at improving forward flow and decreasing the regurgitant fraction of stroke volume. Afterload reduction with nitroprusside and intra-aortic balloon pump are temporizing measures until definitive surgical therapy can be performed.

Septal defects. Acute rupture of the intraventricular septum usually occurs several days after infarction in the left anterior descending distribution. Physical examination reveals a pansystolic murmur. Measurement of oxygen saturation from the proximal and distal ports of the PAC reveals an increase of hemoglobin oxygen saturation of blood in the pulmonary artery relative to the right atrium indicating a left-to-right shunt. Right ventricular cardiac output is greater than left ventricular output. Diagnosis is confirmed with echocardiogram. The amount of left to right shunting is dependent on the resistance to outflow from the left ventricle. The goal of medical management is to improve left ventricular output, which can be accomplished by the use of inotropes, nitrates, or intra-aortic balloon pump before definitive surgical treatment.

Minimize myocardial oxygen demand

This goal should be accomplished only when it is clear that other vital organ oxygen delivery is not compromised. Use of opiates for pain control decreases sympathetic stimulation. Assuming normotension, administration of β-blockers can decrease the heart rate, decrease myocardial oxygen demand, and increase supply by lengthening diastole. Nitroglycerin decreases preload and left ventricular afterload, increases coronary artery vasodilatation resulting in decreased oxygen demand, and possibly increased delivery.

Prevent recurrent thrombosis-propagation

Aspirin inhibits prostaglandin mediated platelet aggregation and has been clearly shown to limit re-infarction and improve mortality in patients with AMI and unstable angina. Although irreversible, it is a relatively mild anti-platelet agent and the reported effects of bleeding in surgical patients are largely anecdotal and generally outweighed by the proven benefit [38–40]. Reports of perioperative bleeding are largely anecdotal and these risks are frequently outweighed by the proved benefits. Cilostazol (Plavix), another antiplatelet agent, is primarily used following percutaneous coronary intervention. Despite a mortality benefit, the risk of bleeding is substantial and its use should generally be avoided in critically ill patients unless the patient has a contraindication to aspirin or if a percutaneous coronary intervention is planned [41,42]. Systemic anticoagulation with unfractionated heparin has demonstrated a consistent mortality benefit over antiplatelet therapy alone [43]. There is a suggestion that use of low-molecular-weight heparin is associated with an increased risk of bleeding and has no significant advantage over unfractionated heparin [44–47]. Direct thrombin inhibitors should only be considered in patients with heparin-induced thrombocytopenia [48].

*Percutaneous coronary intervention, revascularization,
and adjuncts for hemodynamic support*

Patients with evidence of myocardial ischemia or infarction should undergo rapid evaluation, in conjunction with cardiology or cardiothoracic surgery consultation, for restoration of coronary perfusion. Options for restoring perfusion include systemic fibrinolytic therapy; percutaneous coronary intervention (selective fibrinolysis, angioplasty, stenting); and surgical revascularization. The specific indications and contraindications for each are beyond the scope of this article, but are outlined in the American College of Cardiology–American Heart Association Guidelines [43,48].

In severe cardiogenic shock, pharmacologic therapy may be inadequate, and mechanical adjucts should be considered when available. These are often performed in conjunction with reperfusion therapy. The most commonly employed measure is the aortic counterpulsation device or balloon pump. This device is deployed percutaneously and rests in the descending thoracic aorta. Inflation during diastole increases coronary perfusion pressure, while deflation during systole reduces left ventricular afterload and augments cardiac output. Other options for supporting a patient unresponsive to pharmacologic treatment include percutaneous cardiopulmonary bypass, extracorporeal membrane oxygenation, and ventricular assist devices.

Vasodilatory shock

Although sepsis is the classic example of vasodilatory shock, prolonged tissue hypoperfusion with subsequent reperfusion from any cause can result in a virtually indistinguishable clinical scenario. Even though the management goals of patients in vasodilatory and cardiogenic shock are similar, the pathophysiology and treatments are different.

Establish diagnosis and initial assessment

In sepsis and other inflammatory states, the body releases numerous cytokines, most notably interleukin-1β and tumor necrosis factor-α, and nitric oxide in response to exposure of an infectious or inflammatory stimulus. These substances cause peripheral vasodilatation and vasoconstriction, microvascular thrombosis, and capillary leak leading to alterations in peripheral oxygen delivery and extraction contributing to multisystem organ failure [49,50]. This results in relative hypovolemia and the classic hemodynamic profile (see Table 3) of high cardiac output, low systemic vascular resistance, and poor end-organ perfusion. The first priority is to restore intravascular volume to ensure adequate preload by administration of isotonic crystalloids. If the patient remains hypotensive after the first 2 to 3 L, consideration should be given to placement of a PAC further to guide therapy. Treatment with vasoactive medications in the early stages of vasodilatory shock is not indicated unless hypoperfusion is so profound that there is immediate concern for ischemic-hypoxic injury to the heart or brain.

Treatment of underlying disorder

Treatment of the underlying disorder should occur simultaneously with initial assessment. Controlling the source of infection and initiating antibiotic therapy is appropriate in septic shock. In other causes of shock (eg, hypovolemic, cardiogenic, or neurogenic) aggressive treatment of the underlying etiology and rapidly ensuring adequate oxygen delivery may prevent prolonged tissue hypoxia and progression to vasodilatory shock.

Ensuring adequate blood oxygenation and vital organ perfusion

Vasodilatory shock results in a decrease in systemic resistance and relative hypovolemia caused by arteriolar and venous vasodilatation and increased capillary permeability. At the tissue level, oxygenated blood is shunted through capillary beds leading to elevated SVo_2 and contributing to end-organ ischemia [49–51]. Because of impaired oxygen delivery and extraction at the tissue level, global indicators of oxygen delivery (acid-base status, lactate, SVo_2) may not accurately reflect tissue perfusion [52]. A low SVo_2 indicates poor oxygen delivery, but a normal or high SVo_2 does not ensure adequate oxygen delivery to the tissues. Elevated lactate levels may result from altered cellular metabolism or decreased hepatic clearance rather than global hypoperfusion [53]. In addition, clinical indicators of specific end-organ perfusion are not sufficiently sensitive to assess adequacy of resuscitation. Attempts to identify end points of resuscitation based on specific end organs (gastric tonometry, transcutaneous and sublingual oxygen saturation monitors) have not been widely accepted into routine practice [53]. Despite extensive evaluation, use of these markers to guide resuscitation has not been demonstrated to improve patient outcomes in the ICU. Ultimately, patient assessment and treatments should be guided by a combination of clinical, hemodynamic, and laboratory findings.

The primary goal in vasodilatory shock is to maximize peripheral oxygen delivery. Global O_2 delivery may be hampered by pulmonary failure, hypotension, anemia, and depressed myocardial function. Many of these factors can be improved with the institution of mechanical ventilation, cardiotonic-vasoactive medications, or transfusions. Early studies proposed the idea that increasing CO and O_2 delivery to supranormal levels by pharmacologic manipulation improved outcomes [54,55]. More recent evidence suggests that this approach may actually be detrimental [56,57]. Instead, hemodynamic variables should be titrated to achieve normalization of end-organ function whenever possible (urine output, creatinine, lactate, mental status). The blood pressures considered to be adequate should be individualized to the patient's response. In general, a systolic blood pressure of at least 90 mm Hg should be adequate for most patients [58]. Patients with comorbidities, such as visceral, cerebral, or coronary vascular disease, may require a higher systolic blood pressure to maintain blood flow beyond fixed arterial stenoses.

The goal of fluid resuscitation is to restore intravascular volume and increase cardiac preload to obtain an adequate cardiac output. If tissue perfusion remains inadequate despite restoration of intravascular volume, pharmacologic support may be indicated. Which vasopressor to use as a first-line agent has been a matter of debate. The same mechanisms that increase blood pressure have the potential to increase myocardial oxygen consumption, decrease cardiac output, and decrease visceral perfusion.

In early vasodilatory shock, NE has emerged as the agent of choice rather than dopamine. NE more reliably reverses hypotension than dopamine, improving urine output and oxygen delivery and consumption [59]. Furthermore, two observational studies of patients in shock have suggested that treatment with NE was associated with lower mortality rates, whereas treatment with dopamine was associated with increased hospital mortality [60,61]. A direct comparison between dopamine and NE showed that the former increased mean arterial pressure primarily by increasing cardiac output, whereas the latter did so by increasing systemic vascular resistance [34]. The former mechanism has the potential to induce tachyarrhythmias and increase myocardial oxygen consumption. Dopamine may also cause an increase in splanchnic oxygen requirements without a concomitant increase in delivery [34].

Epinephrine is theoretically attractive because it has the potential to increase both myocardial contractility and systemic vascular resistance. Despite this, studies have shown that its use is associated with decrease in splanchnic perfusion, increase in lactate levels, and a decrease in gastric mucosal pH [35,36]. Epinephrine has a very limited role in the treatment of septic shock. Phenylephrine, a pure α agonist without any β activity, can lead to excessive peripheral vasoconstriction, an increase in left ventricular afterload, and an overall decrease in cardiac output. Dopamine and epinephrine are more likely to produce tachyarrhythmias than NE.

Late stages of vasodilatory shock may be associated with myocardial depression. Tumor necrosis factor-α, interleukin-1β, and nitric oxide are the most likely agents causing myocardial depression [62–64]. Both left and right ventricular systolic and diastolic function may be depressed [65–71]. In these cases an inotrope or more often a combination of vasopressor and inotrope is needed. Epinephrine seems to be an ideal single agent, but this agent alone has been associated with a more unpredictable and often detrimental change in splanchnic perfusion [35,72]. The authors consider dobutamine as the first-line inotrope. It may be combined with a second agent, usually NE or dopamine, to counter its vasodilating properties.

Some patients may be resistant to escalating doses of catecholamines, increasing the likelihood of adverse effects, such as arrhythmias and myocardial and splanchnic ischemia. There is evidence to suggest that in the early stages of shock AVP levels are elevated, but in advanced vasodilatory shock levels are inappropriately low [24,73]. Low levels of AVP may be related to depletion of stores, inadequate secretion, or an inappropriate autonomic response [21]. Several trials have shown that administration of AVP in catecholamine-dependent vasodilatory shock improves blood pressure and allows for tapering of catecholamines doses [25,74,75]. Administration of AVP in catecholamine-dependent vasodilatory shock is associated with less tachyarrhythmia, improved global hemodynamics, and improved gut perfusion [76]. In addition, there are reports of success with the use of AVP in other causes of shock including anaphylactic, hemorrhagic, and cardiogenic shock [77–81].

Septic shock may be associated with relative adrenal insufficiency resulting in a decrease in production, secretion, or systemic response to cortisol [13]. Because of cortisol's integral role in maintenance of vascular tone, relative adrenal insufficiency in vasodilatory shock is associated with vascular collapse and increased mortality [11]. Several studies have shown the administration of physiologic doses of CS to patients with evidence of adrenal insufficiency (an increase of less than 9 μg/dL 30 or 60 minutes after 250 μg cosyntropin stimulation test) improves mortality in patients with septic shock [11,15,16,18]. A recent meta-analysis of five studies confirms that a 5- to 7-day course of physiologic doses of CS results in a more rapid reversal of shock and improves survival [82].

Summary

Cardiovascular failure in critically ill patients carries a high mortality. Identification of the underlying etiology and prompt therapy are indicated to avoid the consequences of prolonged shock. Patient assessment should use all available clinical, radiologic, and laboratory data to avoid the pitfalls associated with use of single measures of regional or global perfusion and their inherent limitations. Treatment aimed at reversal of the immediate physiologic derangement should be coupled with efforts to correct the underlying etiology. Finally, the dynamic nature of physiology in critically ill patients requires constant patient reassessment and flexibility in treatment to tailor therapy individually as the pathologic state evolves.

References

[1] Rivers E, Ander D, Powell D. Central venous oxygen saturation monitoring in the critically ill patient. Curr Opin Crit Care 2001;7:204–11.

[2] Zipes DP, Bonow LP, Braunwald R. Braunwald's heart disease: a textbook of cardiovascular medicine, vol. 2. 7th edition. Philadelphia: Elsevier Saunders; 2005.

[3] Guyton AC, Hall JE. Textbook of medical physiology. 11th edition. Philadelphia: Elsevier Saunders; 2006.

[4] Swan HJ, Ganz W, Forrester J, et al. Catheterization of the heart in man with use of a flow-directed balloon-tipped catheter. N Engl J Med 1970;283:447–51.

[5] Gore JM, Goldberg RJ, Spodick DH, et al. A community-wide assessment of the use of pulmonary artery catheters in patients with acute myocardial infarction. Chest 1987;92: 721–7.

[6] Rhodes A, Cusack RJ, Newman PJ, et al. A randomised, controlled trial of the pulmonary artery catheter in critically ill patients. Intensive Care Med 2002;28:6–64.

[7] Binanay C, Califf RM, Hasselblad V, et al. Evaluation study of congestive heart failure and pulmonary artery catheterization effectiveness: the ESCAPE trial. JAMA 2005;294: 1625–33.

[8] Richard C, Warszawski J, Anguel N, et al. Early use of the pulmonary artery catheter and outcomes in patients with shock and acute respiratory distress syndrome: a randomized controlled trial. JAMA 2003;290:2713–20.

[9] Sandham JD, Hull RD, Brant RF, et al. A randomized, controlled trial of the use of pulmonary-artery catheters in high-risk surgical patients. N Engl J Med 2003;348:5–14.

[10] Ullian ME. The role of corticosteriods in the regulation of vascular tone. Cardiovasc Res 1999;41:55–64.

[11] Annane D, Sebille V, Troche G, et al. A 3-level prognostic classification in septic shock based on cortisol levels and cortisol response to corticotropin. JAMA 2000;283:1038–45.

[12] Sam S, Corbridge TC, Mokhlesi B, et al. Cortisol levels and mortality in severe sepsis. Clin Endocrinol (Oxf) 2004;60:29–35.

[13] Schroeder S, Wichers M, Klingmuller D, et al. The hypothalamic-pituitary-adrenal axis of patients with severe sepsis: altered response to corticotropin-releasing hormone. Crit Care Med 2001;29:310–6.

[14] Marik PE, Zaloga GP. Adrenal insufficiency during septic shock. Crit Care Med 2003;31: 141–5.

[15] Annane D, Sebille V, Charpentier C, et al. Effect of treatment with low doses of hydrocortisone and fludrocortisone on mortality in patients with septic shock. JAMA 2002;288: 862–71.

[16] Yildiz O, Doganay M, Aygen B, et al. Physiological-dose steroid therapy in sepsis [ISRCTN36253388]. Crit Care 2002;6:251–9.

[17] Keh D, Boehnke T, Weber-Cartens S, et al. Immunologic and hemodynamic effects of low-dose hydrocortisone in septic shock: a double-blind, randomized, placebo-controlled, crossover study. Am J Respir Crit Care Med 2003;167:512–20.

[18] Briegel J, Forst H, Haller M, et al. Stress doses of hydrocortisone reverse hyperdynamic septic shock: a prospective, randomized, double-blind, single-center study. Crit Care Med 1999; 27:723–32.

[19] Bollaert PE, Charpentier C, Levy B, et al. Reversal of late septic shock with supraphysiologic doses of hydrocortisone. Crit Care Med 1998;26:645–50.

[20] Dunser MW, Wenzel V, Mayr AJ, et al. Management of vasodilatory shock: defining the role of arginine vasopressin. Drugs 2003;63:237–56.

[21] Holmes CL, Patel BM, Russell JA, et al. Physiology of vasopressin relevant to management of septic shock. Chest 2001;120:989–1002.

[22] van Haren FM, Rozendaal FW, van der Hoeven JG. The effect of vasopressin on gastric perfusion in catecholamine-dependent patients in septic shock. Chest 2003;124:2256–60.

[23] Dunser MW, Mayr AJ, Tur A, et al. Ischemic skin lesions as a complication of continuous vasopressin infusion in catecholamine-resistant vasodilatory shock: incidence and risk factors. Crit Care Med 2003;31:1394–8.

[24] Landry DW, Levin HR, Gallant EM, et al. Vasopressin deficiency contributes to the vasodilation of septic shock. Circulation 1997;95:1122–5.

[25] Patel BM, Chittock DR, Russell JA, et al. Beneficial effects of short-term vasopressin infusion during severe septic shock. Anesthesiology 2002;96:576–82.

[26] Walsh TS, McClelland DB, Lee RJ, et al. Prevalence of ischaemic heart disease at admission to intensive care and its influence on red cell transfusion thresholds: multicentre Scottish Study. Br J Anaesth 2005;94:445–52.

[27] Lim W, Qushmaq I, Cook DJ, et al. Elevated troponin and myocardial infarction in the intensive care unit: a prospective study. Crit Care 2005;9:R636–44.

[28] Stone PH, Thompson B, Anderson HV, et al. Influence of race, sex, and age on management of unstable angina and non-Q-wave myocardial infarction: the TIMI III registry. JAMA 1996;275:1104–12.

[29] Hochman JS, Boland J, Sleeper LA, et al. Current spectrum of cardiogenic shock and effect of early revascularization on mortality: results of an International Registry. SHOCK Registry Investigators. Circulation 1995;91:873–81.

[30] Alpert JS, Thygesen K, Antman E, et al. Myocardial infarction redefined–a consensus document of The Joint European Society of Cardiology/American College of Cardiology Committee for the redefinition of myocardial infarction. J Am Coll Cardiol 2000;36:959–69.

[31] Balk EM, Ioannidis JP, Salem D, et al. Accuracy of biomarkers to diagnose acute cardiac ischemia in the emergency department: a meta-analysis. Ann Emerg Med 2001;37:478–94.

[32] Vitarelli A, Tiukinhoy S, Di Luzio S, et al. The role of echocardiography in the diagnosis and management of heart failure. Heart Fail Rev 2003;8:181–9.

[33] Naughton MT, Rahman MA, Hara K, et al. Effect of continuous positive airway pressure on intrathoracic and left ventricular transmural pressures in patients with congestive heart failure. Circulation 1995;91:1725–31.

[34] Marik PE, Mohedin M. The contrasting effects of dopamine and norepinephrine on systemic and splanchnic oxygen utilization in hyperdynamic sepsis. JAMA 1994;272:1354–7.

[35] Levy B, Bollaert PE, Charpentier C, et al. Comparison of norepinephrine and dobutamine to epinephrine for hemodynamics, lactate metabolism, and gastric tonometric variables in septic shock: a prospective, randomized study. Intensive Care Med 1997;23:282–7.

[36] Meier-Hellmann A, Reinhart K, Bredle DL, et al. Epinephrine impairs splanchnic perfusion in septic shock. Crit Care Med 1997;25:399–404.

[37] Zehender M, Kasper W, Kauder E, et al. Right ventricular infarction as an independent predictor of prognosis after acute inferior myocardial infarction. N Engl J Med 1993;328:981–8.

[38] Lewis HD Jr, Davis JW, Archibald DG, et al. Protective effects of aspirin against acute myocardial infarction and death in men with unstable angina: results of a Veterans Administration Cooperative Study. N Engl J Med 1983;309:396–403.

[39] Collaborative meta-analysis of randomised trials of antiplatelet therapy for prevention of death, myocardial infarction, and stroke in high risk patients. BMJ 2002;324:71–86.

[40] Risk of myocardial infarction and death during treatment with low dose aspirin and intravenous heparin in men with unstable coronary artery disease: the RISC Group. Lancet 1990;336:827–30.

[41] Chu MW, Wilson SR, Novick RJ, et al. Does clopidogrel increase blood loss following coronary artery bypass surgery? Ann Thorac Surg 2004;78:1536–41.

[42] Yusuf S, Zhao F, Mehta SR, et al. Effects of clopidogrel in addition to aspirin in patients with acute coronary syndromes without ST-segment elevation. N Engl J Med 2001;345:494–502.

[43] Braunwald E, Antman EM, Beasley JW, et al. ACC/AHA guidelines for the management of patients with unstable angina and non-ST-segment elevation myocardial infarction. A report of the American College of Cardiology/American Heart Association Task Force on Practice Guidelines (Committee on the Management of Patients With Unstable Angina). J Am Coll Cardiol 2000;36:970–1062.

[44] Le Nguyen MT, Spencer FA. Low molecular weight heparin and unfractionated heparin in the early pharmacologic management of acute coronary syndromes: a meta-analysis of randomized clinical trials. J Thromb Thrombolysis 2001;12:289–95.

[45] Husted S, Becker R, Kher A. A critical review of clinical trials for low-molecular-weight heparin therapy in unstable coronary artery disease. Clin Cardiol 2001;24:492–9.

[46] Ferguson JJ, Califf RM, Antman EM, et al. Enoxaparin vs unfractionated heparin in high-risk patients with non-ST-segment elevation acute coronary syndromes managed with an intended early invasive strategy: primary results of the SYNERGY randomized trial. JAMA 2004;292:45–54.

[47] Petersen JL, Mahaffey KW, Hasselblad V, et al. Efficacy and bleeding complications among patients randomized to enoxaparin or unfractionated heparin for antithrombin therapy in non-ST-Segment elevation acute coronary syndromes: a systematic overview. JAMA 2004;292:89–96.

[48] Antman EM, Anbe DT, Armstrong PW, et al. ACC/AHA guidelines for the management of patients with ST-elevation myocardial infarction–executive summary. A report of the American College of Cardiology/American Heart Association Task Force on Practice Guidelines (Writing Committee to revise the 1999 guidelines for the management of patients with acute myocardial infarction). J Am Coll Cardiol 2004;44:671–719.

[49] Bateman RM, Sharpe MD, Ellis CG. Bench-to-bedside review: microvascular dysfunction in sepsis–hemodynamics, oxygen transport, and nitric oxide. Crit Care 2003;7:359–73.

[50] Vincent JL, De Backer D. Microvascular dysfunction as a cause of organ dysfunction in severe sepsis. Crit Care 2005;9(Suppl 4):S9–12.

[51] De Backer D, Creteur J, Preiser JC, et al. Microvascular blood flow is altered in patients with sepsis. Am J Respir Crit Care Med 2002;166:98–104.

[52] Cohen ES, Hollenberg SM. Tissue oxygenation and sepsis. Crit Care Med 2001;29:1479–80.

[53] Beale RJ, Hollenberg SM, Vincent JL, et al. Vasopressor and inotropic support in septic shock: an evidence-based review. Crit Care Med 2004;32(11 Suppl):S455–65.

[54] Shoemaker WC, Appel PL, Kram HB, et al. Prospective trial of supranormal values of survivors as therapeutic goals in high-risk surgical patients. Chest 1988;94:1176–86.

[55] Tuchschmidt J, Fried J, Astiz M, et al. Elevation of cardiac output and oxygen delivery improves outcome in septic shock. Chest 1992;102:216–20.

[56] Hayes MA, Timmins AC, Yau EH, et al. Elevation of systemic oxygen delivery in the treatment of critically ill patients. N Engl J Med 1994;330:1717–22.

[57] Gattinoni L, Brazzi L, Pelosi P, et al. A trial of goal-oriented hemodynamic therapy in critically ill patients. SvO2 Collaborative Group. N Engl J Med 1995;333:1025–32.

[58] Holcroft J. Shock. In: Fink JG, Kaiser MP, Pearce LR, et al, editors. ACS surgery: principles and practice, vol. 1. New York: WebMD; 2005. p. 1624.

[59] Martin C, Papazian L, Perrin G, et al. Norepinephrine or dopamine for the treatment of hyperdynamic septic shock? Chest 1993;103:1826–31.

[60] Sakr Y, Reinhart K, Vincent JL, et al. Does dopamine administration in shock influence outcome? Results of the Sepsis Occurrence in Acutely Ill Patients (SOAP) Study. Crit Care Med 2006;34:589–97.

[61] Martin C, Viviand X, Leone M, et al. Effect of norepinephrine on the outcome of septic shock. Crit Care Med 2000;28:2758–65.

[62] Kumar A, Thota V, Dee L, et al. Tumor necrosis factor alpha and interleukin 1 beta are responsible for in vitro myocardial cell depression induced by human septic shock serum. J Exp Med 1996;183:949–58.

[63] Cain BS, Meldrum DR, Dinarello CA, et al. Tumor necrosis factor-alpha and interleukin-1beta synergistically depress human myocardial function. Crit Care Med 1999;27:1309–18.

[64] Kumar A, Brar R, Wang P, et al. Role of nitric oxide and cGMP in human septic serum-induced depression of cardiac myocyte contractility. Am J Physiol 1999;276(1 Pt 2):R265–76.

[65] Dhainaut JF, Brunet F, Monsallier JF, et al. Bedside evaluation of right ventricular performance using a rapid computerized thermodilution method. Crit Care Med 1987;15:148–52.

[66] Poelaert J, Declerck C, Vogelaers D, et al. Left ventricular systolic and diastolic function in septic shock. Intensive Care Med 1997;23:553–60.

[67] Parker MM, Shelhamer JH, Bacharach SL, et al. Profound but reversible myocardial depression in patients with septic shock. Ann Intern Med 1984;100:483–90.

[68] Monsalve F, Rucabado L, Salvador A, et al. Myocardial depression in septic shock caused by meningococcal infection. Crit Care Med 1984;12:1021–3.

[69] Munt B, Jue J, Gin K, et al. Diastolic filling in human severe sepsis: an echocardiographic study. Crit Care Med 1998;26:1829–33.

[70] Dhainaut JF, Lanore JJ, de Gournay JM, et al. Right ventricular dysfunction in patients with septic shock. Intensive Care Med 1988;14(Suppl 2):488–91.

[71] Vincent JL, Thirion M, Brimioulle S, et al. Thermodilution measurement of right ventricular ejection fraction with a modified pulmonary artery catheter. Intensive Care Med 1986;12:33–8.

[72] De Backer D, Creteur J, Silva E, et al. Effects of dopamine, norepinephrine, and epinephrine on the splanchnic circulation in septic shock: which is best? Crit Care Med 2003;31:1659–67.

[73] Landry DW, Oliver JA. The pathogenesis of vasodilatory shock. N Engl J Med 2001;345:588–95.

[74] Landry DW, Levin HR, Gallant EM, et al. Vasopressin pressor hypersensitivity in vasodilatory septic shock. Crit Care Med 1997;25:1279–82.

[75] Malay MB, Ashton RC Jr, Landry DW, et al. Low-dose vasopressin in the treatment of vasodilatory septic shock. J Trauma 1999;47:699–703 [discussion: 703–5].

[76] Dunser MW, Mayr AJ, Ulmer H, et al. Arginine vasopressin in advanced vasodilatory shock: a prospective, randomized, controlled study. Circulation 2003;107:2313–9.

[77] Sharma RM, Setlur R. Vasopressin in hemorrhagic shock. Anesth Analg 2005;101:833–4.

[78] Krismer AC, Wenzel V, Voelckel WG, et al. Employing vasopressin as an adjunct vasopressor in uncontrolled traumatic hemorrhagic shock: three cases and a brief analysis of the literature. Anesthetist 2005;54:220–4.

[79] Kill C, Wranze E, Wulf H. Successful treatment of severe anaphylactic shock with vasopressin: two case reports. Int Arch Allergy Immunol 2004;134:260–1.

[80] Jolly S, Newton G, Horlick E, et al. Effect of vasopressin on hemodynamics in patients with refractory cardiogenic shock complicating acute myocardial infarction. Am J Cardiol 2005; 96:1617–20.

[81] Tsuneyoshi I, Onomoto M, Yonetani A, et al. Low-dose vasopressin infusion in patients with severe vasodilatory hypotension after prolonged hemorrhage during general anesthesia. J Anesth 2005;19:170–3.

[82] Minneci PC, Deans KJ, Banks SM, et al. Meta-analysis: the effect of steroids on survival and shock during sepsis depends on the dose. Ann Intern Med 2004;141:47–56.

ELSEVIER
SAUNDERS

SURGICAL
CLINICS OF
NORTH AMERICA

Surg Clin N Am 86 (2006) 1523–1539

Management of Sepsis

Gina Howell, BA[a], Samuel A. Tisherman, MD[b,c],*

[a]University of Pittsburgh School of Medicine, Pittsburgh, PA 15261, USA
[b]Department of Surgery, University of Pittsburgh, 638 Scaife Hall,
3550 Terrace Street, Pittsburgh, PA 15261, USA
[c]Department of Critical Care Medicine, University of Pittsburgh, 638 Scaife Hall,
3550 Terrace Street, Pittsburgh, PA 15261, USA

Sepsis is defined as the systemic inflammatory response to infection. Clinical criteria for the diagnosis of sepsis include the presence or suspicion of infection in addition to the systemic inflammatory response syndrome, which includes hypothermia or hyperthermia, tachycardia, tachypnea or hyperventilation, and leukocytosis, a leftward shift of the differential, or leukopenia. When sepsis progresses to organ dysfunction or failure it is classified as severe sepsis, and when severe sepsis progresses to hypotension despite adequate fluid resuscitation it is classified as septic shock [1].

Severe sepsis is the tenth most common cause of death in the United States [2]. Twenty percent of patients who develop severe sepsis are surgical patients, and severe sepsis is a major cause of both preoperative and postoperative morbidity and mortality [3]. It is estimated that more than 750,000 cases of severe sepsis occur each year leading to approximately 225,000 deaths [2]. In addition, the incidence of sepsis seems to be increasing because of many factors, including an increasing number of elderly and immunocompromised patients, antibiotic resistance to an increasing number of pathogens, and increasing use of invasive procedures for diagnosis and patient management [1].

Despite tremendous advances in the understanding of the pathophysiologic alterations that occur during activation of the inflammatory cascade during sepsis, in-hospital mortality associated with severe sepsis remains at 30% to 50%. The importance of both the coagulation and inflammation pathways in the disease process has shifted the focus away from efforts specifically to modify mediators of the inflammatory response, which were almost uniformly unsuccessful, toward manipulation of both systems. An

* Corresponding author. Departments of Surgery and Critical Care Medicine, University of Pittsburgh, 638 Scaife Hall, 3550 Terrace Street, Pittsburgh, PA 15261.
E-mail address: tishermansa@upmc.edu (S.A. Tisherman).

0039-6109/06/$ - see front matter © 2006 Elsevier Inc. All rights reserved.
doi:10.1016/j.suc.2006.08.001   surgical.theclinics.com

example of such a strategy, which has proved to be successful, is the use of recombinant human activated protein C (APC).

The mainstay of management of sepsis remains eradication of the septic source. The increasing understanding of the pathophysiology of sepsis, however, may allow clinicians to modulate the body's response to the inciting agent. Novel management strategies and pharmacologic agents now hold promise for substantially decreasing mortality in septic patients.

Pathophysiology

The pathophysiologic mechanisms that underlie severe sepsis are complex and beyond the scope of this article, but involve an excessive proinflammatory and procoagulant responses to infection that are intricately linked to one another [4,5]. The body's response to any of various infectious stimuli results in the release of tumor necrosis factor-α (TNF-α) and interleukin (IL)-1, which in turn trigger a cascade of proinflammatory cytokines responsible for the systemic inflammatory response syndrome observed in the septic state. Additionally, TNF-α and IL-1 stimulate leukocytes to release anti-inflammatory cytokines and neutralizing molecules, which comprise the body's compensatory anti-inflammatory response syndrome (CARS). The function of CARS is to counteract the excessive release and action of proinflammatory cytokines so as to balance and attenuate what could otherwise become an uncontrolled systemic proinflammatory state leading to endothelial damage, hypotension, and organ dysfunction, such as that observed in severe sepsis. An excessive CARS, however, has the potential to induce a state of immune suppression, rendering patients incapable of clearing infections and increasing their susceptibility to subsequent infectious insults. A delicate balance exists between these two opposing mechanisms [4].

Inflammation related to sepsis is an acquired state of dysregulated coagulation, which can range from a mild reduction in platelet counts to widespread microvascular thromboses resulting in tissue hypoxia and ultimately organ dysfunction. The procoagulant pathway that results in fibrin clot formation is normally regulated by the fibrinolytic system, which involves plasmin-mediated degradation of cross-linked fibrin and the natural anticoagulants, tissue-factor pathway inhibitor (TFPI), antithrombin III (ATIII), and APC, which act to prevent widespread thrombosis. Many of these regulatory molecules are suppressed in severe sepsis, impairing fibrinolysis and promoting a procoagulant environment [6]. For example, TNF-α and IL-1 activate platelets, decrease activity of anticoagulants, stimulate tissue factor–mediated activation of the coagulation cascade, and increase production of plasminogen-activator inhibitor [4–6]. Conversely, components of the coagulation cascade, such as thrombin, factor Xa, and the tissue factor-factor VIIa complex, have potent inflammatory effects through the stimulation of proinflammatory cytokine release and stimulation of neutrophil migration [5]. These are but a few of the complex and synergistic pathways by which coagulation and inflammation initiate and perpetuate organ injury in patients with severe sepsis.

Intensive care management

Traditionally, care of the septic patient focused on antimicrobials and, if possible, removal or drainage of the septic source. Organ system function was supported in a nonstandardized way. Specific protocols for therapy, however, as outlined later, may prove to be beneficial.

Early goal-directed resuscitation therapy

Early goal-directed therapy (EGDT) refers to the early protocol-driven resuscitation of patients with severe sepsis or sepsis-induced hypoperfusion to attain predefined resuscitation end points by adjusting cardiac preload, afterload, and contractility. Hemodynamic resuscitation is necessary to combat the circulatory abnormalities that accompany the transition from sepsis to severe sepsis and septic shock in response to proinflammatory cytokines and other mediators in the septic cascade. Decreased systemic vascular resistance, increased venous capacitance, myocardial depression, intravascular volume depletion, and increased metabolism can lead to an imbalance between systemic oxygen delivery and oxygen demand, which can eventually result in tissue hypoxia and irreversible organ dysfunction or failure.

The current consensus guidelines for initial resuscitation are based on the results of a recent single-institution study that found that severely septic patients treated with 6 hours of EGDT before admission to the ICU had a significant decrease in in-hospital and 60-day mortality compared with patients assigned to receive standard treatment [7,8]. Resuscitation was guided by central venous oxygen saturation ($Scvo_2$) $\geq 70\%$, in addition to central venous pressure 8 to 12 mm Hg, mean arterial pressure 65 to 90 mm Hg, and urine output >0.5 mL/kg/h. The predefined target end points were accomplished by sequential institution of fluid administration, vasopressors and vasodilators, packed red blood cell transfusion, and dobutamine [7].

Because this study is the only one to demonstrate significant mortality benefit from EGDT, its protocol as a whole has been included in the consensus guidelines [8], because no subsequent investigations have yet dissected out which particular aspects of this protocol provide benefit. There is an ongoing debate, for example, over the end points of resuscitation, specifically with the use of $Scvo_2$, and the means by which to attain these end points. Although it is generally believed that $Scvo_2$ is a sensitive indicator of the adequacy of tissue oxygenation [9], it has been questioned whether the use of $Scvo_2$ is essential to the success of the EGDT approach or if there are other indices of resuscitation that may serve as well or better [10]. Additionally, regarding specific interventions in the initial trial with EGDT, the use of blood transfusions may be the most controversial, because a restricted blood transfusion policy seems to have benefit in a general population of critically ill patients [11].

There seems to be agreement that goal-directed resuscitation should begin as early as possible on presentation to the emergency department, and that resuscitative efforts should not be delayed until admission to the ICU. Optimization of hemodynamics before the onset of organ system dysfunction seems to be critical, because early hemodynamic intervention may be able to restore perfusion before the transition from reversible to irreversible cellular dysfunction occurs, thus preventing organ failure or death [12].

Glycemic control

Hyperglycemia associated with insulin resistance is common among critically ill patients with severe sepsis, and occurs in patients with or without a history of diabetes mellitus. It is postulated that the disruption in glucoregulation during sepsis involves stress-induced elevations in catecholamines, glucagon, and cortisol that promote glycogenolysis and gluconeogenesis, in addition to proinflammatory cytokine-mediated insulin resistance [13]. Recent studies suggest that the normalization of blood glucose levels (80–110 mg/dL) with intensive insulin therapy significantly reduces mortality among patients with critical illness, such as severe sepsis, by 30% to 40%, with the greatest reduction in mortality among patients suffering multiple organ failure with a documented septic focus [14]. Intensive insulin therapy was also shown significantly to decrease the incidence of complications common to patients requiring intensive care, such as significant infections, acute renal failure requiring dialysis, median number of red cell transfusions, duration of mechanical ventilation, and critical illness polyneuropathy [14]. Furthermore, the mortality and morbidity benefits seem to be greater in surgical patients as compared with medical patients [14,15].

The morbidity and mortality benefit of achieving normoglycemia with intensive insulin therapy in critically ill patients is thought to result, in part, from the prevention of immune cell dysfunction, reduction in systemic inflammation, and protection of the endothelium [16,17]. Additional studies are needed to determine whether the benefits of intensive insulin therapy are derived from normoglycemia, insulin, or both. It seems that the control of blood glucose concentration may be more important than the quantity of insulin infused [18,19]. In response to these findings the Surviving Sepsis Campaign recommends that blood glucose levels should be maintained below 150 mg/dL following initial stabilization of the patient [8]. Although trial data suggest that even moderate hyperglycemia between 110 and 150 mg/dL is associated with a worse outcome as compared with normoglycemia, it is thought that a goal of 150 mg/dL still confers a significant benefit while also decreasing the risk of hypoglycemia [18,20].

Renal replacement therapy

Renal replacement therapy, such as plasmapheresis, plasma exchange, and hemofiltration, in the management of severe sepsis is currently not recommended for patients without sepsis-induced acute renal failure [8], but is nonetheless currently under active investigation. Hemofiltration and plasma therapies are both nonspecific, immunomodulatory strategies that seek to purify the circulation of bacterial products and inflammatory mediators, thereby restoring immunologic stability and homeostasis. In theory, plasma exchange, if using fresh frozen plasma as a replacement fluid, could have additional beneficial effects through the replenishment of immunoglobulins, coagulation factors, and anticoagulants, addressing the clotting abnormalities and diminished opsonic capacity commonly observed in severe sepsis [21].

Both hemofiltration and plasma therapies have been shown to effectively remove various septic mediators from the circulation [22–25]. There is wide variation, however, in the reported pattern of mediator removal depending on the technique used [26]. Most importantly, the impact of these interventions on relevant clinical outcomes, such as mortality, is unproved and uncertain. For example, one study reported significant improvements in hemodynamics without a concomitant decrease in measurable plasma cytokine levels, casting doubt on the value of plasma cytokine levels as a relevant outcome measure [27]. To date, there is a lack of controlled clinical trial data in humans to support the use of these modalities in the treatment of patients with severe sepsis [28–30].

Pharmacologic strategies

Corticosteroids

The use of corticosteroids in the management of severe sepsis has been investigated for many years. The fundamental role of glucocorticoids in the normal response to stress underlies the rationale for its use in sepsis trials. An early conception of sepsis as a primarily proinflammatory state in which the body's response was more deleterious than the inciting pathogen fueled interest in the use of high-dose corticosteroids aimed at suppressing the body's inflammatory response to infection. After several trials failed to demonstrate any benefit from this approach, and showed a possible trend toward harm, this practice of administering supraphysiologic doses of steroids was largely abandoned [31].

Recently, there has been a reconsideration of the use of corticosteroids at lower doses in response to evidence of transient adrenal dysfunction during severe sepsis. The reported incidence of adrenal insufficiency varies between 50% and 75% in patients with severe sepsis or septic shock, and has been independently correlated with an increased mortality risk in these patients [32–34]. Under normal conditions, activation of the hypothalamic-pituitary-adrenal axis plays a pivotal role in the body's response to stress and results in a rise in blood cortisol concentration. In patients with severe sepsis, however, glucocorticoid insufficiency, as a result of adrenal failure and decreased synthesis, is common. Lack of glucocorticoids can result in the loss of beneficial modulation of the immune response and vascular reactivity to catecholamines [35].

The beneficial effects of low, replacement doses of steroids have been investigated in many recent sepsis trials. Evidence suggests that low-dose treatment with hydrocortisone can reduce severe systemic inflammatory response syndrome [34,36] and prevent an overwhelming CARS, as evidenced by a reduction in measured cytokine profiles, without inducing widespread immune suppression [36]. In addition, treatment with low-dose steroids also seems to improve hemodynamic status and restore vascular responsiveness to catecholamines in patients with septic shock. In recent trials, septic patients who were treated with a single dose of hydrocortisone had a significant increase in mean arterial pressure after vasopressor treatment [37,38]. Patients who were treated for longer courses of low-dose corticosteroids also demonstrated improvement in hemodynamic parameters with significantly shorter time to cessation of vasopressor support and increased rate of shock reversal [34,36,39–41]. These trials further suggest that the hemodynamic effects of glucocorticoids are primarily mediated through an increase in peripheral vascular tone, because the increase in mean arterial pressure observed was associated with a decrease in vasopressor requirement, increased systemic vascular resistance, and decreased cardiac index and heart rate [36].

In addition to attenuation of the immune response and improvement in vascular reactivity, a recent review and meta-analysis found that there was a significant reduction in 28-day, ICU, and in-hospital mortality in those trials using a long course (≥ 5 days) of low-dose (≤ 300 mg hydrocortisone or equivalent per day) corticosteroids among patients with severe sepsis or septic shock, without an increase in the incidence of adverse events, such as gastroduodenal bleeding, superinfection, or hyperglycemia [39]. One trial in particular reported that 7-day treatment with low doses of hydrocortisone and fludrocortisone significantly reduced 28-day mortality rate (53% treatment versus 63% placebo), but that this mortality benefit was only observed in patients with relative adrenal insufficiency, or nonresponders, defined as a <9 μg/dL increase in blood cortisol concentration 30 to 60 minutes after a short corticotropin stimulation test. Steroid-replacement therapy had no significant beneficial effect on outcome in patients with severe sepsis or septic shock who did not demonstrate relative adrenal insufficiency [32]. Based on the results of this study, the authors' recommendations have been incorporated into management guidelines that advocate the administration of steroid treatment immediately after performance of corticotropin stimulation test to patients demonstrating septic shock, with withdrawal of treatment in responders and continuance of low-dose steroid treatment for up to 7 days in nonresponders [8].

Despite inclusion of corticosteroids in recommended management guidelines, there are a number of issues that remain controversial, including the definition of adrenal insufficiency, how best to test for adrenal dysfunction, and whether adrenal-insufficient patients are the only subset of septic shock patients to benefit from therapy [42]. Even the appropriate way to measure cortisol levels (ie, free versus total) has stirred controversy because the hormone circulates primarily bound to plasma proteins, which are uniformly low in the most severely ill patients [43]. In addition, there continues to be discussion regarding dosage reduction after shock reversal [40], the need to taper the dosage at the end of therapy to avoid detrimental rebound effects [36], and the necessity of fludrocortisone as part of the treatment regimen [32].

Targeted anti-inflammatory therapy

Efforts to reduce the mortality associated with severe sepsis by modifying specific proinflammatory mediators of the systemic inflammatory response, such as endotoxin [44], IL-1 [45], platelet-activating factor [46], and TNF-α [47–51], have been largely unsuccessful (Table 1). Manipulating the inflammatory response in individual patients to improve survival is difficult in part because of the complex role of these mediators in the septic response. Further, attenuating inflammation without suppressing it altogether is a difficult and necessary balancing act because the proinflammatory state is a vital response to invading organisms and is essential for survival, but in excess, is likely a key element in the development of organ dysfunction that is associated with severe sepsis.

TNF-α has been one of the more extensively studied inflammatory agents. Along with IL-1, TNF-α serves as a proximal mediator of the inflammatory cascade with the ability to activate multiple downstream inflammatory pathways. Several trials have attempted to block or neutralize TNF-α activity through the use of monoclonal antibodies and soluble TNF-α receptors with no demonstrable mortality benefit [47–51]. A recent study, however, was able to show a modest but significant reduction in 28-day mortality with a target population of patients with elevated IL-6 levels who were treated with afelimomab, an anti-TNF F(ab')₂ monoclonal antibody fragment, as compared with placebo (see Table 1) [52], confirming a similar trend observed in a previous study [49]. Elevated IL-6 levels serve as an indicator of hyperinflammation, are associated with higher severity of illness at baseline, and are observed more commonly in surgical patients as compared with nonsurgical patients [53]. Targeting the specific subpopulation of patients with elevated levels of IL-6, use of a multiple-dosing regimen versus single-dose administration, and use of an antibody fragment versus a complete antibody have all been cited as important differences in this trial as compared with others [52]. One or more of these factors may account for the observed mortality benefit.

Targeted antithrombotic therapy

Attention was directed toward modifiers of the coagulation system in severe sepsis trials after it was discovered that serum concentrations of

Table 1
Pharmaceutical clinical trials in severe sepsis

Drug	Trials	Reference	Number of patients	Mortality[a]				P value	Comments
				Treatment %	Placebo %	Relative risk	95% confidence interval		
HA-IA antiendotoxin monoclonal antibody	CHESS (Centocor: HA-IA Efficacy in Septic Shock)	44	2199	38	36	1.08	0.97–1.21	0.186	Trial assessed 14-day mortality rates.
rhIL-1ra	rhIL-1ra	45	696	33.1	36.4	nr	nr	0.360	Trial stopped early after interim analysis revealed unlikelihood of meeting primary efficacy end point.
PAF-AH	PAF-AH	46	1261	25	24	1.03	0.85–1.25	0.800	Trial stopped early after second planned interim analysis revealed unlikelihood of meeting primary efficacy end point
Anti TNF-α	INTERSEPT (murine monoclonal antibody to human TNF-α)	50		44.6 (15 mg/kg)	42.9	nr	nr	0.670	Reported more rapid reveral of shock, delay in time to onset of first organ failure, and decreased likelihood of organ failure in both treatment groups as compared with placebo in patients who survived for 28 days.
		50	420	36.7 (3 mg/kg)	42.9	nr	nr	0.340	

Intervention	Trial							Comments
	NORASEPT II (murine monoclonal antibody to human TNF-α)	51	1879	40.3	42.8	nr	nr	0.270	No association between treatment and rapidity of shock reversal, shock prevention, or organ failure. No observed mortality benefit for patients in treatment group with elevated interleukin-6.
	MONARCS (afelimomab = anti-TNF antibody F[ab'] 2 fragment)	52	998	43.6	47.6	0.74	0.559–0.998	0.410	Primary target population was patients with elevated Interleukin 6-levels.
Antithrombin III	KyberSept	55	2314	38.9	38.7	1.01	0.91–1.11	0.940	
Tissue-factor-pathway inhibitor	OPTIMIST	58	1754	34.2	33.9	1.01	0.89–1.15	0.880	
Drotrecogin alfa (activated)/recombinant human activated protein C	PROWESS	62	1690	24.7	30.8	0.80	0.69–0.94	0.005	
	ENHANCE	65	2375	25.3	n/a	n/a	n/a	n/a	Single-arm, open-lable trial to provide further evidence of safety and efficacy of activated protein C.

Abbreviations: n/a, not applicable; nr, not reported; PAF-AH, platelet-activating factor acetylhydrolase; rhIL-1ra, recombinant human interleukin-1 receptor antagonists; TNF-α, tumor necrosis factor-α.

[a] 28-day mortality except as noted.

anticoagulants and markers of coagulopathy, such as D dimer, which rises with increasing fibrinogen degradation, are often markedly deranged during sepsis, particularly among surgical patients. For example, some data suggest that D dimer levels, prothrombin time, and activated partial thromboplastin time are significantly higher, and APC, protein S, and ATIII are significantly lower at baseline for surgical patients as compared with nonsurgical patients [53]. Further, it is this coagulopathy and microthrombus formation that is thought to play a central role in the development of tissue ischemia and ultimately organ dysfunction observed in patients with severe sepsis. The three natural anticoagulant proteins (ATIII, APC, and TFPI) have all been tested in phase III clinical trials. Despite promising preliminary data for all three agents only treatment with APC has demonstrated a significant mortality benefit thus far (see Table 1).

ATIII has antithrombotic and anti-inflammatory properties through the direct suppression of thrombin formation, inactivation of several factors of the coagulation cascade, and stimulation of prostacyclin release from endothelial cells [6]. Initial trials comparing ATIII treatment with placebo in patients with severe sepsis demonstrated a considerable trend toward improved survival [54]. Although a follow-up randomized, controlled trial with greater power failed to demonstrate a decrease in overall 28-day mortality with high-dose ATIII treatment as compared with placebo [55], a subsequent retrospective analysis of the data revealed a possible survival benefit up to 90 days in a subgroup of patients with severe sepsis and a moderate predicted mortality between 30% and 60% [56], suggesting that further investigation with this particular subgroup may be justified.

TFPI has anticoagulant activity primarily through suppression of tissue factor–mediated activation of the extrinsic pathway of the coagulation cascade. The septic state often leads to truncation of the TFPI protein, which diminishes its anticoagulant activity and predisposes the patient toward a prothrombotic state [57]. Of interest, although the Optimized Phase 3 Tifacogin in Multicenter International Sepsis Trial [58] evaluating the effects of TFPI failed to show improved overall outcome at study completion, there was a significant mortality benefit observed after a planned interim analysis of 722 patients that fell just shy of predefined termination rules (29.1% TFPI versus 38.9% placebo, $P = .06$). For reasons unknown, the latter half of the trial demonstrated complete reversal of the initial favorable results with a trend toward a decrease in mortality with placebo and an increase in mortality with TFPI, which ultimately resulted in a neutral final outcome [58]. Further studies are evaluating the potential use of TFPI in subgroups of patients with severe sepsis.

Drotrecogin alfa (activated) (DAA), recombinant human APC, is an endogenous vitamin K–dependent serine protease that is converted from its inactive, zymogen form by thrombin bound to endothelial cell thrombomodulin, especially when facilitated by the endothelial protein C receptor. APC is thought to play a pivotal role in the septic cascade because it modulates both the procoagulant and inflammatory responses that characterize severe sepsis. Antithrombotic and profibrinolytic activity is accomplished through the inactivation of factors Va and VIIIa, and the inhibition of plasminogen activator inhibitor-1, respectively. In addition, by limiting thrombin generation, APC also exhibits profibrinolytic activity by reducing thrombin-activatable fibrinolysis inhibitor. Originally, it was thought that the anti-inflammatory effects of APC were limited to its ability to reduce thrombin, which is capable of stimulating multiple inflammatory pathways. It is now thought, however, that APC may also exhibit direct anti-inflammatory properties by inhibiting the production of inflammatory cytokines, such as TNF-α, by macrophages, and by reducing leukocyte adhesion and rolling through the down-regulation of selectin expression on endothelial cells [59,60].

Patients with severe sepsis often have low levels of protein C and an impaired ability to convert protein C to its active form. Several studies support the fact that approximately 90% of patients with severe sepsis have an acquired protein C deficiency, and that this is associated with poorer outcomes, including an increased risk of death [61–64]. Recent studies evaluating the efficacy of recombinant human APC, or DAA, in patients with severe sepsis have had promising results. A phase II clinical trial demonstrated that use of DAA resulted in a dose-dependent reduction in plasma levels of D dimer and IL-6, markers of sepsis-induced coagulopathy and inflammation, respectively, providing confirmatory evidence for its ability to affect both pathways [61]. A subsequent phase III trial, Protein C Worldwide Evaluation in Severe Sepsis (PROWESS), also demonstrated a significant reduction in both IL-6 and D dimer levels in patients treated with DAA. In addition, PROWESS demonstrated a significant difference in 28-day mortality between the DAA group and the placebo group (24.7% versus 30.8%), corresponding to an absolute risk reduction of 6.1% ($P = .005$) [62]. Further evidence for improved outcomes with DAA treatment comes from a single-arm, open-label trial, ENHANCE, that was recently conducted to provide further efficacy and safety information. ENHANCE demonstrated similar mortality as in the PROWESS trial (25.3% ENHANCE, 24.7% PROWESS) [65]. Retrospective subgroup analyses of the data suggest that the greatest mortality benefit is obtained in those patients at highest risk for death at baseline [62,66].

The major safety issue that has been raised surrounding the use of DAA is the increased risk of bleeding, as might be expected because of its anticoagulant properties. In PROWESS, there was a small but significant increase in the incidence of serious bleeding events (intracranial hemorrhage, life-threatening bleeding, or blood loss requiring transfusion of more than three units of packed red blood cells on two consecutive days) among patients in the DAA group than in the placebo group (3.5% versus 2%, $P = .06$). This difference was observed only during the infusion period and tended to occur in patients with an identifiable predisposition to hemorrhage [62]. There was an even higher rate of serious bleeding events, including intracranial hemorrhage, reported among the DAA arm in the ENHANCE trial as compared with PROWESS (6.5% versus 3.5%). In addition, unlike PROWESS, this increase in bleeding risk was observed during both the infusion period and the postinfusion period. In theory, many believe that the risk of bleeding with DAA should be limited to the immediate peri-infusion period because of an extremely short half-life that allows rapid termination of anticoagulant effects once infusion is discontinued. To account for the observed increase in bleeding during the postinfusion period, the authors propose that there may have been a higher background risk of bleeding among ENHANCE patients possibly caused in part by the larger number of surgical patients [65].

A PROWESS Surgical Evaluation Committee was formed to assess further the safety and efficacy of DAA in the surgical cohort through a retrospective analysis of PROWESS data [67]. The investigators confirmed that approximately 30% of the patients in PROWESS were surgical patients, and that approximately two thirds of these surgical patients underwent an intra-abdominal operation. Consistent with the overall PROWESS trial results, the use of DAA in surgical patients resulted in an absolute reduction in mortality risk that was within the 95% confidence interval for the trial as a whole (3.2% surgical cohort versus 6.1% overall). It was further noted that the absolute risk reduction in surgical patients was most pronounced in those who underwent an intra-abdominal operation (9.1%), and especially in those who also had an Acute Physiology and Chronic Health Evaluation (APACHE) II score greater than 25 (18.2%). In contrast, it was observed that the subgroup of patients who underwent non–intra-abdominal operations actually demonstrated increased mortality in the DAA arm as compared with placebo. The authors noted, however, that this sample of patients is likely too small and heterogeneous to allow for meaningful interpretation [67].

As for the associated bleeding risks observed within the surgical cohort in PROWESS, it was concluded that the safety profile of DAA seems to be similar in both medical and surgical patients [67,68]. Serious bleeding rates during the infusion and 28-day study period were higher in the DAA arm as compared with placebo arm for both medical and surgical patients, but there were no statistically significant differences in serious bleeding rates observed between the medical and surgical patients receiving treatment with DAA [68]. Although the authors expected a higher risk of bleeding among surgical patients, there was actually a trend toward a lower overall number of emergent, nonserious bleeding events in surgical patients as compared with medical patients for both treatment groups, although surgical patients were significantly more likely to receive transfusions of packed red blood cells and fresh frozen plasma. The authors postulate that the latter observation could reflect the replacement of operative blood losses, or differences in approach to the use of blood products for resuscitation between medical and surgical patients [68].

Based on the observed mortality benefit and relatively small increase in bleeding risk, DAA was approved and recommended for use in patients with severe sepsis who are at high risk of death (APACHE II ≥25, sepsis-induced multiple organ failure, septic shock, or sepsis-induced acute respiratory distress syndrome) and who have no contraindications related to bleeding risk [8]. There are currently no recommendations regarding time to treatment initiation, although both PROWESS and ENHANCE began treatment within a maximum of 48 hours after diagnosis of organ dysfunction. Of interest, data from ENHANCE suggested that earlier treatment with DAA could be associated with increased survival, an observation that could have significant implications for optimal future use. Patients who were treated within 24 hours were found to have significantly lower 28-day all-cause mortality than those treated after 24 hours (22.9% versus 27.4%, $P = .01$), although the mortality rate in the latter group was still lower as compared with PROWESS placebo patients, indicating that patients treated later may still receive benefit [65].

At the time of approval, use of DAA was not recommended for patients at a low risk of death (APACHE II score <25 or single organ failure) because of subgroup analyses that suggested that these patients demonstrated a nominal and insignificant reduction in mortality [66]. This observation was confirmed by a recent trial in low-risk patients that found no statistically significant differences between the placebo group and the DAA group in 28-day mortality (17% placebo, 18.5% DAA, $P = .34$) or in-hospital mortality (20.5% placebo, 20.6% DAA, $P = .98$) [69]. Further, an exploratory post hoc analysis of the surgical cohort in this study actually revealed a higher 28-day and in-hospital mortality rate in surgical patients with single organ dysfunction who received DAA than those who received placebo [69]. Together, the absence of a beneficial treatment effect, particularly among surgical patients, in addition to an increased incidence in bleeding complications, confirms current treatment recommendations advising that DAA should not be used in patients with severe sepsis and a low risk of death.

Combination therapies

The pathophysiology of sepsis is complex, involving many molecular, biochemical, vascular, and organ system alterations. It seems almost naive to believe that focusing a therapeutic intervention on one system can improve outcome. This issue is further complicated clinically if one considers the great heterogeneity in patients. As a result, combination therapies are appealing for their potential to produce more robust and consistent benefits. One recent, single-center, retrospective study [70] used a treatment pathway incorporating early empiric antibiotic coverage, EGDT, steroids, DAA, glycemic control, and a lung-protective strategy. This treatment plan resulted in more aggressive fluid resuscitation, earlier empiric antibiotic administration, greater use of vasopressors, tighter glucose control, and more frequent assessments of adrenal function, but produced only a nonsignificant trend toward decreased mortality (29% before, 20% after implementation). In another single-center, retrospective study [71] that examined the impact of implementing a "standard operating procedure" for patients with septic shock, including EGDT, glycemic control, steroid replacement, and DAA, mortality decreased significantly, however, from 53% before implementation of the protocol to 27% afterward.

Summary

Severe sepsis remains a common cause of death in surgical patients. Eradication of the septic source and supportive care have long been the mainstay of treatment. In recent years, however, EGDT, tighter glucose control, administration of DAA, and steroid replacement have produced improved morbidity and mortality. In the future, a better understanding of the pathophysiology of sepsis and clinical studies may further improve outcomes from severe sepsis.

References

[1] Balk RA. Severe sepsis and septic shock: definitions, epidemiology, and clinical manifestations. Crit Care Clin 2000;16:179–92.

[2] Minino AM, Arias E, Kochanek KD, et al. Deaths: final data for 2000. Natl Vital Stat Rep 2002;50:1–16.

[3] Angus DC, Linde-Zwirble WT, Lidicker J, et al. Epidemiology of severe sepsis in the United States: analysis of incidence, outcome, and associated costs of care. Crit Care Med 2001;29: 1303–10.

[4] Dellinger RP. Inflammation and coagulation: implications for the septic patients. Clin Infect Dis 2003;36:1259–65.

[5] Esmon CT. The interactions between inflammation and coagulation. Br J Haematol 2005; 131:417–30.

[6] Jagneaux T, Taylor DE, Kantrow SP. Coagulation in sepsis. Am J Med Sci 2004;328: 196–204.

[7] Rivers E, Nguyen B, Havstad S, et al. Early goal-directed therapy in the treatment of severe sepsis and septic shock. N Engl J Med 2001;345:1368–77.

[8] Dellinger RP, Carlet JM, Masur H, et al. Surviving Sepsis Campaign guidelines for management of severe sepsis and septic shock. Intensive Care Med 2004;30:536–55.

[9] Reinhart K, Bloos F. The value of venous oximetry. Curr Opin Crit Care 2005;11:259–63.

[10] Gunn SR, Fink MP, Wallace B. Equipment review: the success of early goal-directed therapy for septic shock prompts evaluation of current approaches for monitoring the adequacy of resuscitation. Crit Care 2005;9:349–59.

[11] Hebert PC, Wells G, Blajchman MA, et al. A multicenter, randomized, controlled clinical trial of transfusion requirements in critical care. N Engl J Med 1999;340:409–17.

[12] Kern JW, Shoemaker WC. Meta-analysis of hemodynamic optimization in high-risk patients. Crit Care Med 2002;30:1686–92.

[13] Brierre S, Kumari R, Deboisblanc BP. The endocrine system during sepsis. Am J Med Sci 2004;328:238–47.

[14] Van den Berghe G, Wouters P, Weekers F, et al. Intensive insulin therapy in critically ill patients. N Engl J Med 2001;345:1359–67.

[15] Van den Berghe G, Wilmer A, Hermans G, et al. Intensive insulin therapy in the medical ICU. N Engl J Med 2006;354:449–61.

[16] Langouche L, Vanhorebeek I, Vlasselaers D, et al. Intensive insulin therapy protects the endothelium of critically ill patients. J Clin Invest 2005;115:2277–86.

[17] Hansen TK, Thiel S, Wouters PJ, et al. Intensive insulin therapy exerts anti-inflammatory effects in critically ill patients and counteracts the adverse effect of low mannose-binding lectin levels. J Clin Endocrinol Metab 2003;88:1082–8.

[18] Van den Berghe G, Wouters PJ, Bouillon R, et al. Outcome benefit of intensive insulin therapy in the critically ill: insulin dose versus glycemic control. Crit Care Med 2004;31:359–66.

[19] Finney SJ, Zekveld C, Elia A, et al. Glucose control and mortality in critically ill patients. JAMA 2003;290:2041–7.

[20] Krinsley JS. Effect of an intensive glucose management protocol on mortality of critically ill adult patients. Mayo Clin Proc 2004;79:992–1000.

[21] Venkataraman R, Subramanian S, Kellum J. Clinical review: extracorporeal blood purification in severe sepsis. Crit Care 2003;7:139–45.

[22] Reeves JH, Butt WW, Shann F, et al. Continuous plasmafiltration in sepsis syndrome. Plasmafiltration in Sepsis Study Group. Crit Care Med 1999;27:2096–104.

[23] Gardlund B, Sjolin J, Nilsson A, et al. Plasma levels of cytokines in primary septic shock in humans: correlation with disease severity. J Infect Dis 1995;172:296–301.

[24] Kellum JA, Johnson JP, Kramer D, et al. Diffusive vs. convective therapy: effects on mediators of inflammation in patient with severe systemic inflammatory response syndrome. Crit Care Med 1998;26:1995–2000.

[25] Cole L, Bellomo R, Journois D, et al. High-volume haemofiltration in human septic shock. Intensive Care Med 2001;27:978–86.

[26] Cole L, Bellomo R, Hart G, et al. A phase II randomized, controlled trial of continuous haemofiltration in sepsis. Crit Care Med 2002;30:100–6.

[27] Heering P, Morgera S, Schmitz G, et al. Cytokine removal and cardiovascular hemodynamics in septic patients with continuous venovenous hemofiltration. Intensive Care Med 1997; 23:288–96.

[28] Kellum H, Angus D, Johnson J, et al. Continuous versus intermittent renal replacement therapy: a meta-analysis. Intensive Care Med 2002;28:29–37.

[29] Reeves JH. A review of plasma exchange in sepsis. Blood Purif 2002;20:282–8.

[30] Busund R, Koukline V, Utrobin U, et al. Plasmapheresis in severe sepsis and septic shock: a prospective, randomized, controlled trial. Intensive Care Med 2002;28:1434–9.

[31] Cronin L, Cook DJ, Carlet J, et al. Corticosteroid treatment for sepsis: a critical appraisal and meta-analysis of the literature. Crit Care Med 1995;23:1430–9.

[32] Annane D, Sebille V, Charpentier C, et al. Effect of treatment with low doses of hydrocortisone and fludrocortisone on mortality in patients with septic shock. JAMA 2002;288: 862–71.

[33] Annane D, Sebille V, Troche G, et al. A 3-level prognostic classification in septic shock based on cortisol levels and cortisol response to corticotropin. JAMA 2000;283:1038–45.

[34] Oppert M, Schindler R, Husung C, et al. Low-dose hydrocortisone improves shock reversal and reduces cytokine levels in early hyperdynamic septic shock. Crit Care Med 2005;33: 2457–64.

[35] Prigent H, Maxime V, Annane D. Science review: mechanisms of impaired adrenal function in sepsis and molecular actions of glucocorticoids. Crit Care 2004;8:243–52.

[36] Keh D, Boehnke T, Weber-Cartens S, et al. Immunologic and hemodynamic effects of "low-dose" hydrocortisone in septic shock. Am J Respir Crit Care Med 2003;167:512–20.

[37] Annane D, Bellisant E, Sebille V, et al. Impaired pressor sensitivity to noradrenaline in septic shock patients with and without impaired adrenal function reserve. Br J Clin Pharmacol 1998;46:589–97.

[38] Bellisant E, Annane D. Effect of hydrocortisone on phenylephrine: mean arterial pressure dose-response relationship in septic shock. Clin Pharmacol Ther 2000;68:293–303.

[39] Annane D, Bellisant E, Bollaert PE, et al. Corticosteroids for severe sepsis and septic shock: a systematic review and meta-analysis. BMJ 2004;329:480–8.

[40] Briegel J, First H, Haller M, et al. Stress doses of hydrocortisone reverse hyperdynamic septic shock: a prospective, randomized, double-blind, single-center study. Crit Care Med 1999;27: 723–32.

[41] Bollaert PE, Charpentier C, Levy B, et al. Reversal of late septic shock with supraphysiologic doses of hydrocortisone. Crit Care Med 1998;25:645–50.

[42] Cooper MS, Stewart PM. Corticosteroid insufficiency in acutely ill patients. N Engl J Med 2003;348:727–34.

[43] Hamrahian AH, Oseni TS, Arafah BM. Measurements of serum free cortisol in critically ill patients. N Engl J Med 2004;350:1629–38.

[44] McCloskey RV, Straube RC, Sanders C, et al. Treatment of septic shock with human monoclonal antibody HA-1A: a randomized, double-blind, placebo-controlled trial CHESS Trial Study Group. Ann Intern Med 1994;121:1–5.

[45] Opal SM, Fisher CJ, Dhainaut JF, et al. Confirmatory interleukin-1 receptor antagonist trial in severe sepsis: a phase III randomized, double-blind, placebo-controlled, multicenter trial. Crit Care Med 1997;25:1115–24.

[46] Opal SM, Laterre PF, Abraham E, et al. Recombinant human platelet-activating factor ace-tylhydrolase for treatment of severe sepsis: results of a phase III, multicenter, randomized, double-blind, placebo-controlled, clinical trial. Crit Care Med 2004;32:332–41.

[47] Abraham E, Wunderink R, Silverman H, et al. Efficacy and safety of monoclonal antibody to human tumor necrosis factor alpha in patients with sepsis syndrome: a randomized, con-trolled, double-blind, multicenter clinical trial. JAMA 1995;273:934–41.

[48] Fisher CJ, Agosti JM, Opal SM, et al. Treatment of septic shock with the tumor necrosis factor receptor: Fc fusion protein. N Engl J Med 1996;334:1697–702.

[49] Reinhart K, Wiegand-Lohnert C, Grimminger F, et al. Assessment of safety and efficacy of the monoclonal anti-tumor necrosis factor antibody-fragment, MAK 195F, in patients with sepsis and septic shock: a multicenter, randomized, placebo-controlled, dose-ranging study. Crit Care Med 1996;24:733–42.

[50] Cohen J, Carlet J. INTERSEPT: an international, multicenter, placebo-controlled trial of monoclonal antibody to human tumor necrosis factor-alpha in patients with sepsis. Crit Care Med 1996;24:1431–40.

[51] Abraham E, Anzueto A, Gutierrez G, et al. Double-blind randomized controlled trial of monoclonal antibody to human tumor necrosis factor in treatment of septic shock. NORASEPT II Study Group. Lancet 1998;351:929–33.

[52] Panacek E, Marshall J, Albertson T, et al. Efficacy and safety of the monoclonal anti-tumor necrosis factor antibody F(ab') 2 fragment afelimomab in patients with severe sepsis and elevated interleukin-6 levels. Crit Care Med 2004;32:2173–82.

[53] Lowry S, Awad S, Ford H, et al. Static and dynamic assessment of biomarkers in surgical patients with severe sepsis. Surg Infect (Larchmt) 2004;5:261–8.

[54] Eisele B, Lamy M, Thijs LG, et al. Antithrombin III in patients with severe sepsis: a random-ized, placebo-controlled, double-blind, multicenter trial plus a meta-analysis on all random-ized, placebo-controlled, double-blind trials with antithrombin III in severe sepsis. Intensive Care Med 1998;24:663–72.

[55] Warren BL, Eid A, Singer P, et al. High-dose antithrombin III in severe sepsis. JAMA 2001; 286:1869–78.

[56] Wiedermann CJ, Hoffmann JN, Juers M, et al. High-dose antithrombin III in the treatment of severe sepsis in patients with a high risk of death: efficacy and safety. Crit Care Med 2006; 34:285–92.

[57] Creasey AA, Reinhart K. Tissue factor pathway inhibitor activity in severe sepsis. Crit Care Med 2001;29(7 Suppl):S126–9.

[58] Abraham E, Reinhart K, Opal S, et al. Efficacy and safety of tifacogin (recombinant tissue factor pathway inhibitor) in severe sepsis. JAMA 2003;290:238–47.

[59] Esmon CT. Protein C pathway in sepsis. Ann Med 2002;34:598–605.

[60] Esmon CT. The anticoagulant and anti-inflammatory roles of the protein C anticoagulant pathway. J Autoimmun 2000;15:113–6.

[61] Bernard GR, Wesley E, Wright TJ, et al. Safety and dose relationship of recombinant human activated protein C for coagulopathy in severe sepsis. Crit Care Med 2001;29:2051–9.

[62] Bernard GR, Vincent J-L, Laterre P-F, et al. Efficacy and safety of recombinant human activated protein C for severe sepsis. N Engl J Med 2001;344:699–709.

[63] Fisher CJ, Yan SB. Protein C levels as a prognostic indicator of outcome in sepsis and related diseases. Crit Care Med 2000;28(9 Suppl):S49–56.

[64] Yan SB, Helterbrand JD, Hartman DL, et al. Low levels of protein C are associated with poor outcome in severe sepsis. Chest 2001;120:915–22.

[65] Vincent J-L, Bernard GR, Beale R, et al. Drotrecogin alfa (activated) treatment in severe sepsis from the global open-label trial ENHANCE: further evidence for survival and safety and implications for early treatment. Crit Care Med 2005;33:2266–77.

[66] Ely EW, Laterre PF, Angus DC, et al. Drotrecogin alfa (activated) administration across clinically important subgroups of patients with severe sepsis. Crit Care Med 2003;31:12–9.

[67] Barie PS, Williams MD, McCollam JS, et al. Benefit/risk profile of drotrecogin alfa (activated) in surgical patients with severe sepsis. Am J Surg 2004;188:212–20.

[68] Fry DE, Beilman G, Johnson S, et al. Safety of drotrecogin alfa (activated) in surgical patients with severe sepsis. Surg Infect (Larchmt) 2004;5:253–9.

[69] Abraham E, Laterre PF, Garg R, et al. Drotrecogin alfa (activated) for adults with severe sepsis and a low risk of death. N Engl J Med 2005;353:1332–41.

[70] Shapiro NI, Howell MD, Talmor D, et al. Implementation and outcomes of the Multiple Urgent Sepsis Therapies (MUST) protocol. Crit Care Med 2006;34:1025–32.

[71] Kortgen A, Niederprum P, Bauer M. Implementation of an evidence-based "standard operating procedure" and outcome in septic shock. Crit Care Med 2006;34:943–9.

SURGICAL
CLINICS OF
NORTH AMERICA

Surg Clin N Am 86 (2006) 1541–1551

Brain Death and Withdrawal of Support

Maxim D. Hammer, MD[a,*], David Crippen, MD[b]

[a]The Stroke Institute, University of Pittsburgh Medical Center, 200 Lothrop Street,
PUH-C-419, Pittsburgh, PA 15213, USA
[b]Neurovascular Critical Care, Department of Critical Care Medicine,
University of Pittsburgh Medical Center, Scaife Hall, 200 Lothrop Street,
Pittsburgh, PA 15213, USA

Critical care medicine has expanded the envelope of debilitating disease through the application of an aggressive and invasive care plan designed to identify and reverse organ dysfunction before it proceeds to organ failure. For a select patient population with a strong potential for reanimation, this care plan has been remarkably successful. But because the patient is given the benefit of any doubt regarding the possibility of reanimation, critical care sometimes creates amalgams of life-in-death: a state of being unable to participate in human life, unable to die. In the new millennium, medical advances have changed the landscape of death by blurring not only the timing but also the nature of death. Before the postmodern technologic revolution, determination of death was simple: a patient was dead when pronounced dead by his or her physician. No one was timing or reversing death. In the age of organ transplantation, however, recovery of viable organs from otherwise dead bodies changes things dramatically.

Resuscitative technology can lead to appearances that are deceiving. Consider the following: in the United States, about 150 legally dead people are suspended in liquid nitrogen, awaiting a nanotechnology that cures their fatal disease and restores them to life [1,2]. The practice of cryopreserving people immediately after they have been pronounced medicolegally dead (almost always according to clinical cardiorespiratory criteria) is called "cryonics" [3,4]. A cryonics patient is first pronounced dead by a physician. At that point the patient is legally dead, and the rules pertaining to procedures that can be performed change radically from those that can be performed on a living patient [5]. In the initial cryopreservation protocol, the patient is intubated and mechanically ventilated and a highly efficient,

---

* Corresponding author.
E-mail address: hammermd@upmc.edu (M.D. Hammer).

mechanical cardiopulmonary resuscitation device takes over circulation. In some cases, the patient begins to show "signs of life" again, including pupillary reaction and spontaneous motion [6]. Are these individuals now alive, and if so, by what criteria? Were these persons ever dead?

The preceding scenario encapsulates the current dilemma of when and how death occurs. Rather than death being defined as "loss of cellular function," a definition that involves a putrefaction criterion, death became defined as "irreversible cessation of the integrated functioning of the organization as a whole," involving a neurologic or cardiorespiratory criterion [7]. This rather obtuse definition simply means that when the entity that integrates the rest of the organism dies, the organism dies with it, even though some of the cellular or tissue components within may remain independently viable if maintained by life support systems. Death of the whole organism is not required for the organism to be pronounced dead; only the organ of integration need be dead. Without this definition, the industry of organ transplantation would be impossible because putrefaction of the whole organism would be the only benchmark of death.

There is confusion, if not controversy, regarding the point at which the brain is dead enough to meet criteria for the dead donor rule. This article explores this dilemma by reviewing the history of the definition of brain death, and by making distinctions between brain death; brainstem death (BSD); and neurologic conditions, such as coma, persistent vegetative state (PVS), and locked-in syndrome.

Historical perspective

The traditional concept of death emphasized cessation of respiration. This idea may have first been challenged by an incident that occurred in 1564, when Andreas Vesalius, the Italian physician and anatomist, is said to have conducted an autopsy on a patient who had just died. When the thorax was opened, the heart was still beating, a situation that produced an uproar [8]. In 1902, Harvey Cushing prolonged cardiac function through the use of artificial ventilation in a patient with a brain tumor who had lost spontaneous respiration (which one may assume resulted from cerebral herniation) [9]. With the advent of life support systems, it became clear that death is not a single event in which the organism fails en bloc, but rather is a fragmented process, such that isolated organ systems can be maintained indefinitely despite the death of the human being.

We now know that ventilation is controlled by the brainstem and that the brainstem relies on circulation to remain viable. This triad—brainstem, ventilation, circulation—is necessary for life; death results from the loss of any of these three systems. In the modern age of medicine, clinicians are able artificially to support both the ventilatory and circulatory systems and sustain life. There is no support system, however, capable of sustaining brain tissue. There arises the necessity to assess brain failure and to define an individual's death in terms of brain death. Sweet [10] stated in the *New England Journal of Medicine*: "It is clear that a person is not dead unless his brain is dead. The time-honored criteria of the stoppage of the heart beat and circulation are indicative of death only when they persist long enough for the brain to die."

The advent of organ transplantation has given the definition of brain death added relevance. Accordingly, "brain death protocols" have evolved to identify medically and legally patients dead enough to bury but with organs viable for transplantation. The clinical determination of brain death was first described in 1957 [11]. Harvard Medical School published its criteria for brain death in 1968, shortly after the first heart transplantation was performed [12]. Numerous other criteria followed [12–16]. The first nation to adopt the brain death as the definition of legal death was Finland in 1971.

Since the introduction of these criteria, the Uniform Determination of Death Act, promulgated in 1981, has served as a model statute for states adopting legislation defining death [17]. The act asserts two possible definitions of death: "An individual who has sustained either (1) irreversible cessation of circulatory and respiratory functions, or (2) irreversible cessation of all functions of the entire brain, including the brain stem, is dead." Scientifically, this distinction is artificial. Cardiopulmonary arrest only causes inevitable death if the brainstem is irreparably damaged because of lack of perfusion with oxygenated blood. The key feature of both mechanisms is irreparable brain damage. The two mechanisms differ only because death is diagnosed in the presence or absence of a beating heart.

Pathophysiology

Relevant brainstem anatomy

The primary ventilatory center is located in the reticular core of the medulla oblongata; the pons might contribute some modulatory effect. In brain death, spontaneous respiration does not occur, even when arterial carbon dioxide (CO_2) tension reaches 55 to 60 mm Hg or when the cough reflex is vigorously stimulated.

The central neurons that control the circulatory system distribute diffusely in the pontine and medullary reticular core. When there is failure of the brainstem, however, autonomic reflex loops may regulate arterial tension and heart rate. Changes in arterial blood pressure and heart rate are not used as measures of brainstem function.

The pupillary reflexes are mediated through the nuclei of cranial nerves II and III in the midbrain. The doll's eye (oculocephalic) reflex and cold caloric (vestibulo-ocular) response are mediated by the same reflex arc by cranial nerves VIII, III, and VI, and the paramedian pontine reticular formation within the pons. It may seem arbitrary to rely on the absence of these reflexes to diagnose brain death. The significance is that these cranial nerve nuclei all lie adjacent to the reticular activating system, however, which spans the midbrain and pons. The reticular activating system is necessary for consciousness; it is the mechanism that activates the cerebral cortex. The reticular activating system is not directly testable, unlike all the adjacent cranial nerve nuclei. If all the adjacent cranial nerve nuclei demonstrate failure, there is no significant possibility of functional integrity of the reticular activating system.

Causes of brain death

Brain death may be caused by two mechanisms: global injury of the entire central nervous system and focal injury of the brainstem. Global injury of the central nervous system may be caused by anoxia from drowning; respiratory failure; or circulatory failure (including cardiac arrest). Carbon monoxide poisoning may also cause anoxia. Focal injury of the brainstem may be primary or secondary. Primary injury may be caused by trauma (eg, direct gunshot wound); ischemia (eg, basilar artery occlusion by thrombus); or intracerebral hemorrhage. Secondary injury usually results from herniation of the brain downward onto the brainstem. Herniation results when an intracerebral mass causes downward displacement of brain tissue. Masses may include neoplasm, ischemia with secondary edema, and hemorrhage. Severe head trauma may induce global cerebral edema, which may also result in brainstem herniation.

Brain death: definition, significance, important distinctions, prognosis

Definitions

Brain death is defined as the complete and irreversible absence of all brain function. The term "brain" in this definition is not defined. Several distinctions may be drawn. Whole-brain death is loss of function of all the central nervous system structures except the spinal cord (ie, the brainstem plus the cerebral cortices). Cortical death means absence of function of the cerebral cortices, with preservation of the brainstem. BSD indicates failure of the brainstem with preservation of the cerebral cortices.

The concept of BSD was demonstrated in a paper by Grigg and coworkers [18] in patients with BSD who underwent electroencephalogram (EEG) testing. Eleven (19.6%) of 56 exhibited electroencephalographic activity, and two patients (3.6%) demonstrated sleeplike cortical EEG activity for as long as 168 hours, although none of the patients recovered. The United Kingdom [19,20] and some other European countries [21] legally distinguish between brain death and BSD.

The clinical criteria for brain death in the United States do not require measurement of cerebral cortical function and do not make a physiologic distinction between brain death and BSD. The rationale is that the brainstem, not the cerebral cortices, controls respiration, circulation, and other homeostatic functions.

Significance

The brain has been defined as the primary integrator of the organism as a whole. The President's Commission for the Study of Ethical Problems in Medicine and Biomedical and Behavioral Research [13] defines integration as "brain function that manifests as physiologic homeostasis." When the brain dies, the rest of the body experiences a loss of integration and can be considered a shell of organs functioning in purposeless disharmony.

Bernat [14] suggested that death occurs when "critical" parts of the brain responsible for integrated functioning of the rest of the body cease functioning. So if every cell in the brain does not have to be dead for a pronouncement of death to be made, then it has been suggested that death of the brain's integrative centers should be sufficient for a pronouncement of death.

This confirmatory evaluation for brain death, however, does not necessarily confirm death of every area of the brain. In fact, some islets of brain activity remain after the criteria for brain death have been met. Many patients who have been certified brain-dead do not show clinical evidence of whole-brain death, for example by maintaining body temperature for variable periods. In addition, some electrical activity may be noted on EEGs.

The brainstem is the keystone of brain function, without which life is not possible. Not only does it integrate the vital functions of respiration and circulation; it also activates consciousness, permitting meaningful function of the cerebral cortices. The brain death criteria in the United States actually are BSD criteria, because they comprise clinical tests of brainstem function but do not require separate tests of cortical viability.

Important distinctions

In brain death, there is failure of the brainstem. There may also be failure of the cerebral cortices. The clinical result is the same: a measurable loss of brainstem reflexes and integrative activity. Other conditions of impairment of consciousness and impairment of brainstem function must not be confused with brain death. These other conditions are defined here.

Coma (from the Greek word koma, meaning "deep sleep") is a state of unconsciousness with total lack of response to any stimulus, no matter how painful. Coma is caused by either impairment of the brainstem consciousness nuclei in the reticular formation spanning the midbrain and pons (usually as a result of some structural problem, such as stroke) or impairment of both cerebral cortices (usually caused by a systemic problem, such as profound ketoacidosis). Comatose patients are still alive; brain-dead patients are not. In many cases, coma is reversible, unlike brain death, which is irreversible.

PVS is the condition in which the brainstem continues to function but the cerebral cortices have failed. PVS is sometimes referred to as cerebral death and is the opposite of BSD. A patient in a PVS is still alive, and the respiratory and circulatory systems continue to function, because of preservation of the brainstem. A patient with PVS may have preservation of sleep-wake cycles and other brainstem-driven behaviors. Although these behaviors may suggest otherwise, there is no interaction with the environment. PVS (or cerebral death) has not been universally accepted as equivalent to death, unlike brain death.

The locked-in syndrome is the condition in which lower brainstem functions of respiration, circulation, and relaying of motor tracts are impaired, whereas upper brainstem functions, especially consciousness, are preserved. At the same time, some cortical function is preserved. The patient cannot breathe or move, save for making limited eye movements. Consciousness can be determined only by examination of voluntary eye movements to command.

Profound hypothermia, whether accidental or iatrogenic, may have clinical manifestations identical to those of brain death. A diagnosis of brain death cannot be made unless the core temperature is at least 32°C.

Prognosis

Patients who fulfill the clinical criteria for brain death have no prospect of survival independent of artificial respiratory and circulatory support, no prospect of recovery of brain function, and no prospect of improvement, even to a comatose state or PVS. Patients who fulfill the criteria for brain death are not alive.

Diagnosis of brain death

Clinical Criteria

Two preconditions must be met [22]. The cause of injury is known: there must be clear evidence of an acute, catastrophic, irreversible brain injury. Reversible conditions that may obfuscate the clinical diagnosis of brain death must be excluded.

Body temperature must be greater than 32°C, to rule out hypothermia. There is no chance of drug intoxication or neuromuscular blockade. The patient is not in shock.

The following test results must be obtained:

1. The patient does not respond to verbal or visual command.
2. The patient makes no movements, no spontaneous movements, or any movement induced by painful reflex.
3. The pupils are fixed and nonreactive.
4. The patient has no oculocephalic reflex. When the patient's eyes are opened and the head is turned from side to side, the eyes remain fixed

in their position. Alternatively, the oculovestibular reflex may be tested. The patient's ear canal is inspected to ensure an intact tympanic membrane. While the eyes are held open, ice water is injected into the ear canal. The eyes of a brain-dead patient remain fixed in their position.

5. The patient has no corneal reflexes when a cotton swab is dragged across the cornea while the eye is held open.
6. The patient has no gag reflex. The movement of the breathing tube (in and out) or insertion of a smaller tube down the breathing tube does not elicit a reflex.
7. The patient has no spontaneous ventilation. The patient is temporarily removed from life support (the ventilator). With the cessation of breathing by the machine, the body immediately starts to build up metabolic waste of CO_2 in the blood. When the CO_2 level reaches 55 mm Hg, an active brain causes the patient to breathe spontaneously. A dead brain gives no response.

If, after this extensive clinical examination, the patient shows no sign of neurologic function and the cause of the injury is known, the patient can be pronounced brain-dead. In some states, more than one physician is required to make this pronouncement for brain death to become legal death.

Although the patient has a dead brain and dead brainstem, spinal cord reflexes (eg, a knee jerk) can sometimes be elicited. In some brain-dead patients, a short reflex movement may occur when the hand or foot is touched in a particular manner.

Many physicians order a confirmatory test for brain death when the clinical examination demonstrates no neurologic function. In many states, however, such confirmatory testing is not required.

Confirmatory testing

Many tests, described in this section, have been used to corroborate brain death. All of these tests, with the exception of brainstem auditory evoked potentials, measure cortical activity in some way. It is possible to meet criteria for brain death when only the brainstem has died and the cortex is preserved (hence the distinction discussed previously). It is possible to meet clinical criteria for brain death but demonstrate some brain activity on confirmatory testing. It is probably for this reason that confirmatory tests are not generally required in the United States, where clinical criteria do not distinguish between brain death and BSD. In contrast, in several European [21], Central American, South American, and Asian countries, confirmatory testing is mandatory [23].

Electroencephalographic recording

Loss of bioelectrical brain activity as shown on the EEG (ie, isoelectric EEG) is a reliable confirmation of whole-brain death. Total electrical silence is not required for brain death. It is important to note that an isoelectric

EEG can be obtained after drug intoxication, such as intoxication with barbiturates [24], and residual electrical activity may persist after BSD [18]. Electrocerebral inactivity or electrocerebral silence is defined as no EEG activity above 2 µV/mm. The specific parameters and EEG settings have been described [25].

Evoked responses

Brainstem auditory evoked potentials and median nerve somatosensory evoked potentials are used for diagnosing brain death. Brainstem auditory evoked potentials are signals generated at the level of the auditory nerves and brainstem in response to an acoustic stimulus. Brainstem auditory evoked potentials consist of five identifiable waves. Wave I represents the vestibular nerve action potential; wave II, the vestibular and cochlear nerves; wave III, the lower pons; and waves IV and V, the upper pons and the midbrain [26]. The loss of waves III to V or II to V, or no reproducible brainstem auditory evoked potentials on both sides, is usually regarded as indicating BSD [27]. Somatosensory evoked potentials are waves of neural activity generated from the neural structures along the afferent somatosensory pathways, which are generated after electrical stimulation of a peripheral nerve. The pathway starts at a peripheral nerve, then ascends by the brachial plexus, upper cervical cord, dorsal column nuclei, ventroposterior thalamus, and sensory cortex. Bilateral absence of specific waves (N20–P22) following median nerve stimulation is consistent with brain death confirmatory laboratory finding [22].

Measurement of blood flow

Absent intracranial circulation indicates irreversible cerebral damage. The following methods are used to measure cerebral blood flow.

Angiography. Absence of blood flow to the brain leads to destruction of brain tissue. The greatest advantage of angiography for the determination of brain death is that it is influenced neither by central nervous system–depressant drugs nor by hypothermia. The American Academy of Neurology has defined specific criteria for confirming brain death by cerebral angiography: absence of intracerebral filling at the level of the carotid bifurcation or circle of Willis; patency of the external carotid circulation; and delayed filling of the superior longitudinal sinus [22].

CT. Various CT techniques may be used, including CT angiography, CT perfusion, and xenon-CT perfusion, to demonstrate absent or nonviable cortical blood flow [28–32].

MRI. MRI and magnetic resonance angiography should be used with caution in confirming brain death. MRI may provide information regarding ultrastructural anatomic injury, especially using diffusion-weighted imaging.

Ultrastructural diffusion-weighted imaging injury is not necessarily equivalent, however, to absent physiologic activity.

Transcranial Doppler sonography. Transcranial Doppler sonography uses a 2-MHz ultrasonic probe affixed to the temporal area, and the flow velocity of each of the major intracranial arteries may be measured. In brain death, cerebral perfusion pressure approaches zero, and transcranial Doppler demonstrates systolic spikes; undetectable flow (ie, no signal); or reversal of blood flow in diastole (ie, to-and-fro or oscillating waveform) [33–35]. These patterns were highly specific for brain death [34,35]. It is recommended that these abnormal transcranial Doppler signals should be recorded from multiple intracranial arteries to rule out the possibility of occlusion of a single artery.

Withdrawing care

Once a patient is declared dead by whatever criteria, the family is advised that the patient is dead and artificial life support will be removed. Surrogates may not refuse to accept brain death as a criterion for death and demand continuance of life support, unless the patient resides in a state that allows such a refusal on religious grounds [36]. The decision to withdraw artificial life support from a brain-dead patient is made before any mention of organ donation (organ donation is a completely separate issue). Because brain death, confirmed by protocol, is synonymous with death, a death certificate is filled out, noting the time of death as the time the protocol was completed. The withdrawal process is simply the removal of the machines. The patient is considered already dead, and there is no "dying process" to palliate.

Summary

This article presents the historical evolution of the concept of death from a cardiorespiratory paradigm to a brain-failure paradigm. The idea that brain death is equivalent to death is now internationally established and codified. Debates continue over how much brain function must be irreversibly injured for a diagnosis of brain death to be made. This debate has resulted in only minor differences between different clinical criteria for brain death. All established criteria require demonstration of failure of the brainstem, the indispensable integrative center for consciousness and vital bodily functions.

References

[1] http://www.cryonics.org/. Accessed June 1, 2006.
[2] http://www.alcor.org/AboutAlcor/index.html.

[3] Wowk B, Darwin M. Realistic scenario for nanotechnological repair of the frozen human brain. In: Cryonics: reaching for tomorrow. Scottsdale (AZ): Alcor Life Extension Foundation; 1991.

[4] Lemler J, Harris SB, Platt C, et al. The arrest of biological time as a bridge to engineered negligible senescence. Ann N Y Acad Sci 2004;1019:559–63.

[5] Wowk B. Cardiopulmonary support in cryonics: does legal death matter? Available at: http://www.alcor.org/Library/html/CardiopulmonarySupport.html.

[6] Darwin MG, Leaf JD, Hixon H. Neuropreservation of Alcor patient A-106. Available at: http://www.alcor.org/Library/html/casereport8504.html#part2.

[7] Bernat JL, Culver CM, Gert B. On the definition and criteria of death. Ann Intern Med 1981; 94:389–94.

[8] O'Malley CD. Andreas Vesalius' pilgrimage, Isis. Available at: en.wikipedia.org.

[9] Cushing H. Some experimental and clinical observations concerning states of increased intracranial tension. Am J Med Sci 1902;124:373–400.

[10] Sweet WH. Brain death. N Engl J Med 1978;299:410–2.

[11] Wertheimer P, Jouvet M, Descotes J. À propos du diagnostic de la mort du système nerveux dans les comas avec arrêt respiratoire traités par respiration artificielle. Presse Med 1959;67:87–8.

[12] A definition of irreversible coma. Report of the Ad Hoc Committee of the Harvard Medical School to Examine the Definition of Brain Death. JAMA 1968;205:337–40.

[13] Guidelines for the determination of death. Report of the medical consultants on the diagnosis of death to the President's Commission for the Study of Ethical Problems in Medicine and Biomedical and Behavioral Research. JAMA 1981;246:2184–6.

[14] Bernat JL. A defense of the whole-brain concept of death. Hastings Cent Rep 1998;28: 14–23.

[15] Izac SM. Quality assurance in determinations of brain death. Am J Electroneurodiagnostic Technol 2004;44:159.

[16] Spoor MT, Sutherland FR. The evolution of the concept of brain death. Ann R Coll Physicians Surg Can 1995;28:30–2.

[17] Uniform Determination of Death Act. 12 Uniform Laws Annotated 320 (1990 Supp).

[18] Grigg MM, Kelly MA, Celesia GG, et al. Electroencephalographic activity after brain death. Arch Neurol 1987;44:948.

[19] Diagnosis of brain death. Statement issued by the honorary secretary of the Conference of Medical Royal Colleges and their faculties in the United Kingdom. BMJ 1976;2:1187.

[20] Diagnosis of death. Memorandum issued by the honorary secretary of the Conference of Medical Royal Colleges and their faculties in the United Kingdom. BMJ 1979;1:322.

[21] Haupt WF, Rudolf J. European brain death codes: a comparison of national guidelines. J Neurol 1999;236:432.

[22] Practice parameters for determining brain death in adults (summary statement). The Quality Standards Subcommittee of the American Academy of Neurology. Neurology 1995;45: 1012–4.

[23] Wijdicks EF. The diagnosis of brain death. N Engl J Med 2001;344:1215.

[24] Segura T, Jimenez P, Jerez P, et al. Prolonged clinical pattern of brain death in patients under barbiturate sedation. Neurologia 2002;17:219.

[25] Guideline Three. Minimum technical standards for EEG recording in suspected cerebral death. J Clin Neurophysiol 1994;11:10.

[26] Ciappa KH, Hock DB. Electrophysiologic monitoring. In: Ropper AH, editor. Neurological and neurosurgical intensive care. New York: Raven Press; 1993. p. 147.

[27] Nau R, Prange HW, Klingelhoéfer J, et al. Results of four technical investigations in fifty clinically brain dead patients. Intensive Care Med 1992;18:82.

[28] Tan WS, Wilbur AC, Jafar JJ, et al. Brain death: use of dynamic CT and intravenous digital subtraction angiography. AJNR Am J Neuroradiol 1987;8:123.

[29] Arnold H, Kuhne D, Rohr W, et al. Contrast bolus technique with rapid CT scanning: a reliable diagnostic tool for the determination of brain death. Neuroradiology 1981;22:129.

[30] Johnson DW, Stringer WA, Marks MP, et al. Stable xenon CT cerebral blood flow imaging: rationale for and role in clinical decision making. AJNR Am J Neuroradiol 1991;12:201.

[31] Pistoia F, Johason DW, Darby JM, et al. The role of xenon CT measurements of cerebral blood flow in the clinical determination of brain death. AJNR Am J Neuroradiol 1991;12:97.

[32] Darby J, Yonas H, Brenner RP. Brainstem death with persistent EEG activity: evaluation by xenon-enhanced computed tomography. Crit Care Med 1987;15:519.

[33] Hassler W, Steinmetr H, Gawlowski J. Transcranial Doppler ultrasonography in raised intracranial pressure and intracranial circulatory arrest. J Neurosurg 1988;68:745.

[34] Feri M, Ralli L, Felici M, et al. Transcranial Doppler and brain death diagnosis. Crit Care Med 1994;22:1120.

[35] Petty GW, Mohr JP, Pedleym TR, et al. The role of transcranial Doppler in confirming brain death: sensitivity, specificity, and suggestions for performance and interpretation. Neurology 1990;40:300.

[36] Olick RS. Brain death, religious freedom, and public policy: New Jersey's landmark legislative initiative. Kennedy Inst Ethics J 1991;4:275–92.

**ELSEVIER
SAUNDERS**

Surg Clin N Am 86 (2006) 1553–1562

**SURGICAL
CLINICS OF
NORTH AMERICA**

Index

Note: Page numbers of article titles are in **boldface** type.

Moving?

Make sure your subscription moves with you!

To notify us of your new address, find your **Clinics Account Number** (located on your mailing label above your name), and contact customer service at:

E-mail: elspcs@elsevier.com

800-654-2452 (subscribers in the U.S. & Canada)
407-345-4000 (subscribers outside of the U.S. & Canada)

Fax number: 407-363-9661

Elsevier Periodicals Customer Service
6277 Sea Harbor Drive
Orlando, FL 32887-4800

*To ensure uninterrupted delivery of your subscription, please notify us at least 4 weeks in advance of move.